T0198198

Orthopedic Emergencies

Editors

MICHAEL C. BOND
ARUN SAYAL

EMERGENCY MEDICINE CLINICS OF NORTH AMERICA

www.emed.theclinics.com

Consulting Editor
AMAL MATTU

February 2020 • Volume 38 • Number 1

ELSEVIER

1600 John F. Kennedy Boulevard • Suite 1800 • Philadelphia, Pennsylvania, 19103-2899

http://www.theclinics.com

EMERGENCY MEDICINE CLINICS OF NORTH AMERICA Volume 38, Number 1
February 2020 ISSN 0733-8627, ISBN-13: 978-0-323-71273-6

Editor: Colleen Dietzler
Developmental Editor: Casey Potter

Emergency Medicine Clinics of North America (ISSN 0733-8627) is published quarterly by Elsevier Inc., 360 Park Avenue South, New York, NY, 10010-1710. Months of issue are February, May, August, and November. Business and Editorial Offices: 1600 John F. Kennedy Boulevard, Suite 1800, Philadelphia, PA 19103-2899. Customer Service Office: 6277 Sea Harbor Drive, Orlando, FL 32887-4800. Periodicals postage paid at New York, NY, and additional mailing offices. Subscription prices are $100.00 per year (US students), $352.00 per year (US individuals), $716.00 per year (US institutions), $220.00 per year (international students), $462.00 per year (international individuals), $882.00 per year (international institutions), $100.00 per year (Canadian students), $411.00 per year (Canadian individuals), and $882.00 per year (Canadian institutions). International air speed delivery is included in all *Clinics*' subscription prices. All prices are subject to change without notice. **POSTMASTER:** Send address changes to *Emergency Medicine Clinics of North America*, Elsevier Periodicals Customer Service, 11830 Westline Industrial Drive, St. Louis, MO 63146. Customer Service (orders, claims, online, change of address): Elsevier Periodicals **Customer Service, 11830 Westline Industrial Drive, St. Louis, MO 63146. Tel: 1-800-654-2452 (U.S. and Canada); 314-453-7041 (outside U.S. and Canada). Fax: 314-453-5170. E-mail: journalscustomerservice-usa@elsevier.com (for print support)**; **journalsonlinesupport-usa@elsevier.com (for online support)**.

Reprints. For copies of 100 or more of articles in this publication, please contact the Commercial Reprints Department, Elsevier Inc., 360 Park Avenue South, New York, NY 10010-1710. Tel.: 212-633-3874; Fax: 212-633-3820; E-mail: reprints@elsevier.com.

Emergency Medicine Clinics of North America is covered in *MEDLINE/PubMed (Index Medicus), Current Contents/Clinical Medicine, EMBASE/Excerpta Medica, BIOSIS, SciSearch, CINAHL, ISI/BIOMED,* and *Research Alert.*

Printed in the United States of America.

Contributors

CONSULTING EDITOR

AMAL MATTU, MD
Professor and Vice Chair of Academic Affairs, Department of Emergency Medicine, University of Maryland School of Medicine, Baltimore, Maryland, USA

EDITORS

MICHAEL C. BOND, MD, FACEP, FAAEM
Associate Professor, Department of Emergency Medicine, University of Maryland School of Medicine, Baltimore, Maryland, USA

ARUN SAYAL, MD, CCFP(EM)
Staff Physician, Emergency Department and Fracture Clinic, North York General Hospital, Associate Professor, Faculty of Medicine, University of Toronto, Toronto, Ontario, Canada

AUTHORS

MICHAEL K. ABRAHAM, MD, MS
Clinical Assistant Professor, Chair, Department of Emergency Medicine, University of Maryland School of Medicine, University of Maryland Upper Chesapeake Health System, Bel Air, Maryland, USA

EVANGELINE ARULRAJA, MD
Resident Physician, Division of Emergency Medicine, Duke University Medical Center, Durham, North Carolina, USA

MICHAEL C. BOND, MD, FACEP, FAAEM
Associate Professor, Department of Emergency Medicine, University of Maryland School of Medicine, Baltimore, Maryland, USA

KATHY BOUTIS, MD, MSc, FRCPC
Staff Emergency Physician, Division of Emergency Medicine, Academic Director, ImageSim, Senior Associate Scientist, Research Institute, The Hospital for Sick Children, Professor of Pediatrics, University of Toronto, Toronto, Ontario, Canada

MAJ JASON V. BROWN, MD, MC, USAF
Staff Physician, Emergency Medical Services, United States Air Force, Eglin AFB, Florida, USA

GEORGE CHIAMPAS, DO
Department of Emergency Medicine, Feinberg School of Medicine, Northwestern University, Chicago, Illinois, USA; Chief Medical Officer, United States Soccer Federation

BRIAN N. CORWELL, MD
Assistant Professor, Departments of Emergency Medicine and Orthopaedics, University of Maryland School of Medicine, Baltimore, Maryland, USA

MOIRA DAVENPORT, MD
Associate Residency Director, Department of Emergency Medicine, Allegheny General Hospital, Temple University School of Medicine, Pittsburgh, Pennsylvania, USA

NATALIE L. DAVIS, MD, MMSc
Assistant Professor, Department of Pediatrics, University of Maryland School of Medicine, Baltimore, Maryland, USA

DENNIS P. HANLON, MD, FAAEM
EM Quality Director, Allegheny General Hospital, Associate Professor of Emergency Medicine, Drexel University, College of Medicine, Pittsburgh, Pennsylvania, USA

TERESITA M. HOGAN, MD
Associate Professor, Department of Medicine, Division of Emergency Medicine, The University of Chicago Pritzker School of Medicine, Chicago, Illinois, USA

PHILLIP D. MAGIDSON, MD, MPH
Assistant Professor, Department of Emergency Medicine, Johns Hopkins School of Medicine, Baltimore, Maryland, USA

SANJEEV MALIK, MD
Department of Emergency Medicine, Feinberg School of Medicine, Northwestern University, Chicago, Illinois, USA

VASILIOS MAVROPHILIPOS, MD
Department of Emergency Medicine, Inova Fairfax Hospital, Virginia, USA

MICHAEL ROBERT MISCH, MD, CCFP-CAC(EM)
Lecturer, Division of Emergency Medicine, Department of Family and Community Medicine, University of Toronto, Toronto, Canada

BRUCE MOHR, BSc, MD, CCFP-EM, Diploma of Sports Medicine, FRRMS
Department of Emergency Medicine, Whistler Health Care Centre, Clinical Instructor, University of British Columbia, Whistler, British Columbia, Canada

NUPUR NISCHAL, DO
Senior Resident Physician, Division of Emergency Medicine, Duke University Medical Center, Durham, North Carolina, USA

MATTHEW P. OCZYPOK, MD
Resident Physician, Department of Emergency Medicine, Allegheny General Hospital, Pittsburgh, Pennsylvania, USA

NEHA P. RAUKAR, MD, MS, FACEP, CAQ Primary Care Sports Medicine
Senior Associate Consultant, Department of Emergency Medicine, Mayo Clinic, Rochester, Minnesota, USA

MARK SANDERSON, BSc, MD
Emergency Department, University of British Columbia, Kelowna General Hospital, Kelowna, British Columbia, Canada

ARUN SAYAL, MD, CCFP(EM)
Staff Physician, Emergency Department and Fracture Clinic, North York General Hospital, Associate Professor, Faculty of Medicine, University of Toronto, Toronto, Ontario, Canada

STEPHEN P. SHAHEEN, MD, CAQSM
Assistant Professor of Emergency Medicine and Orthopedic Surgery, Division of Emergency Medicine and Department of Orthopedic Surgery, Duke University Medical Center, Durham, North Carolina, USA

ROBERT SIMARD, MD, FRCPC
Clinical Associate, Emergency Department, Sunnybrook Health Sciences Centre, Staff Physician, Emergency Department, North York General Hospital, Toronto, Ontario, Canada

JACOB STELTER, MD
Department of Emergency Medicine, Feinberg School of Medicine, Northwestern University, Chicago, Illinois, USA

ALLISON K. THOBURN, MD
Geriatrics Fellow, Department of Medicine, Section of Geriatrics and Palliative Medicine, The University of Chicago Medicine, Chicago, Illinois, USA

GEORGE C. WILLIS, MD, FACEP, FAAEM
Assistant Professor, Department of Emergency Medicine, University of Maryland School of Medicine, Baltimore, Maryland, USA

SHARLEEN YUAN, MD, PhD
Resident, Department of Emergency Medicine, University of Maryland Medical Center, Baltimore, Maryland, USA

Contents

> Acute musculoskeletal injuries are commonly seen in our emergency depart-ments, and are commonly missed. There are many reasons for more missed injures and a significant one is over-reliance on radiographs. An emergency department orthopedic assessment goes far beyond the radiographs. A focused, yet comprehensive history is vital to understand the forces and mechanism of injury. That injury must be understood in the context of the pa-tient, because older and much younger patients have weaker bone. Finally, the physical examination is instrumental in localizing the pathology and is essential to put radiograph results in the proper clinical context.

> Appropriate recognition of the physiologic, psychological, and clinical dif-ferences among geriatric patients, with respect to orthopedic injury and disease, is paramount for all emergency medicine providers to ensure they are providing high-value care for this vulnerable population.

> Approximately one-third of children sustain a fracture before the age of 16 years; however, their unique anatomy and healing properties often result in a good outcome. This article focuses on the diagnosis and management of pediatric extremity injuries. The article describes the anatomic features and healing principles unique to children and discusses pediatric upper and lower extremity fractures and presents evidence-based and standard practice for their management. Finally, the article describes the conditions under which emergency physicians are likely to miss pediatric fractures by highlighting specific examples and discussing the general factors that lead to these errors.

> Injury patterns of the hand and wrist can be complex and challenging for the emergency physician to diagnose and treat. The ability of the hand

to perform delicate maneuvers requires a very intricate interplay of bones, ligaments, and tendons. Unfortunately, due to the omnipresence of the hand, the hand and wrist are commonly injured. These injuries can be debilitating if not treated correctly and can be both time-consuming and fraught with medicolegal risk. This article provides the necessary knowledge to diagnose and treat common hand and wrist injuries encountered in the emergency department.

This article provides an updated review of the emergent evalution and treatment of elbow and forearm injuries in the emergency department. Clinically necessary imaging is discussed. Common and uncommon injuries of the elbow and forearm are reviewed with an emphasis on early recognition, efficient management, and avoidance of complications. The astute emergency physician will rely on a focused history and precise examination, applied anatomic knowledge, and strong radiographic interpretative skills to avoid missed injuries and complications.

Shoulder pain is a common presentation in the emergency department. The list of differential diagnoses is broad. This article summarizes common diagnoses of shoulder pain, including bony, infectious, and connective tissue pathologies and their proper treatment. It also reviews which shoulder pain conditions are emergency diagnoses and need immediate treatment and which diagnoses need conservative management and outpatient follow-up.

Traumatic injuries of the hip and pelvis are commonly encountered in the emergency department. This article equips all emergency medicine practitioners with the knowledge to expertly diagnose, treat, and disposition these patients. Pelvic fractures occurring in young patients tend to be associated with high-energy mechanisms and polytrauma. Pelvic and hip fractures in the elderly are often a result of benign trauma but are associated with significant morbidity and mortality.

Knee and leg injuries are extremely common presentations to the emergency department. Understanding the anatomy of the knee, particularly the vasculature and ligamentous structures, can help emergency physicians (EPs) diagnose and manage these injuries. Use of musculoskeletal ultrasonography can further aid EPs through the diagnostic process. Proper use of knee immobilizers can also improve long-term patient outcomes.

Neck and back pain are among the most common symptom-related complaints for visits to the emergency department (ED). They contribute to high levels of lost work days, disability, and health care use. The goal of ED assessment of patients with neck and back pain is to evaluate for potentially dangerous causes that could result in significant morbidity and mortality. This article discusses the efficient and effective evaluation, management, and treatment of patients with neck and back pain in the ED. Emphasis is placed on vertebral osteomyelitis, epidural abscess, acute transverse myelitis, epidural compression syndrome, spinal malignancy, and spinal stenosis.

Many orthopedic injuries can have hidden risks that result in increased liability for the emergency medicine practitioner. It is imperative that emergency medicine practitioners consider the diagnoses of compartment syndrome, high-pressure injury, spinal epidural abscess, and tendon lacerations in the right patient. Consideration of the diagnosis and prompt referrals can help to minimize the complications these patients often develop.

A systematic approach is required for patients with a suspected concussion. Although standardized tools can aid in assessment, the diagnosis of concussion remains a clinical one. At the time of diagnosis, patients should be given both verbal and written review of the common symptoms of concussion, expected course of recovery, as well as strategies to manage symptoms. Most patients benefit from a brief period of rest, followed by a gradual reintroduction of activities, and a graduated return-to-sport protocol. Patients with prolonged recovery from a concussion may benefit from exercise, vestibular, and cognitive rehabilitation programs.

Pain management in acute orthopedic injury needs to be tailored to the presentation and patient. Subjective and objective assessment, in conjunction with pathophysiology, should be used to provide symptom control. Ideally, treatment should be administered in an escalating fashion, attempting to manage pain with the lowest dose of the safest medication available. There are also adjunctive therapies, including those that are nonpharmacologic, that can provide additional relief.

Video content accompanies this article at http://www.emed.
theclinics.com.

With the high cost and limited availability of gold standard imaging modalities, ultrasound has become an alternative in many musculoskeletal (MSK) injuries. Ultrasound has become increasingly portable and readily available in many acute care settings. Its ability to diagnose MSK injuries and help guide management has the potential to improve patient safety and flow. Ultrasound has been shown to diagnose fractures, dislocations, and tendon and ligament injuries. It helps guide fracture and dislocation reductions and aids in regional anesthesia for pain management. This article reviews the common MSK injuries that can be diagnosed with ultrasound with a focus on point-of-care ultrasound.

EMERGENCY MEDICINE CLINICS OF NORTH AMERICA

SERIES OF RELATED INTEREST

Orthopedic Clinics
https://www.orthopedic.theclinics.com/

THE CLINICS ARE NOW AVAILABLE ONLINE!
Access your subscription at:
www.theclinics.com

Foreword

Orthopedic Emergencies

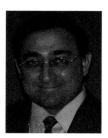

Amal Mattu, MD
Consulting Editor

Emergency orthopedics is the "bread and butter" of emergency medicine. This area of emergency medicine constitutes everything from mild bumps and bruises all the way through major traumatic injuries, which can result in hemorrhagic shock. It includes injuries to every region of the body, and these injuries, no matter how mild or severe, are among the most common reasons patients present to emergency departments (EDs) and urgent care centers around the world.

Despite the frequency with which we see orthopedic emergencies in the ED, it seems that many training programs are often deficient in teaching the proper skills to deal with these conditions. Training programs often emphasize higher-profile conditions in their curricula, such as cardiovascular and neurologic disease, and neglect emergency orthopedics. The result is that many current graduates of training programs report a subjective sense of unease when dealing with orthopedic emergencies in actual practice, leading to many unnecessary imaging studies, unnecessary consultations, and frequent misdiagnoses.

For readers of *Emergency Medicine Clinics of North America* who have ever felt uncertain about how to care for orthopedic conditions, this issue is written just for you. Guest Editors Drs Sayal and Bond have created an outstanding curriculum in emergency orthopedics, and they have recruited an expert group of authors to provide the education. Articles cover orthopedic injuries from head to foot, including discussions of patients at the extremes of age. Separate articles cover pain management, legal pitfalls in orthopedics, and also the hot topic of bedside ultrasound diagnosis of these injuries.

This issue of *Emergency Medicine Clinics of North America* should be considered must-reading for every trainee in emergency medicine, and it serves as an invaluable

Emerg Med Clin N Am 38 (2020) xiii–xiv
https://doi.org/10.1016/j.emc.2019.10.002
0733-8627/20/© 2019 Published by Elsevier Inc.

emed.theclinics.com

resource for routine clinical practice in emergency medicine. Kudos to the editors and authors for this excellent work!

Amal Mattu, MD
Department of Emergency Medicine
University of Maryland School of Medicine
110 South Paca Street
6th Floor, Suite 200
Baltimore, MD 21201, USA

E-mail address:
amattu@som.umaryland.edu

Preface

Orthopedic Emergencies

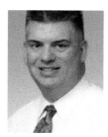
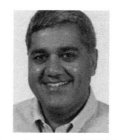

Michael C. Bond, MD, FACEP, FAAEM   Arun Sayal, MD, CCFP(EM)
Editors

Patients with orthopedic complaints in the emergency department (ED) are very commonly seen, and their injuries are of widely variable significance. The spectrum runs from injuries that are relatively minor to serious injuries that can compromise function, and rarely, can be limb or even life threatening. Many of the serious injuries are clinically obvious. But some are fairly occult, especially on plain radiographs. These subtle but serious complaints are commonly missed and can be easily mismanaged due to a variety of factors. Medical students typically receive minimal training on how to perform a musculoskeletal exam. Exposure during an Emergency Medicine residency is also variable. If any of the following components of an ED orthopedic assessment are omitted, then important clinical clues can be missed: an accurate history, an adequate physical exam, important patient factors (eg, age, occupation, comorbidities), limitations of radiographs, understanding of the mechanics and importance of the injury, understanding of the natural history of the injury, and ideal management. These facts along with the realization that immediate orthopedic consultation in the ED can often be difficult to impossible to obtain in some communities require that the emergency provider be comfortable and competent with the initial stabilization and management of orthopedic injuries. The American Association of Orthopaedic Surgeons also recognizes this and released a position statement in 2008 that acknowledges, "access to emergency orthopaedic care in the United States is problematic and may get worse. At present, there is variable access to orthopaedic emergency care in many communities in the United States."[1] The availability of orthopedic consultations can be even a bigger challenge when dealing with pediatric, hand, or uninsured cases.

In this issue of *Emergency Medicine Clinics of North America*, we have asked the authors to focus on the pearls and pitfalls of making the correct diagnosis in the ED along with providing up-to-date treatment recommendations. This issue starts with an article on how to approach the orthopedic patient and prevent some of the biases that occur in our busy everyday practice. There are also articles on using point-of-care ultrasound

Emerg Med Clin N Am 38 (2020) xv–xvi
https://doi.org/10.1016/j.emc.2019.10.001
0733-8627/20/© 2019 Published by Elsevier Inc.

as an aid in diagnosing musculoskeletal complaints that can often be missed on plain radiographs, high-risk injuries, and risk management, and in the era of the opioid crisis, an article on pain management options. Other notable areas to mention are the articles on geriatrics, where expert guidance is provided on pain control, prevention of delirium, prevention of hip fractures, and dealing with the unique pathophysiology of the elderly patient, and the article on mild traumatic brain injury (eg, concussions), where the treatment and screening recommendations seem to be changing on a weekly basis.

We hope you find this issue of the *Emergency Medicine Clinics of North America* to be highly educational and stimulating and a useful resource as you deal with those challenging orthopedic cases. We would like to thank all the authors, who spent endless hours scouring through the literature and writing their articles.

Michael C. Bond, MD, FACEP, FAAEM
Department of Emergency Medicine
University of Maryland School of Medicine
Paca-Pratt Building
110 South Paca Street
6th Floor, Suite 200
Baltimore, MD 21201, USA

Arun Sayal, MD, CCFP(EM)
Emergency Department and Fracture Clinic
North York General Hospital
Faculty of Medicine
University of Toronto
Room NW-126
4001 Leslie Street
Toronto, Ontario M2K 1E1, Canada

E-mail addresses:
mbond007@gmail.com (M.C. Bond)
arun.sayal@utoronto.ca (A. Sayal)

REFERENCE

1. Emergency Orthopaedic Care Position Statement. American Academy of Orthopaedic Surgeons and the American Association of Orthopaedic Surgeons. 2015. Available at: https://www.aaos.org/uploadedFiles/PreProduction/About/Opinion_Statements/position/1172%20Emergency%20Orthopaedic%20Care.pdf. Accessed July 4, 2019.

Emergency Medicine Orthopedic Assessment
Pearls and Pitfalls

Arun Sayal, MD, CCFP(EM)

KEYWORDS

- Emergency orthopedic assessment • History • Physical examination

KEY POINTS

- The history is as important for acute orthopedic injuries as it is for chest pain, abdominal pain, etc - determine as best as possible the mechanism of injury, the forces involved, and the events that occurred after the injury.
- Patient factors such as age, bone quality, past medical history, medications, previous injuries, occupational/recreational demands, hand dominance affect ED diagnosis, management and disposition.
- On physical examination, it is important to localize the point of maximal tenderness and focus on 'look, feel, and move'.
- Emergency department extremity radiographs are far from perfect, therefore, a sound history and physical are vital for the optimal ED diagnosis and management of injuries that are radiographically occult.

INTRODUCTION

Acute orthopedic injuries are a large component of emergency medicine comprising 10% to 20% of emergency department (ED) visits. Emergency physicians (EPs) treat a wide variety of acute orthopedic conditions from life- and limb-threatening trauma to relatively minor injuries.

Despite the relatively high volume of orthopedic injuries seen, studies have shown that EPs have decreased confidence in their musculoskeletal (MSK) skills. EPs perform relatively poorly on standardized tests of MSK knowledge.[1] Medical school curricula contain relatively minuscule amounts of dedicated MSK education.

MSK injuries remain the most common cause of litigation and misdiagnosis for EPs.[2-5] Given that orthopedic injuries are commonly seen, and commonly missed, it seems that there is a void that needs to be filled. There is a need to improve our ED orthopedic diagnostic and management skills.

Disclosure Statement: None.
Emergency Department and Fracture Clinic, North York General Hospital, Faculty of Medicine, University of Toronto, Room NW-126, 4001 Leslie Street, Toronto, Ontario M2K 1E1, Canada
E-mail address: arun.sayal@utoronto.ca

Emerg Med Clin N Am 38 (2020) 1–13
https://doi.org/10.1016/j.emc.2019.09.001
emed.theclinics.com

Studies looking at missed ED orthopedic diagnoses reveal that the missed injury is most commonly a fracture. Reasons for missing fractures include misinterpretation of radiographs, the presence of occult fractures, improper views obtained, and the presence of multiple fractures. Actually, 13% of the fractures that were missed were because radiographs were not ordered in the first place![5]

A diagnostic challenge of emergency medicine is identifying those that are sick or potentially sick from all the patients we assess with their myriad of complaints. Some patients with significant illness may be relatively easy to detect. Obvious aspects of the history, physical examination, and tests ordered indicate the level of clinician concern. However, the detection of severe but subtle cases requires a high index of suspicion. A worrisome history is often enough to prompt further investigation. A 69-year-old man with the sudden onset of severe, tearing chest pain going straight through to his back is a worrisome story without even performing an examination. In addition to the history of present illness, the index of suspicion changes with several patient factors: age, past medical history, medications, risk factors for disease, physical examination findings, test results, the age-related prevalence of the diagnosis considered, and their clinical course during their ED stay.

For patients with headache, chest pain, or fever, EPs generally understand the importance of the history and physical and place test results in the proper clinical context. For a variety of reasons, EPs tend to do things differently for orthopedic patients. These patients are often seen in fast track or urgent care centers. So the EPs are primed to move quickly and often assume that the patient is of low acuity (ie, triage bias). The radiographs are often done first, and if negative, it is common for the EP to default to a diagnosis of a soft tissue injury, glossing over the history and physical. This over-reliance on a negative radiographs can lead to missing subtle diagnoses. Diagnoses that could be made if a detailed history, physical examination, or review of the radiographs was done to look for subtle clues. However, because the EPs often do not examine the patient before reviewing the radiographs, they are not clued into the area of clinical concern. A major pitfall in the ED management of acutely injured MSK patients is the over-reliance on radiographs, and the failure to identify critical red flags on the history or physical examination.

Missing occult fractures is a concern in the ED. In most patients with a significant fracture, their injury will be apparent on the radiographs and examination. Although many occult fractures have a relatively benign natural history, some occult fractures (eg, scaphoid, cervical spine, femoral neck) are at risk of complications if undiagnosed and mismanaged.

Although the most concerning ED orthopedic conditions are fractures, the spectrum of injury includes operative soft tissue conditions (eg, patellar tendon rupture, quadriceps tear, distal biceps rupture, compartment syndrome), infections (eg, septic joints, necrotizing fasciitis), and dislocations/subluxations that have spontaneously reduced before presenting to the ED. Therefore, the orthopedic differential must expand beyond a search for fractures alone.

This article discusses key aspects of an efficient and comprehensive ED orthopedic assessment.

HISTORY

The general principles of an ED assessment are germane to orthopedic patients. Look for immediate life-threatening conditions that require simultaneous assessment, diagnosis, and management. In their absence, perform a detailed history and a physical examination to develop a provisional diagnosis, then order tests as necessary to alter the likelihood of a diagnosis or assist in the management of the patient. Finally, based on pretest probability, the test results, and the patient's clinical course in the ED, determine a final diagnosis, ED management plan, and disposition.

Obtaining a detailed history and physical examination should have the same importance for orthopedic patients as it is for other complaints (ie, chest pain, abdominal pain). A good orthopedic history does not necessarily need to be long and exhaustive, but the answers to a number of key questions are necessary for the history to be comprehensive. A focused, history must include consideration of the following factors.

1. Age
2. Hand dominance if applicable
3. Trauma, present or not
4. If a fall, was it caused by some medical issue (ie, syncope) or mechanical (ie, a mechanical fall)
5. Forces involved
6. Mechanism of injury
7. Events after injury
8. Quality of the bone to which the force was applied (ie, prior fracture, osteoporosis)
9. Previous injuries to that joint or the comparison, opposite side
10. Past medical history
11. Medications
12. Occupation/recreation demands

A fracture occurs because of an abnormal force on a normal bone, or a normal force on an abnormal bone. As such, the EP needs to understand both the force that was applied and consider the quality of bone to which it was applied. Knowledge of both the forces and the bone quality helps predict the likelihood of fracture or other significant injuries.

For nonfracture orthopedic conditions (eg, operative soft tissue injuries, infections, dislocations), the patient's history is instrumental in directing attention to the respective diagnoses. Failure to appreciate any of these components can result is missing subtle clues to both the diagnosis and the optimal management strategy.

1. Age

The relative strength of the bone is determined in large part by the patient's age. Both the relatively young (<15 years) and relatively old (>55 years) have weaker bone. So after trauma, the pretest probability for a fracture is greater for these groups.

Children have open growth plates, which tend to be weaker than ligaments, and softer bone that is more likely to buckle. Thus, although there is an increased tendency to fracture, many childhood injuries, in fact, are soft tissue injuries. Older patients tend to have osteoporosis with structurally weaker bone and are more likely to fracture with relatively less force. In between these ages, mid-teens to 55 years, it takes significantly more force to fracture.

A similar force can have different outcomes depending on the age of the patient. In the 25-year-old, young adult (**Fig. 1**A), the bone is stronger and a valgus stress results in pressure on the lateral tibial plateau, which is solid and the force exits through the medial knee resulting in a medial collateral ligament injury. A similar force in a 14-year-old patient (**Fig. 1**B) results in pressure on the lateral tibial plateau, which exits through the distal femoral growth plate.

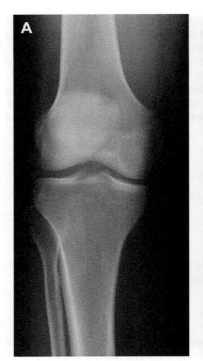

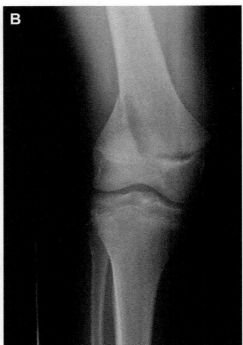

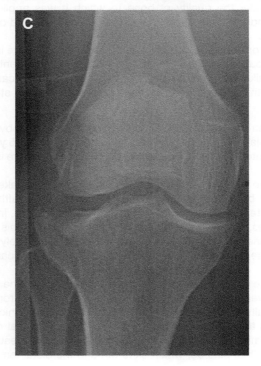

The same force in a 73-year-old patient (**Fig. 1**C) results in compression of the lateral tibial plateau owing to the weaker osteoporotic bone in this age range. Therefore, the same mechanism of injury, in 3 different age groups, results in 3 different injuries, and these injuries are predictable based on the age of the patient.

2. Trauma: In the ED, most fractures involve a traumatic injury. The absence of significant trauma makes a fracture much less likely to have occurred. However, pathologic fractures, a fracture that occurs in a bone that is weakened by another condition (eg, osteoporosis, tumor, infection), can occur without trauma. For instance, older patients can fracture their femoral neck by merely rotating on an osteoporotic arthritic hip without a fall. Therefore, EPs should have a relatively lower threshold to obtain radiographs in older and younger patients owing to their increased risk fracture even with mild trauma.

If nontraumatic MSK symptoms persist, the EP must consider other bone pathology that can cause the pain (eg, infection, tumor, pathologic fractures, stress fractures). Therefore, if MSK pain persists for weeks in a younger adult, even in the absence of trauma, plain radiographs are needed to evaluate for these other causes.

A careful review of the patient's past medical history and medications can also provide clues about possible pathologic fracture such as:

1. Falls

   It is not unusual for a patient to get triaged to the lower acuity side of the ED with an extremity injury from a fall, who had a medical condition (eg, presyncope, syncope, seizure) that precipitated the fall. In cases of a significant fall from height; EPs need to ensure self-harm was not intended. A proper ED orthopedic assessment includes a consideration of all factors that may have contributed to the fall (eg, medical issues, unsteady gait, need for cane/walker, home safety).

2. Forces involved

   For low-energy and medium-energy forces, consider the weakest link in the chain. This area is typically where injuries will occur. For the young and old, the weak link tends to be the bone. For high-energy forces, the chain can break at any link, so high-energy forces can cause fractures in any age group.

   A chain is only as strong as its weakest link. For an elderly patient, a minor twist of the ankle can cause an impressive lower leg fracture through an osteoporotic tibia, whereas young adults would require significant force to suffer a fracture.

   For patients involved in motor vehicle collisions, EPs are typically comprehensive in detailing all the forces and factors (eg, speed, seat belt use, air bag deployment, amount of intrusion, rollover, degree of damage) that could contribute to an injury. EPs should be similarly thorough in detailing the specifics of other traumatic injuries.

   It is important to determine the relative magnitude of the force involved because it is one of the critical determinants in predicting resultant injuries. A fall from ground level versus a fall from a ladder 12 feet up will have different injuries.

Fig. 1. The same mechanism, a valgus stress to the knee, is shown in 3 different age groups resulting in 3 significantly different knee pathologies. (*A*) In a 25-year-old patient, a medial collateral ligament strain. (*B*) In a 14-year-old patient, a Salter II fracture of the distal femur. (*C*) In an 73-year-old patient, a lateral tibial plateau fracture.

3. Mechanism of injury

Details of the mechanism of injury help to predict injury patterns. In addition to the magnitude of the force, knowledge of the direction the force was applied can further refine the likely diagnosis.

For example, with knee injuries, a valgus strain (a force impacting on the lateral side and directed medially) is the common mechanism of an medial collateral ligament injury in a young adult and suggestive of a lateral tibial plateau in an older adult. A sudden deceleration or change of direction is typical of an anterior cruciate ligament (ACL) injury, whereas a significant twist is more typical of meniscal pathology.

For ankle injuries, forced inversion often injures the lateral structures alone. Whereas an eversion–external rotation mechanism is likely to cause a syndesmosis injury, or a Maisonneuve fracture in a young adult, and a Tillaux fracture in the early teenager. Knowledge of axially loading from a height onto both feet should prompt consideration of injury to the calcaneus, talus, the opposite foot, distal tibia, knee, hip, or spine.

4. Events surrounding the injury

EPs should inquire about events preceding and following an injury because this information can help to predict the more likely injuries. For instance, if an athlete was able to continue playing after an injury, the chance of a fracture is less likely. Immediate pain after a motor vehicle collision is more likely to denote a fracture, whereas delayed pain makes a significant fracture less likely and soft tissue injury (eg, muscle strain, whiplash) more likely.

In patients with acute knee injuries, immediate joint swelling is suggestive of a hemarthrosis (which suggests a fracture or ACL tear). In contrast, delayed swelling over 12 to 24 hours is suggestive of inflammation from an intra-articular soft tissue source (eg, meniscus injury). Finally, the absence of joint swelling should heighten one's concern for an alternative diagnosis as significant intra-articular pathology is unlikely.

5. Previous injuries to that joint or the comparison side.

This establishes a baseline (pre-injury) status of the joint and denotes if the opposite joint can serve as a normal comparison. If a patient has a previous tear of the ACL on the affected knee, then a positive Lachman may be reflective of a previous injury. If the other knee has a torn ACL, then a reliable comparison end point of ACL function is not available. In this case, symmetric findings may be indicative of pathology.

6. Past medical history: Current and past medical illnesses (eg, gout, diabetes, cancer, osteoporosis) can alter both the pretest probability and presentation of illness. A history of cancer should prompt one to consider metastases, whereas patients on long-term bisphosphonates are at risk for atypical femur fractures. Peripheral neuropathy affects sensation and proprioception, which make injuries less painful to patients. This lack of pain may give EPs a false sense of security. It may also prevent patients from being able to protect injuries because the pain may not discourage them from using the injured extremity. Have a low threshold to protect and arrange close follow-up in patients with injured extremities and preexisting altered sensation.

7. Medications: A growing list of medications (eg, prednisone, disease-modifying antirheumatic drugs, immunosuppressants, bisphosphonates) can alter both the pretest probability and presentation of illness. For example, patients on immunosuppressants may not have clinically apparent septic joints so a higher index of suspicion is mandated.

8. Occupation/recreation demands: The more physically demanding a patient is due to work/play demands, the more anatomically aligned fractures need to be. Hand dominance and occupation also play a significant role in how upper extremity injuries are treated.

Therefore, a thorough and targeted history can reveal small but important details that will help to develop an appropriate differential that can than direct the physical examination and testing of the patient.

PHYSICAL EXAMINATION

Some orthopedic injuries can be quite impressive and clinically obvious; however, it is imperative that these obvious injuries do not distract EPs from a second, potentially higher priority concern. EPs need to have the discipline to briefly ignore the clinically obvious injury, and search for life-threatening conditions (eg, head, neck, spine), and manage them emergently. Finally, careful examination of the injured extremity must be conducted to ensure there are no limb-threatening conditions and that the limb is neurovascularly intact with unremarkable compartments.

Develop the habit of examining the joint above and below as a second, more subtle injury may be noted. Finally, once life- and limb-threatening injuries have been considered, the local injury can be addressed.

The orthopedic physical examination is a critical step to making an accurate diagnosis. There is a tendency to shortchange the physical examination owing to the patient's pain or their reluctance to cooperate with the examination. However, one should not default to ordering radiographs without performing an examination. Adequate pain control can help to decrease their pain and anxiety and allow them to better participate in their evaluation. Bypassing important parts of the physical examination increases the risk of missing vital clues to important diagnoses. The path to an accurate orthopedic diagnosis, especially subtle diagnoses, often travels through the physical examination.

A few simple, yet mandatory aspects of an ED orthopedic assessment are look, palpate, and move.

Look
- Look for alignment and swelling. Compare with the opposite side.
- Look for redness, erythema, as a sign of infection or inflammation.
- Disrobe the patient and remove any prehospital splints so you can look at the skin when you assess the patient.

It is appropriate for prehospital personnel to splint injuries before transport, but the splint must be removed to get a 360° look of the limb and ensure there is no compromise of the skin. Occasionally, displaced fractures will pinch the skin and can develop into a open fracture if the fracture is not reduced quickly. Tenting of the skin, stretching of the skin so tightly it is on the verge of opening, is a clinical diagnosis that is only appreciated by examining the skin.

Palpate
- Localize pain. Ideally, start your examination by examining the opposite side or away from the suspected injury first, and examine the suspected painful area last.
  - In children, this order allows for a more accurate assessment of the rest of the extremity. Children may seem to have pain later owing to fear if the injury is palpated first.
  - In adults, eliciting pain often causes muscle spasm that can affect the accurate assessment of other ligaments.

- If a positive finding is noted, compare with the opposite side to know if it is a true finding. For example, it is common to have snuffbox tenderness as a normal finding in the absence of scaphoid pathology.
- Find the point of maximal tenderness.
  - This point is important because you have localized the source of the pain to somewhere below your examining finger. Failure to reproduce the pain around the joint is a red flag that the source of the pain may be referred pain from a more proximal source (eg, a hip source in patients who complain of knee pain).
  - Maximal tenderness reminds us that the goal is not only to find a point of tenderness, but to find a point of maximal tenderness because they might have multiple points of pain. Be sure to palpate all areas or risk missing a second injury. An astute clinician will examine a patient carefully, and look for additional painful areas, and then review the radiographs with a keen eye focused on the area(s) of clinical tenderness identified on their examination. This practice improves detection of the second fracture, and the reason why radiographs should be reviewed after the patient has been examined.
- Assess and document the patient's distal neurovascular status.
  - Palpate pulses and compare with the opposite side. Assess distal motor and sensory function and clearly document for each nerve of concern (eg, radial, ulnar, and median for the hand).
- Assess for warmth, always considering infection as a possible cause.
- Palpate the compartments and document your assessment.
  - Compartment syndrome is rare but it is a limb and potentially life-threatening condition that is commonly missed. Palpating compartments regularly will develop a sense of what normal feels like because there are differences between male and female, and young and old patients. A true sense of normal makes it easier to recognize abnormal.

Move
- Assess active and passive range of motion (ROM).

Several keys to missed diagnoses are found when assessing movement. Failure to assess for active movement of a limb risks missing an operative soft tissue injury. If there is a fracture suspected the assessment of ROM can be deferred until after radiographs can be reviewed. The evaluation should include active and passive ROM.

For example, a posterior shoulder dislocation is missed 50% to 80% of the time by the first examiner.[6–8] The clinical clue on physical examination is the arm is locked in internal rotation. Failure to passively external rotate the shoulder means missing this clue. In knee injuries, an extensor mechanism disruption of the knee is commonly missed, but this can be diagnosed if the patient fails in an attempt to complete a straight leg raise.

In certain instances, even in the presence of a fracture, ROM testing affects management decisions. Undisplaced patellar fractures require an assessment of the extensor mechanism via a straight leg raise test to ensure the extensor mechanism is intact. Undisplaced olecranon fractures require evaluation of the integrity of the extensor mechanism of the elbow. If either extensor mechanism is disrupted the patient will require surgical repair, but would often be managed non-operatively if intact.

Investigations
- Obtain appropriate radiographs.
- Obtain appropriate laboratory studies if infection is suspected.

- Consider joint aspiration in patients suspected of having crystal-induced arthritis (eg, gout, pseudogout) and septic joints.

For orthopedic injuries, radiographs are often obtained. Several clinical decision rules have been developed to safely reduce the number of radiographs obtained in the ED, without missing significant fractures. These include the Ottawa Ankle Rules,[9] The Ottawa Knee Rules,[10] and the Pittsburgh Knee Rules.[11] When implementing these rules, care must be taken to ensure that an appropriately comprehensive history and physical examination are performed to fully develop a differential diagnosis and that there is not just a simple application of the rules and review of the radiographs being done.

For example, the Ottawa Ankle Rules only require palpation of the posterior 6 cm of both the lateral and medial malleolus, the navicular and the base of the fifth metatarsal to determine if radiographs are needed.[9] However, a more complete history and physical examination are needed to accurately interpret the radiographs and come to a more precise diagnosis. Knowledge of the mechanism (eg, inversion, external rotation, axial loading), footwear (eg, presence of a boot, skate, or cleats), tenderness over other areas (eg, Achilles, calcaneus, syndesmosis, deltoid ligament, etc) are all crucial to making an accurate diagnosis. Therefore, the importance a complete history and physical can not be overstated, and sole application of the rule can miss significant injuries.

In addition to radiographs, additional testing may be needed to secure the correct diagnosis. Ultrasound imaging may have a role in diagnosing fractures and soft tissue injuries and is covered in Robert Simard's article, "Ultrasound Imaging of Orthopedic Injuries," in this issue of *Emergency Medicine Clinics of North America*. Computed tomography scanning provides 3-dimensional information on alignment as well as having increased sensitivity for fractures and dislocations. Computed tomography scanning is of limited value for soft tissue assessment, but it tends to be more readily available than MRI.

MRI has the greatest sensitivity for soft tissue and fractures, but has limited availability in most ED settings. MRI is the preferred modality for soft tissues injuries (eg, ligamentous injury), and spinal cord injuries (eg, herniated disk, epidural abscess).

Laboratory evaluations can include white blood count, C-reactive protein, erythrocyte sedimentation rate, creatine kinase, lactate, and myoglobin. White blood count, C-reactive protein, and erythrocyte sedimentation rate can be elevated in infectious and inflammatory conditions and, although they may have limited usefulness acutely, they are often trended to assess response to treatment. Creatine kinase, lactate, and myoglobin injuries are useful for the assessment of muscle damage, as is seen in compartment syndrome and rhabdomyolysis.

RADIOGRAPHS

Treat the patient, and not the x-ray.

Imaging is an important aspect of ED MSK assessments, and there are many pitfalls to avoid. In a UK study looking at missed fractures in the ED, 13% were missed because a radiograph was not obtained.[4] In malpractice cases of missed ED diagnoses, a failure to order the right test was the problem cited in 58% of cases (with radiographs being at the top of the list).[2] And a misinterpretation of a test was cited in 37% of cases, with radiographs being the most common.[2]

Order appropriately specific series. Wider is not better because fine detail is sacrificed. The objective is to center the x-ray beam close to the location of the injury. For example, if a distal radius is injured, it is better to order a wrist radiograph, rather than a forearm series (even though a forearm series still provides a view of the wrist). If worried about both the elbow and wrist, order both studies separately. Do not only order a forearm series to cover both joints because forearm views provide suboptimal views of both the elbow and wrist.

Ensure an adequate number of views are obtained. A minimum of 2 views at 90° is required. The lateral view is the main view in orthopedics so it is essential that a proper lateral view is obtained. Oblique and other special views can be of value in understanding the injury and increasing chances that a fracture is visualized because subtle fractures may only be seen on a single view (**Fig. 2**).

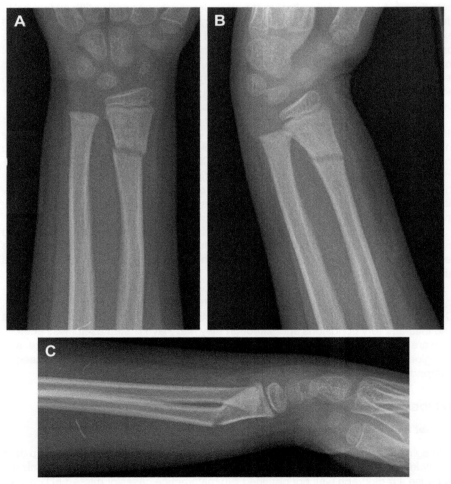

Fig. 2. Importance of adequate views. A minimum of 2 views at 90° should be obtained. (*A*, *B*) The original 2 views provided by radiology for a 4-year-old girl who fell and injured her wrist. Image (*A*) is an anteroposterior view and (*B*) is an attempt at a lateral view. The patient was sent back to the radiology department to get a true lateral (*C*), which revealed a significantly angulated fracture not appreciated on the original (suboptimal) attempt at a lateral.

Additional views can provide a different angle to better visualize a fracture. For example, a scaphoid view helps to detect a scaphoid fracture; an oblique wrist view helps detect a distal radius fracture, and oblique knee views are best for tibial plateau fractures.

Radiographically occult fractures are well-known within some anatomic regions (eg, scaphoid, radial head, talar dome, hip) and are possible with any injured area, given the correct clinical context. The clinical probability of a fracture is based on the patient's age, mechanism of injury, events after injury, past medical history, degree and rapidity of swelling, ROM, and focal tenderness. A high clinical probability of a fracture with normal radiographs often requires treatment for an occult fracture. Treatment can include immobilization and follow-up with orthopedics for relatively minor injuries with less acute concerns (eg, occult scaphoid fractures, occult distal radius fractures) or may warrant further investigation in the ED with bone scan, computed tomography scanning, or MRI for more serious injuries (eg, occult hip fractures, suspected cervical spine fractures) (**Fig. 3**).

Radiologists will often remind us that, "The most commonly missed fracture is the second fracture." With this comes the warning that, if a fracture is seen, carefully look for a second fracture (**Fig. 4**).

Contrary to the radiologists' well-known mantra, EPs are more likely to miss the first fracture than have a case where the second fracture was missed. In one ED-based UK study of 727 missed fractures that were visible on plain radiographs, only 11 cases (1.5%) were for a second fracture being missed.[4] In 716 cases (98.5%), it was the first fracture that went undetected. So the most commonly missed fracture is the first fracture!

Be aware of normal variants and common accessory ossicles, especially in the feet, because these are often mistaken for fractures. There are often bilateral variations, so comparison films can be helpful. A textbook of normal radiologic variants can serve to reassure in suspicious cases. Clinically correlate any suspicious radiograph findings; if it is nontender, it is unlikely to be acute.

It is important for EDs to have a radiograph recall system to identify missed or possible missed findings that are subsequently detected by the radiologist. It is expected that radiologists will detect abnormalities we miss. EPs have the advantage of a history and physical examination to help with the interpretation of the radiographs. So even if a radiologist's report is ready in real time, it is important to view the plain films because there is a chance that the treating providers may detect an abnormality the radiologist has missed, especially because most of our ED radiology requests do

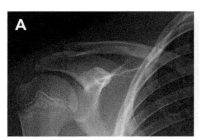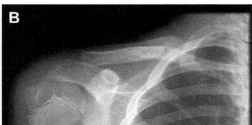

Fig. 3. Plain radiographs are not 100% sensitive for fracture. Plain film on (*A*) and day 19 (*B*) for a 12-year-old boy who fell into the boards playing hockey. Initial radiographs were negative. This patient was diagnosed with a probable occult midshaft clavicle fracture (based on the clinical assessment) and follow-up was arranged. Radiographs on day 19 confirmed the fracture.

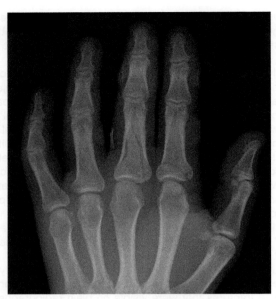

Fig. 4. Plain radiographs demonstrating fractures of the proximal phalanges of digits 2 and 3. A closer look reveals a third fracture at the base of digit 4.

not offer specific clinical information that could assist radiology in the interpretation of the radiographs.

If the radiographs are interpreted as normal in the ED, advise the patients that a fracture was not seen, but that it will be read again later by a radiologist and they will be notified of any changes. Depending on the clinical scenario, it may also be advisable to inform the patients whose radiographs are negative that they have:

- Significant soft tissue injuries and though the bone is not broken or dislocated they have a significant injury.
- A clinically suspected fracture is still possible and although the fracture cannot be seen today, repeat radiographs may need to be done if symptoms persist.

These discussions should be dictated by the level of clinical concern, and not by the results of imaging studies.

SUMMARY

Proper management of ED orthopedic patients mandates a thorough history and physical examination, along with an understanding of the limitations of radiographs and laboratory testing. A comprehensive risk assessment can be made when we have a good knowledge of the following:

- The injury/complaint (ie, history of present illness)
- the patient (eg, age, past medical history, occupation, medications, physical demands)
- the effect the injury (ie, physical examination).

This risk assessment determines the pretest probability of radiographs and laboratory testing while predicting any limitations the diagnostic studies might have. Finally,

EPs can then review the radiographs with the proper clinical context. This leads to less reliance on the imaging and a greater reliance on the complete assessment. The end result is a more accurate clinical diagnosis, fewer missed injuries, better ED management of orthopedic injuries, and more appropriate dispositions.

REFERENCES

1. Comer GC, Liang E, Bishop JA. Lack of proficiency in musculoskeletal medicine among emergency medicine physicians. J Orthop Trauma 2014;28:e85–7.
2. Kachalia A, Gandhi TK, Puopolo AL, et al. Missed and delayed diagnoses in the emergency department: a study of closed malpractice claims from 4 liability insurers. Ann Emerg Med 2007;49:196–205.
3. Brown TW, McCarty ML, Kelen GD, et al. An epidemiologic study of closed emergency department malpractice claims in a national database of physician malpractice insurers. Acad Emerg Med 2010;17(5):553–60.
4. Selbst SM, Friedman MJ, Singh SB. Epidemiology and etiology of malpractice lawsuits involving children in US Emergency Departments and Urgent Care Centers. Pediatr Emerg Care 2005;21:165–9.
5. Guly H. Diagnostic errors in an accident and emergency department. Emerg Med J 2001;18(4):263–9.
6. Robinson CM, Seah M, Akhtar MA. The epidemiology, risk of recurrence, and functional outcome after an acute traumatic posterior dislocation of the shoulder. J Bone Joint Surg Am 2011;93:1605–13.
7. Clough TM, Bale RS. Bilateral posterior shoulder dislocation: the importance of the axillary radiographic view. Eur J Emerg Med 2001;8(2):161–3.
8. Xu W, Huang LX, Guo JJ, et al. Neglected posterior dislocation of the shoulder: a systematic literature review. J Orthop Translat 2015;3(2):89–94.
9. Stiell IG, Greenberg GH, McKnight RD, et al. Decision rules for the use of radiography in acute ankle injuries: refinement and prospective validation. JAMA 1993; 269:1127–32.
10. Stiell IG, Greenberg GH, Wells GA, et al. Prospective validation of a decision rule for use of radiography in acute knee injury. JAMA 1996;275:611–5.
11. Seaberg DC, Jackson R. Clinical decision rule for knee radiographs. Am J Emerg Med 1994;12:541–3.

Emergency Orthogeriatrics
Concepts and Therapeutic Considerations for the Geriatric Patient

Phillip D. Magidson, MD, MPH[a],*, Allison K. Thoburn, MD[b], Teresita M. Hogan, MD[c]

KEYWORDS

- Older adult • Orthopedics • Hip fractures • Pain management
- Multidisciplinary care

KEY POINTS

- Aging increases the likelihood of orthopedic injuries, atypical presentations, and the need for special management and transitions of care.
- These issues should be understood when determining treatment strategies for orthopedic injuries in older adults.
- Patient baseline functionality should guide management for orthopedic care in older adults.
- Multidisciplinary team care models improve system and patient-centered outcomes in older adults with acute orthopedic issues.

INTRODUCTION

Older adults sustain frequent orthopedic injuries that may result in devastating consequences to their overall health, quality of life, function, mobility, and independence, and even in death. Appropriate emergency care can avoid this downward spiral through early recognition, appropriate treatment, and improved collaborative systems of care. Emergency medicine providers (EMPs) should prepare themselves to meet the demands of the large and complex population of elders requiring emergency treatment. Such preparation can help to achieve the triple aim of improving the health of individuals and populations while saving costs. This article highlights orthopedic

Disclosure Statement: The authors have no financial disclosures.
[a] Department of Emergency Medicine, Johns Hopkins University School of Medicine, 4940 Eastern Avenue, A1 East Suite 150, Baltimore, MD 21224, USA; [b] Department of Medicine, Section of Geriatrics and Palliative Medicine, University of Chicago Medicine, 5841 South Maryland Avenue, MC 6098, Chicago, IL 60637, USA; [c] Department of Medicine, Division of Emergency Medicine, University of Chicago School of Medicine, 5841 South Maryland Avenue, MC 6098, Chicago, IL 60637, USA
* Corresponding author.
E-mail address: pmagidson@jhmi.edu

injuries in older adults and describes optimal concepts in emergency orthopedic care for this unique population.

GERIATRIC ANATOMIC AND PHYSIOLOGIC DIFFERENCES

The biological and physiologic changes of aging play a significant role in the injury patterns, presentations, evaluation, and treatment of older patients with orthopedic disease and injuries. It is important for EMPs to recognize these critical differences because they the guide clinical care of older adult patients with such injuries.

Osteoporosis, the loss of bone mass and strength, contributes to more than 2 million fractures in older adults annually.[1] The primary mechanism of osteoporosis in women is related to decreased estrogen production and accelerated bone resorption that affects up to 25% of women 80 years of age and older. The primary causes in men, and secondary causes in women, are hypogonadism, medications such as steroids and proton pump inhibitors, nutritional deficits as well as renal, thyroid and gastrointestinal diseases.[1,2] In addition to increasing the likelihood of fractures, bone fragility also affects bone healing. Nonunion, delayed union, and failures of operative fixation are all more common in patients with osteoporosis and osteopenia. EMPs should carefully individualize care plans for these patients.[3,4]

Sarcopenia, or the decrease in skeletal muscle mass, results in functionally less strength, balance, coordination, and overall endurance. More than 50% of patients over the age of 80 have a skeletal muscle mass index that is more than 2 standard deviations below the mean of a younger reference group.[5,6] This significant sarcopenia contributes to injuries and delays recovery.

The concept of fragility fracture defines how these conditions, combined with standing height falls or repetitive physiologic loading, results in significant fractures from even insignificant mechanisms.[7] Fragility fractures occur in the vertebrae, proximal femur, and distal radius of 40% of women over the age of 50.[8] Fragility fractures often result in prolonged pain and disability, and may reduce quality of life. Work by Gosch and associates[9] showed that 29.4% of patients with fragility fractures died within 1 year and 70.6% of patients died within 2.1 years of the event. The mean life expectancy of patients after a fragility fracture was only 527 days.[9]

Comorbidities affect most geriatric patients with nearly 75% having 2 or more preexisting conditions.[10] Preexisting conditions impact the type of orthopedic injuries sustained, the emergency treatment of these injuries, and potential recovery to the preinjury state. For example, cardiopulmonary disease impacts sedation techniques and operative risk. Neurologic disorders, including Parkinson's and Alzheimer's diseases, hinder pain identification and management, as well as rehabilitation efforts. Baseline functional impairments impact decisions to undertake specific reductions, splinting, or operative interventions.[3,11] Liver or kidney disease and peripheral vascular disease increase bleeding risks, impact medication metabolism, and impair wound healing.[12]

The decision of if and when to proceed with operative intervention needs to be well understood by all EMPs. Any preoperative optimization of comorbid conditions must be balanced with the knowledge that operative delays strongly increase morbidity and mortality. A 2010 meta-analysis evaluating surgical timing in older patients with acute hip fractures found a 19% decrease in mortality, a 41% decrease in pneumonia, and a 52% reduction in pressure ulcers in patients with early operative intervention.[13] These findings have been replicated in other systemic reviews and meta-analyses.[14,15] Proximal humeral fractures that require operative intervention can also be significantly complicated by a delay in surgical fixation.[16]

Traditionally, expensive and unnecessary tests are ordered in preoperative geriatric patients. However, studies show there is no need for routine echocardiography or pulmonary function testing in elders undergoing noncardiac procedures.[17] Therefore, it is incumbent on the EMP to advocate for rapid evaluation by the orthopedic team and if necessary, obtaining formal geriatrics or internal medicine preoperative evaluation, to speed time to safe surgical intervention.

GERIATRIC FRACTURE SPECIFICS

In older adults, standing height falls are the primary precipitating event for fractures.[3,18] These falls can cause serious injury in older patients, including intracranial hemorrhage, spinal fractures, and pelvic fractures that may have significant hemorrhagic complications.[19–21]

Functional impairments and slowed reflexes, such as lack of trunk rotation and delayed hand outstretch, lead to hip fractures being far more common in older patients versus wrist fractures, which are more common in younger patients who fall. **Table 1** summarizes key differences in specific fracture patterns between younger and older adults.

GERIATRIC BACK PAIN

Lower back pain (LBP) is one of the most common medical complaints among older adults with a 1-year prevalence of 50%.[40] Some authors have suggested classifying patients with LBP into 1 of 4 categories as a means of guiding the EMPs diagnostic and treatment decisions: (1) LBP and red flag symptoms, (2) LBP and radicular symptoms, (3) nonspecific LBP, and (4) those with referred back pain. **Table 2** outlines these categories as well as the next important actions suggested for EMP.

For patients with acute or subacute nonspecific or radicular, pain, management of pain is an essential part of the emergency department course and likely discharge plan. In the yes column, generally start with acetaminophen owing to its favorable safety profile in older adults. However, effectiveness is modest and some trials have shown no difference in symptoms when compared with placebo.[46] Nonsteroidal anti-inflammatory drugs and muscle relaxants should be used with caution and only for short periods in older adults. However, nonsteroidal anti-inflammatory drugs may offer temporary improvement in back pain.

In the no column, steroids are no more effective than placebo and carry an increased risk of bleeding and hyperglycemia. Therefore, steroids should be avoided for routine relief of nonspecific LBP in older adults.[47] Opioids and benzodiazepines have consistently been associated with adverse events in older adults and do not show sustainable effectiveness in acute or subacute back pain and, therefore, should be avoided for this specific type of LBP in older adults.[48]

Although conventional teaching has led to an earlier is better in imaging for LBP older adults, a 2015 study suggests early imaging may not be necessary. This study concluded, in the absences of red flags, that older patients with back pain who received early imaging had no better 1-year outcomes than patients who had delayed imaging.[49]

GERIATRIC PHARMACOLOGIC CONSIDERATIONS

Pain management is an essential component of care for all patients with orthopedic emergencies.[50] However, geriatric pain control presents particular challenges because of the physiologic changes of aging, the high prevalence of comorbidities

Table 1
Unique characteristics in geriatric fracture patterns

Fracture Type	Epidemiology/Presentation	Evaluation	Treatment
Proximal humerus	1 in 8 older adults will have at least 1 additional fracture when a proximal humerus fracture is found[16]	Loss of sensation over the lateral deltoid and inability to abduct shoulder, suggests axillary nerve injury[15]	Operative and nonoperative management (sling with range of motion exercises) have similar outcomes[17]
Distal radius	Incidence increases with age, especially in woman[3]	Nearly 1 in 10 older adults sustain concurrent median nerve injury and should be evaluated for acute carpal tunnel syndrome[18]	Functional outcomes in less active older adults is similar in both operative and nonoperative management[19]
Vertebral body	Two-thirds are asymptomatic and incidentally diagnosed Can occur after minor movements such as sitting, coughing, or lifting[20]	Low threshold for CT evaluation in older adults with acute back pain and point tenderness[21]	Little evidence for thoracic lumbar sacral orthosis brace Consider calcitonin for pain control, 200 IU intranasally shown to be more effective for pain relief than acetaminophen[22,23]
Pelvic	At risk for pelvic injury from high and low impact trauma Mortality is 4–5 times higher than younger patients with similar injury[24,25]	More likely to require embolization and blood transfusion than younger patients[26] Physical examination in alert patient without other injuries has outstanding sensitivity (98%) and specificity (100%) for pelvic injury[27]	Even with stable nonoperative fractures, admission for physical and occupational therapy and multidisciplinary discharge planning is warranted
Hip	The 30% 1 y mortality is more than twice that of younger patients Decrease in reaction time results in failure to protectively outstretch a hand, increasing hip injuries[28–32]	Two-view radiographs for acute hip fracture has good sensitivity (90%) 2%–4% of negative hip films will still have occult fractures CT scan sensitivity (87%) and specificity (100%) for occult fractures but MRI is gold standard[21,33–35]	Even minor delay in operative repair is associated with worse outcomes/more complications
Ankle	More closely associated with obesity than osteoporosis[36]	Most Ottawa Ankle Rule studies were done in younger patients (mean age of 28.3) so applicability to older adults unclear[37] Have a low threshold for radiographs	Only ambulatory patients have favorable risk profile as mortality rate is 3% for ankle open reduction internal fixation[38,39]

Abbreviation: CT, computed tomography.

Table 2
LBP approach in the older adult

	1: Red Flag Symptoms	2: Radicular Pain	3: Nonspecific	4: Referred Pain
History	Cancer history Unexplained weight loss Night sweats/fevers Bacteremia Urinary retention Bowel incontinence	Leg pain > back pain Buttock pain Worse with standing/movement and improves with rest Previously diagnosed spinal stenosis	Worse with movement Long-standing pain Recent increase in physical activity	Associated abdominal pain Dermatomal distribution Associated with eating, nausea or vomiting, Urinary symptoms
Physical examination	Progressive motor/sensory neurologic deficit Saddle anesthesia Loss of rectal tone Spinal point tenderness	Positive straight leg raise Isolated motor, sensory, or reflex abnormality	May or may not have point tenderness Generally normal examination	Pulsatile abdominal mass or abdominal tenderness Rash Costovertebral angle tenderness Pulse deficits
Differential	Cancer history Epidural abscess Osteomyelitis/discitis Cauda equina symptoms	Spinal stenosis Herniated discs or facet joints Arthropathy	Myofascial pain Muscle sprain/strain	Abdominal aortic aneurysm Herpes zoster Pyelonephritis/nephrolithiasis Gastritis Pancreatitis
Next steps	Emergent computed tomography scan and/or MRI	Ensure no red flags Pain control Physical therapy Outpatient orthopedic or primary care	Primary care referral Physical therapy	Systemic laboratory values including liver and pancreas function Dedicated abdominal imaging Urinalysis

Data from Refs.[41–45]

and the risks of polypharmacy. Across care settings, the oldest old and those with cognitive impairment are at highest risk of pain undertreatment.[51,52] Undertreatment increases the development of delirium,[53] and may lead to increased frailty and functional decline.[54] Conversely, overtreatment of pain places older patients at higher risk of oversedation and confusion,[55] as well as respiratory depression[56] and falls.[57] When adequate pain control is achieved, older orthopedic patients ambulate earlier and have improved outcomes.[58]

Older adults have decreased renal[59] and hepatic[60] function that affect the absorption, distribution, metabolism, and elimination of many drugs. Aging brings an increase in body fat, while lean body mass and total body water decrease.[61] This can change the concentration or half-life of many pain medications. Therefore, pain medications must be dosed carefully in older patients. **Table 3** provides an overview of pain medication dosing considerations.

MULTIMODAL PAIN CONTROL

Given the many risks opioids carry, including dependency, misuse, respiratory depression, and falls, multimodal pain control is now the standard of care. In the setting of orthopedic injury, regional nerve blocks are central to multimodal analgesia. Regional nerve blocks improve analgesia,[70,71] decrease opioid use,[72–74] and decrease the length of hospital stay.[75,76] With the placement of indwelling catheters as opposed to single anesthetic injections, nerve blocks can provide excellent analgesia from the emergency department to the operating room, and even into the postoperative period.[77,78]

Femoral nerve and fascia iliaca block techniques have been described extensively and are used frequently for hip fracture in the emergency department in the United Kingdom,[79] but are used far less often in North America.[80] This difference may be related to fewer EMPs trained in these techniques.[73] Although regional blocks are relatively safe, clinicians should be aware of possible adverse events with femoral nerve blocks including quadriceps weakness, femoral neuropathy and neuritis, postoperative falls, and masking of compartment syndrome.[81]

Regional analgesia techniques for the upper extremities such as intra-articular lidocaine,[82] or interscalene nerve block for shoulder dislocation,[83] brachial plexus block for dislocation or fracture,[84] or hematoma block for proximal humeral fracture[85] have been studied in the emergency department. Furthermore, regional analgesia has shown benefit in shoulder,[86] hand,[87] knee,[88] and ankle[89] surgeries. Improvements in pain control and decreased length of stay are noted. Given the benefits of regional analgesia seen for geriatric patients with hip fractures, these techniques deserve further study of their application in the emergency setting.

DISPOSITION CONSIDERATIONS

To date, no formalized criteria exist for emergency department disposition decisions in orthogeriatric patients. In addition to the presenting pathology, EMPs must take into account underlying frailty, ability to comprehend discharge instructions, and level of social support when deciding whether or not to admit these patients. Hospital admission itself poses many risks for the older adult.[90] Therefore, EMPs must understand that discharge may improve outcomes in some patients as long as appropriate transitions of care are arranged.[91]

Comprehensive geriatric assessment has been shown to improve outcomes for vulnerable elders after an emergency department visit.[92] However, it is too resource intensive to be performed regularly in the emergency department. Recognizing the

Table 3
Systemic options for pain control in older adults

Drug	Indications	Considerations	Dosing Recommendations
Nonopioids			
Acetaminophen	First line for acute or chronic mild to moderate pain[56]	Use with caution in liver dysfunction or alcohol use.	3 g maximum daily dose[57]
NSAIDs	Appropriate for acute, mild to moderate pain	On Beers list of potentially inappropriate medications for older adults owing to well-established gastrointestinal and renal toxicities[58] Avoid in patients with renal dysfunction	Use lowest possible dose for shortest possible duration Consider topical NSAIDs such as diclofenac gel, which have a lower risk of side effects[59]
Opioids			
Tramadol	Appropriate for moderate to severe pain[56] Should be used as only one part of multimodal pain control strategy	Weak potency with similar side effect burden as other opioids Lowers seizure threshold[60] May lead to hyponatremia[61]	Starting doses for older adults should be 25%–50% of typical dose to allow for differences in metabolism, distribution, and elimination associated with aging[62]
Codeine		High variability in metabolism, avoid in older adults Weak potency with similar side effect burden as other opioids	Initiate and titrate 1 agent at a time to accurately monitor for side effects[58]
Hydrocodone		Formulated in combination with acetaminophen, which limits maximum dose	
Oxycodone		Safer than morphine in renal dysfunction[63–69]	
Morphine		Avoid in renal dysfunction owing to toxic metabolites Effective concentration higher in older adults with decreased lean body mass	
Hydromorphone		Safer than morphine in renal dysfunction[63]	

(continued on next page)

Table 3 (continued)			
Drug	**Indications**	**Considerations**	**Dosing Recommendations**
Fentanyl		Use with caution in opioid-naïve patients Lipid soluble, effective half-life may increase in older adults	

Abbreviation: NSAIDs, nonsteroidal anti-inflammatory drugs.

challenge of identifying high-risk elder patients, several screening tools have been developed to quickly assess the risk of geriatric syndromes in the emergency department, including the Identification of Seniors at Risk tool from the Geriatric Emergency Department Guidelines,[93] and the Emergency Geriatric Assessment tool.[94] For falls specifically, which increase future risk of orthopedic injury, many screening tools exist; however, there is little evidence to support the use of a definitive tool.[95] Using these tools to stratify older patients at high risk for poor outcomes can identify those requiring extra assistance at the transition of care.

MULTIDISCIPLINARY MANAGEMENT

For older adults admitted after a hip fracture, several different models of care exist. Historically, hip fractures were the purview of orthopedic surgeons until the idea of comanagement between orthopedics and medicine or geriatrics developed in the UK in the 1980s and 1990s.[96] Since this time, 4 main models of care have emerged.[97]

- Orthopedic admission with geriatric or medicine consult as needed
- Orthopedic admission with daily geriatric or medicine consult
- Geriatric or medicine admission with daily orthopedic consult
- Orthopedic and geriatric or medicine comanagement

Data regarding benefits of the first 3 models are variable,[96] whereas the fourth model of integrated orthopedic and geriatric comanagement has shown consistent benefit. Benefits include decreased complication rates,[98,99] mortality,[100,101] length-of-stay,[99,102] and costs,[103,104] as well as improved functional outcomes.[105]

One of the largest and most studied orthogeriatric comanagement programs in the United States, the Geriatric Fracture Center, was developed at Highland Hospital in Rochester, New York.[106] The care provided in this model is governed by 5 principles[107]:

- Most patients benefit from surgical stabilization of their fracture.
- The sooner patients have surgery, the less time they have to develop iatrogenic illness.
- Comanagement with frequent communication avoids common medical and functional complications.
- Standardized protocols decrease unwarranted variability.
- Discharge planning begins at admission.

A true comanagement model requires significant interdisciplinary coordination and cooperation, which is difficult to implement. However, the practice of this model has increased in recent years. By collecting data as they switched from a geriatric consult model to a fully integrated comanagement model, one orthopedic trauma unit in the UK was able to show a direct improvement in mortality, length of stay, and time to surgery with the comanagement.[108] These results could likely be replicated in other orthopedic trauma units making a similar transition. In 2017, the American Geriatric Society launched AGS CoCare: Ortho, which is a geriatrics–orthopedics comanagement model for the care of older adults with hip fractures.[109] It includes evidence-based educational curriculum and an implementation toolkit for institutions to adopt a comanagement model for their hip fracture patients.

SUMMARY

The biological and physiologic changes of aging, coupled with an increase in comorbid conditions and impacts the presentation, diagnosis, and treatment of orthopedic disease in older adults. It is imperative for the EMP to recognize the many key differences in geriatric patients to provide high-value, timely care. Much of this care should be provided by a multidisciplinary team, of which the EMP is a critical constituent. These multidisciplinary care team models have consistently shown improvement in health system and patient-centered outcomes in older adults with orthopedic disease and injury. Knowledge gained through this article can help EMPs to develop systems of care to improve the management and outcomes of orthogeriatric conditions in the emergency department.

REFERENCES

1. Siris ES, Adler R, Bilezikian J, et al. The clinical diagnosis of osteoporosis: a position statement from the National Bone Health Alliance Working Group. Osteoporos Int 2014;25(5):1439–43.
2. Bellantoni MF. Osteoporosis and other metabolic bone disorders. In: Busby-Whitehead J, Arenson C, Durso SC, et al, editors. Reichel's care of the elderly: clinical aspects of aging. New York: Cambridge University Press; 2016. p. 446–52.
3. Danna NR, Zuckerman JD. Musculoskeletal injuries in the elderly. In: Busby-Whitehead J, Arenson C, Durso SC, et al, editors. Reichel's care of the elderly: clinical aspects of aging. New York: Cambridge University Press; 2016. p. 462–76.
4. Hung WW, Egol KA, Zuckerman JD, et al. Hip fracture management: tailoring care for the older patient. JAMA 2012;307(20):2185–94.
5. Ogawa S, Yakabe M, Akishita M. Age-related sarcopenia and its pathophysiological bases. Inflamm Regen 2016;36:17.
6. Baumgartner RN, Koehler KM, Gallagher D, et al. Epidemiology of sarcopenia among the elderly in New Mexico. Am J Epidemiol 1998;147(8):755–63.
7. National Institute for Health and Care Excellence. Osteoporosis: assessing the risk of fragility fracture, clinical guidelines. 2012. Available at: https://www.nice.org.uk/guidance/cg146/resources/osteoporosis-assessing-the-risk-of-fragility-fracture-pdf-35109574194373. Accessed February 11, 2019.
8. Cummings SR, Melton LJ. Epidemiology and outcomes of osteoporotic fractures. Lancet 2002;359(9319):1761–7.
9. Gosch M, Hoffmann-Weltin Y, Roth T, et al. Orthogeriatric co-management improves the outcomes of long-term care residents with fragility fractures. Arch Orthop Trauma Surg 2016;136(10):1403–9.

10. Anderson G. Chronic care: making the case for ongoing care. Robert Wood Johnson Foundation, Princeton, New Jersey: 2010. Available at: https://www.rwjf.org/en/library/research/2010/01/chronic-care.html. Accessed August 17, 2018.

11. Potter JF. The older orthopaedic patient. Clin Orthop Relat Res 2004;425:44–9.

12. Blanda MP. Pharmacologic issues in geriatric emergency medicine. Emerg Med Clin North Am 2006;24(2):449–65.

13. Simunovic N, Devereaux P, Sprague S, et al. Effect of early surgery after hip fracture on mortality and complications: a systemic review and meta analysis. CMJA 2010;182(15):1609–16.

14. Moja L, Piatti A, Pecoraro V, et al. Timing matters in hip fracture surgery: patients operated within 48 hours have better outcomes. A meta-analysis and meta-regression of over 190,000 patients. PLoS One 2012;7(10):e46175.

15. Khan S, Kalra S, Khanna A, et al. Timing of surgery in hip fractures: a systemic review of 52 published studies involving 291,413 patients. Injury 2009;40(7): 692–7.

16. Siebenburger G, Van Delden D, Helfen T, et al. Timing of surgery for open reduction and internal fixation of displaced proximal humeral fractures. Injury 2015;46(Suppl 4):S58–62.

17. Ikpeze TC, Mohney M, Elfar JC. Initial preoperative management of geriatric hip fractures. Geriatr Orthop Surg Rehabil 2017;8(1):64–6.

18. Clement ND, Duckworth AD, McQueen MM, et al. The outcome of proximal humeral fractures in the elderly. Bone Joint J 2014;96-B(7):970–7.

19. Timler D, Dworzynski MJ, Szarpak L, et al. Head trauma in elderly patients: mechanisms of injuries and CT findings. Adv Clin Exp Med 2015;24(6):1045–50.

20. Hall S, Myers AM, Sadek A, et al. Spinal fractures incurred by a fall from standing height. Clin Neurol Neurosurg 2019;177:106–13.

21. Dietz SO, Hofmann A, Rommens PM. Haemorrhage in fragility fractures of the pelvis. Eur J Trauma Emerg Surg 2015;41(4):363–7.

22. Schumaier A, Grawe B. Proximal humerus fractures: evaluation and management in the elderly patient. Geriatr Orthop Surg Rehabil 2018;9:1–11.

23. Olerud P, Ahrengart L, Ponzer S, et al. Internal fixation versus nonoperative treatment of displaced 3-part proximal humeral fractures in elderly patients: a randomized controlled trial. J Shoulder Elbow Surg 2011;20(5):747–55.

24. Niver GE, Ilyas AM. Carpal tunnel syndrome after distal radius fracture. Orthop Clin North Am 2012;43(4):521–7.

25. Egol KA, Walsh M, Romo-Cardoso S, et al. Distal radial fractures in elderly: operative compared with nonoperative treatment. J Bone Joint Surg Am 2010;92(9): 1851–7.

26. Wong AYL, Karppinen J, Samartzis D. Low back pain in older adults: risk factors, management options and future directions. Scoliosis Spinal Disord 2017; 12:14.

27. Fink HA, Milavetz DL, Palermo L, et al. What proportion of incident radiographic vertebral deformities is clinically diagnosed and vice versa? J Bone Miner Res 2005;20(7):1216–22.

28. Shah LM, Jennings JW, Kirsch CFE, et al. ACR appropriateness criteria management of vertebral compression fractures. J Am Coll Radiol 2018;15(11S): S347–64.

29. McCarthy J, Davis A, Grant D. Diagnosis and management of vertebral compression fractures. Am Fam Physician 2016;94(1):44–50.

30. Lyritis GP, Ioannidis GV, Karachalios T, et al. Analgesic effect of salmon calcitonin suppositories in patients with acute pain due to recent osteoporotic vertebral crush fracture: a prospective double-blind, randomized, placebo-controlled clinical study. Clin J Pain 1999;15(4):284–9.

31. Borczuk P. An evidence-based approach to the evaluation and treatment of low back pain in the emergency department. Emerg Med Pract 2013;15(7):1–23.

32. Casazza B. Diagnosis and treatment of acute low back pain. Am Fam Physician 2012;85(4):343–50.

33. Henry SM, Pollak AN, Jones AL, et al. Pelvic fracture in geriatric patients: a distinct clinical entity. J Trauma 2002;53(1):15–20.

34. O'Brien DP, Luchette FA, Pereira SJ, et al. Pelvic fracture in the elderly is associated with increased mortality. Surgery 2002;132(4):710–5.

35. Pehle B, Nast-Kolb D, Oberbeck R, et al. Significance of physical examination and radiography for the pelvis during treatment in the shock emergency room. Unfallchirurg 2003;106(8):642–8 [in German].

36. Tajeu GS, Delzell E, Smith W, et al. Death, debility, and destitution following hip fracture. J Gerontol A Biol Sci Med Sci 2014;69(3):346–53.

37. Keene GS, Parker MJ, Pryor GA. Mortality and morbidity after hip fractures. BMJ 1993;307(6914):1248–50.

38. Nevitt MC, Cummings SR. Type and fall and risk of hip and wrist fractures: the study of osteoporotic fractures. J Am Geriatr Soc 1994;42(8):909.

39. Dominguez S, Liu P, Roberts C, et al. Prevalence of traumatic hip and pelvic fractures in patients with suspected hip fracture and negative initial standard radiographs—a study of emergency department patients. Acad Emerg Med 2005;12(4):366–9.

40. Bressler HB, Keyes WJ, Rochon PA, et al. The prevalence of low back pain in the elderly: a systematic review of the literature. Spine 1999;24(17):1813–9.

41. Hossain M, Barwick C, Sinha AK, et al. Is magnetic resonance imaging (MRI) necessary to exclude occult hip fracture? Injury 2007;38(10):1204–8.

42. Haubro M, Stougaard C, Torfing T, et al. Sensitivity and specificity of CT- and MRI-scanning in evaluation of occult fracture of proximal femur. Injury 2015; 46(8):1557–61.

43. Mears SC, Kates SL. A guide to improving the care of patients with fragility fractures, edition 2. Geriatr Orthop Surg Rehabil 2015;6(2):58–120.

44. Beckenkamp PR, Chung-Wei CL, Macaskill P, et al. Diagnostic accuracy of the Ottawa Ankle and Midfoot Rules: a systemic review with meta-analysis. Br J Sports Med 2017;51(6):504–10.

45. Srinivasan CMS, Moran CG. Internal fixation of ankle fractures in the very elderly. Injury 2001;32(7):559–63.

46. Williams CM, Maher CG, Latimer J, et al. Efficacy of paracetamol for acute lowback pain; a double-blind, randomized controlled trial. Lancet 2014;384(9954): 1586–96.

47. Friedman BW, Holden L, Esses D. Parenteral corticosteroids for emergency department patients with non-radicular low back pain. J Emerg Med 2006; 31(4):365–70.

48. Qassem A, Wilt TJ, McLean RM, et al. Noninvasive treatments for acute, subacute and chronic low back pain: a clinical practice guidelines from the American College of Physicians. Ann Intern Med 2017;166(7):514–30.

49. Jarvik JG, Gold LS, Comstock BA, et al. Association of early imaging for back pain with clinical outcomes in older adults. JAMA 2015;313(11):1143–53.

50. Jones J, Southerland W, Catalani B. The importance of optimizing acute pain in the orthopedic trauma patient. Orthop Clin North Am 2017;48(4):445–65.
51. Ko A, Harada MY, Smith EJT, et al. Pain assessment and control in the injured elderly. Am Surg 2016;82(10):867–71.
52. Platts-Mills TF, Esserman DA, Brown DL, et al. Older US emergency department patients are less likely to receive pain medication than younger patients: results from a national survey. Ann Emerg Med 2012;60(2):199–206.
53. Morrison RS, Magaziner J, Gilbert M, et al. Relationship between pain and opioid analgesics on the development of delirium following hip fracture. J Gerontol A Biol Sci Med Sci 2003;58(1):M76–81.
54. Shega JW, Dale W, Andrew M, et al. Persistent pain and frailty: a case for home-ostenosis. J Am Geriatr Soc 2012;60(1):113–7.
55. Karani R, Meier DE. Systemic pharmacologic postoperative pain management in the geriatric orthopaedic patient. Clin Orthop Relat Res 2004;425:26–34.
56. Mckeown JL. Pain management issues for the geriatric surgical patient. Anesthesiol Clin 2015;33:563–76.
57. Rolita L, Spegman A, Tang X, et al. Greater number of narcotic analgesic prescriptions for osteoarthritis is associated with falls and fractures in elderly adults. J Am Geriatr Soc 2013;61(3):335–40.
58. Siu A, Penrod J, Boockvar K, et al. Early ambulation after hip fracture. Arch Intern Med 2006;166(7):766–71.
59. Davies DF, Shock NW. Age changes in glomerular filtration rate, effective renal plasma flow, and tubular excretory capacity in adult males. J Clin Invest 1950; 29(5):496–507.
60. Zeeh J, Platt D. The aging liver. Gerontology 2002;48(3):121–7.
61. Forbes GB, Reina JC. Adult lean body mass declines with age: some longitudinal observations. Metabolism 1970;19(9):653–63.
62. American Geriatric Society. Pharmacological management of persistent pain in older persons American Geriatrics Society panel on the pharmacological management of persistent pain in older persons. J Am Geriatr Soc 2009;57:1331–46.
63. Malec M, Shega JW. Pain management in the elderly. Med Clin North Am 2015; 99:337–50.
64. Samuel MJ. American Geriatrics Society 2015 updated beers criteria for potentially inappropriate medication use in older adults. J Am Geriatr Soc 2015; 63(11):2227–46.
65. Zeng C, Wei J, Persson MSM, et al. Relative efficacy and safety of topical non-steroidal anti-inflammatory drugs for osteoarthritis: a systematic review and network meta-analysis of randomised controlled trials and observational studies. Br J Sports Med 2018;52:642–50.
66. Talaie H, Panahandeh R, Fayazonouri MR, et al. Dose-independent occurrence of seizure with tramadol. J Med Toxicol 2009;5(2):63–7.
67. Fournier JP, Yin H, Nessim SJ, et al. Tramadol for noncancer pain and the risk of hyponatremia. Am J Med 2015;128(4):418–25.
68. Gupta DK, Avram MJ. Rational opioid dosing in the elderly: dose and dosing interval when initiating opioid therapy. Clin Pharmacol Ther 2012;91(2):339–43.
69. Pergolizzi J, Böger RH, Budd K, et al. Opioids and the management of chronic severe pain in the elderly: consensus statement of an international expert panel with focus on the six clinically most often used world health organization step III opioids. Pain Pract 2008;8(4):287–313.
70. Elkassabany N, Cai LF, Mehta S, et al. Does regional anesthesia improve the quality of postoperative pain management and the quality of recovery in patients

undergoing operative repair of tibia and ankle fractures? J Orthop Trauma 2015; 29(9):404–9.

71. Abou-Setta AM, Beaupre LA, Rashiq S, et al. Comparative effectiveness of pain management interventions for hip fracture: a systematic review. Ann Intern Med 2011;155(4):234–45.

72. Unneby A, Svensson O, Gustafson Y, et al. Femoral nerve block in a representative sample of elderly people with hip fracture: a randomised controlled trial. Injury 2017;48:1542–9.

73. Ritcey B, Pageau P, Woo MY, et al. Regional nerve blocks for hip and femoral neck fractures in the emergency department: a systematic review. Can J Emerg Med 2016;18(1):37–47.

74. Beaudoin FL, Haran JP, Liebmann O. A comparison of ultrasound-guided three-in-one femoral nerve block versus parenteral opioids alone for analgesia in emergency department patients with hip fractures: a randomized controlled trial. Acad Emerg Med 2013;20(6):584–91.

75. Hunt KJ, Higgins TF, Carlston CV, et al. Continuous peripheral nerve blockade as postoperative analgesia for open treatment of calcaneal fractures. J Orthop Trauma 2010;24(3):148–55.

76. Lees D, Harrison WD, Ankers T, et al. Fascia iliaca compartment block for hip fractures: experience of integrating a new protocol across two hospital sites. Eur J Emerg Med 2016;23(1):12–8.

77. Arsoy D, Huddleston JI III, Amanatullah DF, et al. Femoral Nerve Catheters Improve Home Disposition and Pain in Hip Fracture Patients Treated With Total Hip Arthroplasty. J Arthroplasty 2017;32:3434–7.

78. Nie H, Yang YX, Wang Y, et al. Effects of continuous fascia iliaca compartment blocks for postoperative analgesia in patients with hip fracture. Pain Res Manag 2015;20(4):210–2.

79. Mittal R, Vermani E. Femoral nerve blocks in fractures of femur: variation in the current UK practice and a review of the literature. Emerg Med J 2014;31(2): 143–7.

80. Haslam L, Lansdown A, Lee J, et al. Survey of current practices: peripheral nerve block utilization by ED physicians for treatment of pain in the hip fracture patient population. Can Geriatr J 2013;16(1):16–21.

81. Lovald ST, Ong KL, Lau EC, et al. Readmission and complications for catheter and injection femoral nerve block administration after total knee arthroplasty in the Medicare population. J Arthroplasty 2015;30(12):2076–81.

82. Fitch RW, Kuhn JE. Intraarticular lidocaine versus intravenous procedural sedation with narcotics and benzodiazepines for reduction of the dislocated shoulder: a systematic review. Acad Emerg Med 2008;15(8):703–8.

83. Raeyat Doost E, Heiran MM, Movahedi M, et al. Ultrasound-guided interscalene nerve block vs procedural sedation by propofol and fentanyl for anterior shoulder dislocations. Am J Emerg Med 2017;35(10):1435–9.

84. Stone MB, Wang R, Price DD. Ultrasound-guided supraclavicular brachial plexus nerve block vs procedural sedation for the treatment of upper extremity emergencies. Am J Emerg Med 2008;26(6):706–10.

85. Lovallo E, Mantuani D, Nagdev A. Novel use of ultrasound in the ED: ultrasound-guided hematoma block of a proximal humeral fracture. Am J Emerg Med 2015; 33(1):130.

86. Borgeat A, Perschak H, Bird P, et al. Patient-controlled interscalene analgesia with intravenous analgesia after major shoulder surgery. Anesthesiology 2000; 92:102–8.

87. Dufeu N, Marchand-Maillet F, Atchabahian A, et al. Efficacy and safety of ultrasound-guided distal blocks for analgesia without motor blockade after ambulatory hand surgery. J Hand Surg Am 2014;39(4):737–43.

88. Hebl JR, Dilger JA, Byer DE, et al. A pre-emptive multimodal pathway featuring peripheral nerve block improves perioperative outcomes after major orthopedic surgery. Reg Anesth Pain Med 2008;33(6):510–7.

89. Goldstein RY, Montero N, Jain SK, et al. Efficacy of popliteal block in postoperative pain control after ankle fracture fixation: a prospective randomized study. J Orthop Trauma 2012;26(10):557–61.

90. Sourdet S, Lafont C, Rolland Y, et al. Preventable Iatrogenic disability in elderly patients during hospitalization. J Am Med Dir Assoc 2015;16(8):674–81.

91. McCusker J, Verdon J, Tousignant P, et al. Rapid emergency department intervention for older people reduces risk of functional decline: results of a multicenter randomized trial. J Am Geriatr Soc 2001;49(10):1272–81.

92. Caplan GA, Williams ÃAJ, Daly ÃB, et al. A randomized , controlled trial of comprehensive geriatric elderly from the emergency department: the DEED II Study. J Am Geriatr Soc 2004;52:1417–23.

93. Rosenberg MS, Carpenter CR, Bromley M, et al. Geriatric emergency department guidelines. Ann Emerg Med 2014;63(5):e7–25.

94. Ke YT, Peng AC, Shu YM, et al. Emergency geriatric assessment: a novel comprehensive screen tool for geriatric patients in the emergency department. Am J Emerg Med 2018;36(1):143–6.

95. Carpenter CR, Avidan MS, Wildes T, et al. Predicting geriatric falls following an episode of emergency department care: a systematic review. Acad Emerg Med 2014;21(10):1069–82.

96. Della Rocca GJ, Crist BD. Hip fracture protocols: what have we changed? Orthop Clin North Am 2013;44(2):163–82.

97. Pioli G, Giusti A, Barone A. Orthogeriatric care for the elderly with hip fractures: where are we? Aging Clin Exp Res 2008;20(2):113–22.

98. Vidán M, Serra JA, Moreno C, et al. Efficacy of a comprehensive geriatric intervention in older patients hospitalized for hip fracture: a randomized, controlled trial. J Am Geriatr Soc 2005;53(9):1476–82.

99. Friedman SM, Mendelson DA, Bingham KW, et al. Impact of a comanaged geriatric fracture center on short-term hip fracture outcomes. Arch Intern Med 2009; 169(18):1712–7.

100. Forni S, Pieralli F, Sergi A, et al. Mortality after hip fracture in the elderly: the role of a multidisciplinary approach and time to surgery in a retrospective observational study on 23,973 patients. Arch Gerontol Geriatr 2016;66(124):13–7.

101. Grigoryan KV, Javedan H, Rudolph JL. Orthogeriatric care models and outcomes in hip fracture patients. J Orthop Trauma 2014;28(3):e49–55.

102. Lynch G, Shaban RZ, Massey D. Evaluating the orthogeriatric model of care at an Australian tertiary hospital. Int J Orthop Trauma Nurs 2015;19(4):184–93.

103. Swart E, Vasudeva E, Makhni EC, et al. Dedicated perioperative hip fracture comanagement programs are cost-effective in high-volume centers: an economic analysis. Clin Orthop Relat Res 2016;474(1):222–33.

104. Kates SL, Mendelson DA, Friedman SM. The value of an organized fracture program for the elderly: early results. J Orthop Trauma 2011;25(4):233–7.

105. Prestmo A, Hagen G, Sletvold O, et al. Comprehensive geriatric care for patients with hip fractures: a prospective, randomised, controlled trial. Lancet 2015; 385(9978):1623–33.

106. Friedman SM, Mendelson DA, Kates SL, et al. Geriatric co-management of proximal femur fractures: Total quality management and protocol-driven care result in better outcomes for a frail patient population. J Am Geriatr Soc 2008;56(7): 1349–56.
107. Mendelson DA, Friedman SM. Principles of comanagement and the geriatric fracture center. Clin Geriatr Med 2014;30(2):183–9.
108. Middleton M, Wan B, Da Assunçao R. Improving hip fracture outcomes with integrated orthogeriatric care: A comparison between two accepted orthogeriatric models. Age Ageing 2017;46(3):465–70.
109. Jacobs L. A Case Study in Moving From Research to Practice: AGS CoCare: Ortho. J Gerontol Nurs 2018;44(9):51–2.

The Emergency Evaluation and Management of Pediatric Extremity Fractures

Kathy Boutis, MD, MSc, FRCPC

KEYWORDS

- Children • Fractures • Diagnosis • Management • Emergency

KEY POINTS

- There are validated clinical decision rules that aim to reduce unnecessary radiographs in children who present with wrist, knee, and ankle injuries.
- Abuse should be considered in any infant who is not walking and presents with a fracture.
- A conservative approach is encouraged that includes immobilization and referral to an orthopedic surgeon (emergency or outpatient depending on the severity of the fracture) if there is radiographic evidence of a fracture or a high clinical suspicion of a fracture without radiographic evidence with the following exceptions: low-risk distal fibular ankle and distal radius buckle fractures; the latter minor fractures can be managed with a removable device, return to activities as guided by the patient's symptoms, and follow-up with a primary care provider.
- Approximately 10% of pediatric fractures are not identified on the initial emergency department visit, and this is particularly true when the emergency department physician has a low suspicion for a fracture or the location of the injury is a joint. Although most missed fractures are minor, the most commonly missed serious fractures are the Tillaux fracture and the Monteggia fracture.

ANATOMIC AND HEALING PRINCIPLES

The anatomy of the pediatric musculoskeletal system changes with the growth and development that occurs in children. The long bones of children consist of discrete anatomic areas. The physis is an area of growth cartilage and may occur at one or both ends of a long bone. The area of bone between the physis and the

Disclosure Statement: Dr K. Boutis is the academic director of ImageSim Continued Professional Development and Training platform (www.imagesim.com). ImageSim operates as nonprofit course under the academic umbrellas of the Hospital for Sick Children and the University of Toronto. Dr K. Boutis does not receive any funds for her participation the management of ImageSim.
Division of Emergency Medicine, ImageSim, Research Institute, The Hospital for Sick Children, University of Toronto, 555 University Avenue, Toronto, Ontario M5G1X8, Canada
E-mail address: Kathy.boutis@sickkids.ca

Emerg Med Clin N Am 38 (2020) 31–59
https://doi.org/10.1016/j.emc.2019.09.003

adjacent joint is the *epiphysis*. The midshaft of a long bone is the *diaphysis*. The *metaphysis* of a long bone is the area between the diaphysis and the physis (**Fig. 1**).

Children's bones, especially in younger children, are softer and more pliable than those of adults, and therefore can respond to mechanical stress by bowing and buckling rather than routinely fracturing through and through like adult bone fractures. The periosteum of the diaphysis and the metaphysis is thick in children, and is continuous from the metaphysis to the epiphysis, surrounding and protecting the mechanically weaker physis. The physis is sensitive to alterations in the blood supply, and physeal injuries can result in a bony bridge resulting in growth arrest.[1] On the other hand, the ligaments of children are stronger and more compliant than in adults, and ligaments tolerate mechanical forces better than the weaker physis.

The pediatric musculoskeletal system also has some distinctive healing features. Remodeling allows for a certain degree of angulation in pediatric fractures, as children can remodel with bone growth to nearly perfect anatomic alignment without any intervention except for immobilization. The degree of remodeling is greatest in young children, if there is a metaphyseal fracture, or if the deformity occurs in the plane of motion of the adjacent joint.[2] Therefore, the acceptable amount of angulation, minimizing the need for reduction, in pediatric fractures is much greater than that in similar adult fractures. In addition, there is often sufficient callus formation such that nonunion almost never occurs in displaced fractures.[3] Therefore, even though fractures occur more frequently in children than they do in adults, they have an exceptional healing capacity and usually have good outcomes.

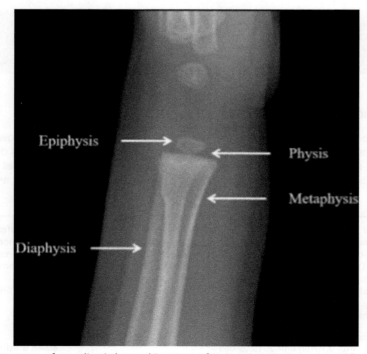

Fig. 1. Anatomy of a pediatric bone. (*Courtesy of* K. Boutis, MD, Toronto, ON.)

FRACTURE PATTERNS
Physeal Fractures

The Salter and Harris classification system classifies physeal fractures with respect to prognosis for growth disturbance. It is important to note that the risk of growth arrest varies with the particular bone as well. That is, the risk for growth arrest in a Type II fracture of the distal fibula is not the same as this risk in Type II fractures of the distal tibia. Differential risks largely relates to the anatomy of the growth plate and its vascular supply. In general, the more linear the growth plate (eg, distal fibula) the less risk for vascular disturbance in the event of a growth plate fracture.[1]

Salter-Harris Type I fractures occur when there is cleavage through the hypertrophic cell zone of the physis, with the reproductive cells of the physis remaining with the epiphysis. There is often separation from the metaphysis, which is often temporary or can result in a displaced epiphysis; however, there are no associated fragments of bone. In the absence of epiphyseal displacement, radiographs only demonstrate soft tissue swelling. The diagnosis is clinical with tenderness and swelling maximal over the physis. Type I injuries have a very low incidence of growth disturbances.

Salter-Harris Type II fractures occur when the fracture line extends along the physis and then out through a part of the metaphyseal bone. Growth is often preserved because the reproductive layers of the physis maintain their position with the epiphysis and the epiphyseal circulation. Diagnosis is made radiographically by noting a triangular-shaped metaphyseal fragment (ie, Thurstan Holland fragment) (**Fig. 2**).

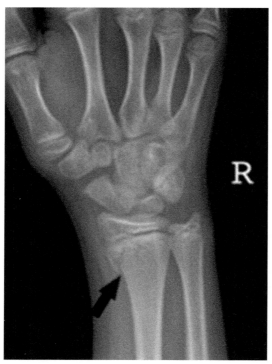

Fig. 2. Salter-Harris II of the distal radius. Arrow points to the fracture in the metaphysis that extends into the growth plate. (*Courtesy of* K. Boutis, MD, Toronto, ON.)

Salter-Harris Type III fractures have a fracture line that extends into the intra-articular area from the epiphysis, through the physis, with the cleavage plane continuing to the periphery. The prognosis for subsequent bone growth relates to the preservation of circulation to the epiphyseal bone fragment; however, the prognosis is usually quite favorable. The diagnosis of a Type III injury is made radiographically (**Fig. 3**). Occasionally, additional imaging with computed tomography (CT) or magnetic resonance imaging (MRI) is used to better evaluate the extent of the fracture and articular surface involvement.

Salter-Harris Type IV fractures have a fracture line that originates at the articular surface and extends through the epiphysis, the entire thickness of the physis, and continues through the metaphysis. The diagnosis of a Type IV injury is made radiographically on identification of epiphyseal and metaphyseal fragments (**Fig. 4**). The risk of growth disturbance with this type of fracture can be significant.

Salter-Harris Type V fractures are rare and typically are the result of a profound compressive force transmitted to the physis. The diagnosis of a Type V injury may be difficult initially, leading to a lack of appreciation of the severity of the injury. The mechanism of injury should point to a Type V injury, as these injuries are typically associated with fall from a great height. Radiographs may appear normal or may demonstrate focal narrowing of the physeal plate and obtaining comparison views of the uninjured side may be beneficial.

Torus and Greenstick Fractures

Compressive forces may result in a bulging or buckling of the periosteum termed a *torus* or *buckle* fracture. Any asymmetry, bulging, or deviation of the cortical margin indicates a torus fracture (**Fig. 5**), although it may be subtle.

A *greenstick* fracture is characterized by cortical disruption on the convex side of the bone, with a buckling or intact cortex on the concave side of the bone. These injuries typically occur at the metaphyseal-diaphyseal junction of a long bone (**Fig. 6**).

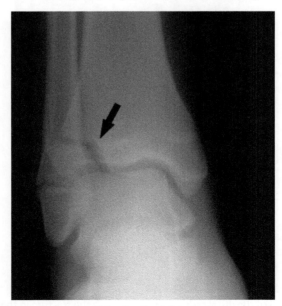

Fig. 3. Salter-Harris III of the distal tibia. Arrow points to the fracture in the epiphysis that extends into the joint. (*Courtesy of* K. Boutis, MD, Toronto, ON.)

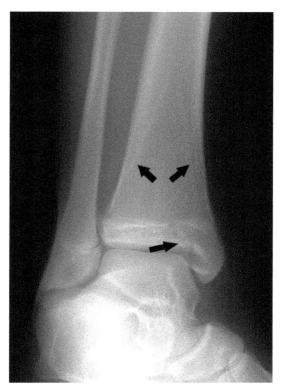

Fig. 4. Salter-Harris IV of the distal tibia. Arrows highlight the fracture in the metaphysis and epiphysis with extension into the joint. (*Courtesy of* K. Boutis, MD, Toronto, ON.)

PLASTIC DEFORMITIES

Plastic deformities are also referred to as *bowing* fractures and typically occur after a fall on the outstretched hand (FOOSH). The classic clinical hallmark is pain out of proportion to the physical examination findings. In forearm bowing fractures, pain is maximal on protonation/supination. The cortex of the diaphysis of the long bone is deformed, but the periosteum along the entire diaphysis is preserved. Moderate-severe plastic deformity is usually obvious clinically. However, in mild cases of bowing injuries, comparison films of the uninvolved extremity can be helpful (**Fig. 7**) to ensure that these injuries are not missed.

UPPER EXTREMITY INJURIES
Clavicle

Clavicle fractures occur during infancy as a result of birth trauma or during childhood as a result of FOOSH or onto the lateral side of the shoulder. Mid-clavicular fractures are the most common, whereas medial and lateral clavicular fractures are relatively rare.

Middle third of clavicle

Most of these injuries can be treated with analgesics, support of the injury with a broad arm sling for 3 to 4 weeks, and follow-up with the primary care physician (PCP).[4]

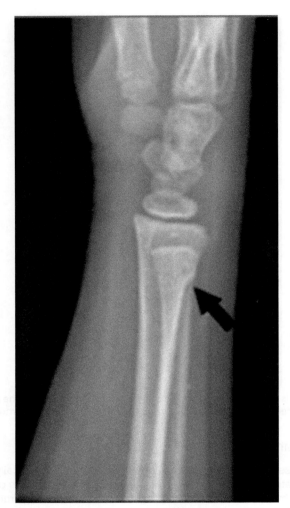

Fig. 5. Buckle fracture of the distal radius. Arrow identifies the buckling in the cortex. (*Courtesy of* K. Boutis, MD, Toronto, ON.)

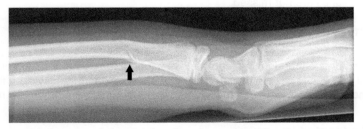

Fig. 6. Greenstick fracture of the distal radius. Arrow identifies the cortical break in the meta-diaphyseal junction. There is also buckling on the opposite of the cortex. (*Courtesy of* K. Boutis, MD, Toronto, ON.)

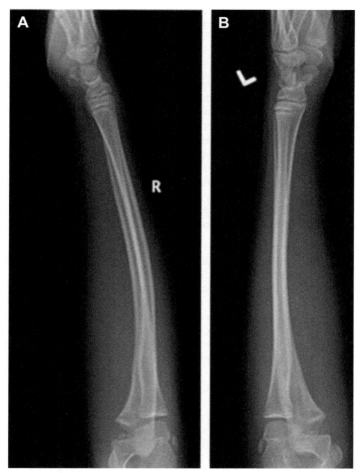

Fig. 7. (*A*) Bowing of the radius and ulna of the injured right arm. (*B*) A normal radius and ulna on the uninjured left arm. (*Courtesy of* K. Boutis, MD, Toronto, ON.)

Urgent orthopedic consultation is indicated when a child is >12 years, the fracture is ≥100% displaced or shortened ≥2 cm, there is skin tenting, neurovascular compromise, or fracture through a pathologic lesion.[5]

Medial clavicle
Given the strong ligamentous attachment of the clavicle to the sternum, injuries to this area are usually epiphyseal disruptions. Urgent orthopedic consultation is recommended for these injuries.

Lateral clavicle
Minimally displaced distal clavicle fractures only need immobilization with a sling or equivalent. Urgent orthopedic consultation is needed for fractures with 100% displacement, ≥2 cm shortening or associated acromioclavicular dislocation.[6]

Humerus

Midshaft humeral fractures typically occur from a FOOSH or a direct blow to the upper arm.

Proximal humerus

These fractures may occur at the physis or the proximal humeral metaphysis, and they have an extraordinary ability to repair themselves. Proximal humeral physeal fractures occur more commonly in adolescence because this area becomes relatively weak during this time of rapid growth. Fractures of the proximal humeral metaphysis are more common in preadolescents. Treatment depends on the age of the child and degree of displacement or angulation. In general, children ≤10 to 12 years with a proximal humeral fracture that is displaced ≤50% and less than 60° angulated can be treated in a broad arm sling for 4 weeks and follow-up in an orthopedics clinic within a week.[7,8] If the child is >10 to 12 years with greater than 50% displacement or greater than 30° angulation, there is a pathologic fracture, or neurovascular compromise then urgent referral to an orthopedic surgeon is indicated.[9,10]

Humeral diaphysis

Direct trauma to the humerus can cause a transverse fracture, and a violent rotation can cause a spiral fracture. Spiral/oblique fractures of the humeral diaphysis in infants and toddlers have been strongly linked to child abuse.[11,12] Rarely, the fracture fragment may injure the radial nerve as it runs in the radial groove. Thus, assess radial nerve function (eg, wrist extensors and supinators, sensation of dorsoradial hand, thumb, and second digits) on initial examination and following any splinting. The potential for healing is good, and treatment is usually immobilization in a long-arm plaster splint with orthopedic follow-up. Orthopedic consultation is recommended for midshaft humeral fractures that present with a clinical deformity or angulation more than 20° in children and 10° in adolescents.[10]

Elbow

Acute pediatric elbow injuries usually are related to falls. The large cartilaginous component of the elbow makes radiograph interpretation difficult.[13] As a result, compared with other fractures, elbow fractures in children are commonly missed in the emergency department (ED).[14] True lateral and anteroposterior radiographs of the elbow are essential to diagnose elbow fractures. Because competency in pediatric elbow interpretation is difficult to achieve, many clinicians obtain comparison radiographs of the uninjured side as a reference to what is normal.[15]

Supracondylar fractures

Most supracondylar fractures occur in children from 3 to 10 years with the peak incidence occurring between ages 5 and 7 years. The extension type supracondylar fracture is by far the most common, accounting for 90% to 98% of cases.

An extension-type supracondylar fracture is caused by a FOOSH with the elbow hyperextended. A flexion-type fracture results from falling on a flexed elbow and is rare. The complications of a supracondylar fracture, although uncommon, range from transient neurapraxia to Volkmann ischemic contracture, with the most common being an injury to the anterior interosseous nerve resulting in the "pointing finger sign."

Type I fractures are displaced ≤2 mm and may have a posterior fat pad sign as the only radiographic finding (**Fig. 8**). Type I supracondylar fractures are inherently stable. The goal of therapy is pain control and immobilization with a long-arm posterior splint with the elbow at 90° and the forearm in protonation or neutral rotation for 3 weeks. Arrange orthopedic follow-up within 2 to 7 days. Although collar and cuff

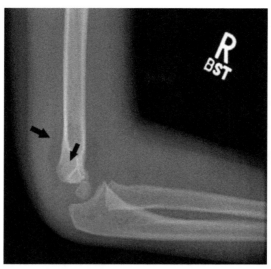

Fig. 8. Type I supracondylar fracture. Smaller arrow points to the posterior fat pad. Larger arrow points to the displaced distal humerus fracture. (*Courtesy of* K. Boutis, MD, Toronto, ON.)

immobilization is used in some centers, it does not offer as good pain management as splinting.[16,17]

Type II fractures are angulated to varying degrees, but the posterior cortex of the humerus is intact (**Fig. 9**).

Type III fractures are completely displaced with no cortical contact (**Fig. 10**). The distal fragment may be posteromedially (Type IIIa) rotated and, as such, can impinge against the radial nerve or be posterolaterally (Type IIIb) rotated. In posterolaterally displaced fractures, the brachial artery and median nerve are at risk for injury, and compartment syndrome can develop.[18,19] Consult orthopedic surgery emergently (within 1 hour) if there is a suspicion of compartment syndrome, if there is loss of radial pulses, or a cool, white hand. Otherwise, Type II and III fractures need urgent orthopedic consultation (within 4 hours) in the ED for definitive management that typically includes operative pinning.[20]

Lateral condylar fractures

These fractures occur when there is varus stress on an extended elbow with the forearm in supination. Swelling and tenderness are usually limited to the lateral elbow, and neurovascular injury is uncommon. The diagnosis can be made with standard anteroposterior and lateral views, but obtain an oblique view if the clinical suspicion is high. In Type 1 lateral condylar fractures, defined by ≤2 mm displacement, the child's elbow injury can be treated in a long-arm backslab with the elbow flexed at 90° and broad arm sling (**Fig. 11**).[21,22] Type 2 lateral condylar fractures occur when there is >2 mm displacement with congruity of the articular surface, whereas Type 3 occur with greater than 2 mm displacement and without congruity of the articular surface. Type 2 and 3 lateral condylar fractures require urgent orthopedic consultation because these fractures often require open reduction and internal fixation (ORIF). Nonunion, malunion, osteonecrosis, cubitus valgus, and ulnar nerve palsy are well-described complications.[23]

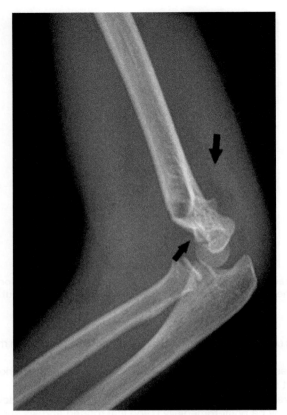

Fig. 9. Type II supracondylar fracture. Larger arrow points to the posterior fat pad and smaller arrow points to the subtle lucency in the cortex. (*Courtesy of* K. Boutis, MD, Toronto, ON.)

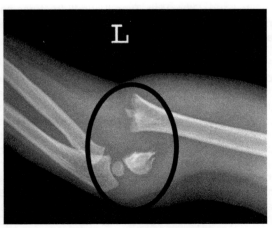

Fig. 10. Type III supracondylar fracture. The area in the circle identifies a markedly displaced supracondylar fracture. (*Courtesy of* K. Boutis, MD, Toronto, ON.)

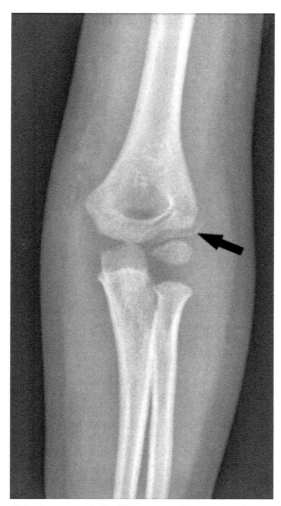

Fig. 11. Lateral condylar fracture of distal humerus. The arrow points to the fragment that represents a lateral condylar fracture. (*Courtesy of* K. Boutis, MD, Toronto, ON.)

Medial epicondyle fractures

These fractures tend to occur in older children, between the ages of 10 and 14 years. Simple fractures of the medial epicondyle are extra-articular injuries with limited soft tissue involvement, but nearly half of these injuries are associated with elbow dislocation; in such injuries, the epicondyle can become entrapped in the joint.[24,25] Fractures are classified by the amount of displacement and associated extremity injuries (**Fig. 12**). Typically, if there is <5 mm of displacement, these fractures can be managed in a long-arm backslab at 90° elbow flexion for 3 weeks and follow-up in orthopedics. More than 5 mm of displacement is an indication for urgent orthopedic consultation. It is important to distinguish between a medial epicondyle fracture from a medial condyle fracture. Medial condyle fractures are intra-articular and require urgent review by an orthopedic surgeon.

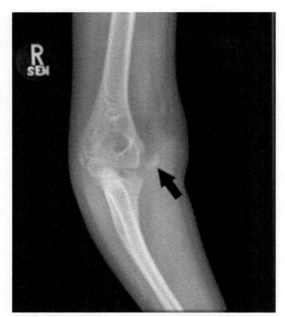

Fig. 12. Medial epicondylar fracture of the distal humerus. The arrow points to the fragment that represents a medial condylar fracture. (*Courtesy of* K. Boutis, MD, Toronto, ON.)

Monteggia fracture dislocation

This injury refers to the dislocation of the radial head (proximal radioulnar joint) with fracture of the ulna. This type of injury is the most commonly missed serious fracture of the elbow. A good general rule to avoid missing this injury is that if there is an ulnar fracture always look for an associated injury in the radius. The Bado classification system identifies 4 types of Monteggia fractures. The most common type occurs when there is an anterior dislocation of the radial head with fracture of the ulna shaft (**Fig. 13**). Emergent orthopedic consultation is indicated for this fracture as reduction is always required for these injuries.

Olecranon fractures

These injuries generally result from a fall on the elbow and are best seen on the lateral view. Orthopedic consultation is best to guide treatment. If the fracture is displaced ≤5 mm, it should be immobilized in the most stable position, usually 90° of elbow flexion, for 3 to 6 weeks.[26] ORIF is indicated for unstable fractures. Olecranon fractures occur in association with fractures of the radial head and neck. A "simple"

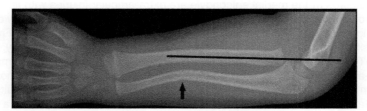

Fig. 13. Monteggia fracture. The transverse line demonstrates a radial head dislocation and the arrow points to the associated ulnar fracture. (*Courtesy of* K. Boutis, MD, Toronto, ON.)

olecranon fracture may be part of a Monteggia lesion, so the radial head position should be carefully evaluated.

Radial head and neck fractures

The radial neck is fractured more frequently than the radial head, and most radial neck fractures occur through the metaphysis (**Fig. 14**). The most common mechanism is a FOOSH. Obtain orthopedic consultation to guide treatment. Reduction is often necessary when angulation is >35^0 or displacement is greater than 60%.[27]

Elbow dislocation

These are uncommon in children, but the most common type of dislocation is posterior and often there are associated fractures of the medial and lateral epicondyle or radial neck. Neurologic injury is associated with approximately 10% of elbow dislocations. Ulnar neuropathy is the most common and is usually associated with medial epicondyle entrapment. Median nerve injury may be caused by entrapment of the nerve inside the joint, behind the medial epicondyle, or in an epicondyle fracture. Radial nerve and arterial injury are both rare. Consult orthopedics emergently if a neurovascular injury is suspected. After reduction and review of postreduction radiographs, immobilize the reduced elbow in a posterior mold and refer for orthopedic follow-up within one week.

Subluxation of the radial head

This is otherwise known as a *pulled elbow* or *nursemaid's elbow*. It is a common injury in young children. It can occur any time from birth to 6 years of age but commonly occurs from 1 to 4 years of age. The mechanism of injury is often a sudden pull on the arm, usually by an adult or taller person. The force pulls the radius through the annular ligament, resulting in subluxation (partial dislocation) of the radial head. The child experiences sudden acute pain and loss of function of the affected arm. On examination, the child holds the involved arm in slight flexion and protonation, and there is no focal swelling or tenderness. However, there is significant pain with protonation/supination of the forearm. This is a clinical diagnosis and should not be confused with other radial head pathology (eg, radial head/neck fractures) or bowing fractures that can also illicit tenderness with protonation/supination. Distinguishing features in favor of a pulled elbow include lack of focal symptoms/signs, younger age, and relatively benign mechanisms. There are 2 favored techniques to reduce a pulled elbow.[28] The first is called the "supination-flexion" method. The provider grasps the humeral epicondyles with their thumb over the radial head, and with the other hand, quickly supinates the forearm and flexes the elbow. An alternative method is called "hyperpronation." Hold the child's hand as if shaking hands, hold the epicondyles with your other hand, extend the forearm, and pronate quickly. If one method is not successful, you can try the alternative method. A recent meta-analysis concluded that hyperpronation was more

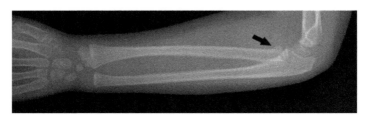

Fig. 14. Radial neck fracture. The arrow points to the lucency located at the radial neck. (*Courtesy of* K. Boutis, MD, Toronto, ON.)

effective in terms of success rate and less painful compared with the supination-flexion maneuver.[29] If successful, the pain resolves after reduction and normal arm movement is quickly regained.

Forearm

Childhood forearm fractures are the most common pediatric fractures,[30] and most often occur after a FOOSH. In general, with the presence of any localized pain, swelling, or limited movement, a radiograph of the affected area is recommended. The Amsterdam Pediatric Wrist rules have been validated in children 3 to 18 years and based on historical and physical examination variables provides a probability for the presence of a fracture and the recommendation to obtain or not to obtain radiographs. These rules have the potential to reduce unnecessary wrist radiographs in children by approximately 20%, with a reported sensitivity of 98%.[31]

Radius and ulna diaphyseal fractures
Injuries of the shaft can remain unstable despite attempts at closed reduction and occasionally require open fixation. Proximal third shaft fractures are relatively uncommon. In skeletally immature children younger than 10 years, angulation less than 10° often does not require anatomic reduction.[32]

Bowing deformities
These injuries can be difficult to diagnose and often missed. Radiologic comparison with the uninjured side may be necessary in mild cases (see **Fig. 7**). Failure to correct bowing (which tends to be along the whole bone) may lead to permanent deformity and disability. Although minimally angulated bowing fractures and those in younger children can often be managed in a splint/cast and follow-up with an orthopedic surgeon, more advanced bowing fractures may require completion of the break to establish proper realignment. Urgent orthopedic consultation is required for any plastic deformities. In general, proper reduction and realignment is recommended for any angulation ≥20° in children younger than 10 years or ≥15° degrees in children older than 10 years.[33]

Isolated ulnar fractures
These are rare and caused by a direct blow. Typically, those that are minimally angulated can be managed with a splint and follow-up in an orthopedic clinic. If caused by an indirect force, typically, there is an associated fracture or dislocation of the radius. As described previously, the combination of an ulnar fracture with a dislocation of the radial head is called *Monteggia fracture* (see **Fig. 13**). *Galeazzi fracture* is a radial shaft fracture with an associated dislocation of the distal radioulnar joint. Although this injury is uncommon, immediate orthopedic consultation is warranted.

Radius/ulna metaphyseal greenstick or complete fractures
Younger children and more distal injuries have a greater capacity for remodeling. In general, in girls younger than 10 years and boys younger than 12 years with fractures that are ≤15° angulated in the sagittal and ≤5 mm displaced in the frontal plane do not need reduction and can be managed in a short arm circumferential cast or splint for 4 weeks to 6 weeks.[33,34] Follow-up with an orthopedic surgeon is still recommended because these fractures can be unstable and can displace further in follow-up regardless of if they are managed in a cast or a splint.[35] For greater degrees of angulation, consult orthopedic surgery to determine the need for urgent reduction.

Radius and ulnar metaphyseal torus fractures
Torus or buckle-type fractures (see **Fig. 5**) of the distal forearm are the most common pediatric fracture. There is point tenderness over the distal radius or ulna, occasionally

with associated localized swelling. Distal radius buckle fractures can be radiologically subtle and therefore can be missed without careful review of both the anteroposterior and lateral radiograph views. In contrast, approximately 10% of cases thought to have a distal radius buckle fracture actually have a more advanced or unstable fracture (eg, distal radius greenstick fracture, distal radius Salter-Harris II fracture).[36] Because errors are likely to occur routinely in these and other pediatric fractures, it is important that EDs have a robust quality assurance program to correct radiograph interpretation errors so that appropriate management can be applied. Correctly diagnosed distal radius buckle fractures are best treated by splinting in a position of function with the PCP within 1 to 3 weeksfunction with follow up at the PCP office within 1 to 3 weeks of the initial injury.[37,38] Three studies have recommended home removal of the splint as safe and cost-effective.[39–41] Regardless, orthopedic surgery referral should does not need to be routine; rather, orthopedic referral should be reserved for cases that are not healing as expected.

Distal radius physical fractures
Salter-Harris I fractures of the distal radial physis are assumed if there is point tenderness or swelling over the distal radius physis and no radiographic evidence of a visible bony fracture. These injuries are rarely associated with growth disturbances. Undisplaced or minimally displaced Salter-Harris I fractures should be immobilized with a below-elbow splint and followed in an orthopedic clinic within 1 week. Significantly displaced Salter-Harris I often require urgent closed reduction in the ED. Consult orthopedic surgery for guidance on when reduction is recommended. Salter-Harris Type II injuries (see **Fig. 2**) can be managed as per Salter-Harris I fractures of the distal radius.[3] For Salter-Harris Type III, IV, and V injuries, urgent orthopedic consultation is necessary.

Carpal bone injuries
Fractures of the carpal bones are quite rare in the skeletally immature child. However, these injuries increase in frequency in the skeletally mature adolescent population. Most are sports-related injuries. Fracture patterns and presentation are similar to the adult, and scaphoid fractures are the most common type, although still relatively rare.[42] However, unlike adults, nonunion is less common in children.[43] Immobilize any suspected fracture of a carpal bone in a thumb spica splint and arrange early orthopedic follow-up, even in the absence of radiographic findings. Repeat plain radiographs, CT, or MRI may be needed at follow-up for further assessment of the injury.

Phalangeal fractures
The most common injury is to the distal phalanx resulting from a crush injury, often when a door has been closed on a child's finger. If there is an associated nail bed injury, the nail bed may need to be repaired, and the fracture is considered "open." The use of prophylactic antibiotics in "open" fractures of the distal tuft remains controversial, with no clear evidence of benefit.[44] Consultation with an orthopedic or plastic surgeon may be appropriate for repair of the nail bed if needed. Immobilize a distal phalanx "tuft" fracture with a finger splint. Phalangeal shaft fractures should be assessed for displacement, rotational deformity, and tendon disruption. Significantly displaced, rotated fractures or those with tendon disruption need orthopedic/plastic surgery consultation for reduction and repair.

LOWER EXTREMITY INJURIES
Pelvis

The immature, relatively cartilaginous pediatric pelvis is somewhat pliable. There are 2 broad categories of pelvic fractures, nonavulsive and avulsive. Nonavulsive pediatric pelvic fractures usually result from significant force, and the most common mechanism is pedestrian versus motor vehicle collisions.[45] A child with a pelvic fracture should be assumed to have multisystem trauma and be transferred to a level 1 pediatric trauma center. Avulsion-type injuries of the pelvis are usually seen in the adolescent and are unusual before 8 years of age (**Fig. 15**). These typically result from sudden contraction of musculature attached to the pelvis and occur during athletic activities. The child will often complain of sudden pain and have point tenderness over the fracture site. Nearly all avulsion fractures can be managed conservatively with rest, limitation of activity until symptoms resolve, and orthopedic follow-up.

Femur

Trauma can result in an epiphyseal disruption or a fracture of the head, neck, trochanteric, or subtrochanteric region of the femur. Proximal fractures involving the femoral head or neck have a high risk of complications (eg, avascular necrosis, growth arrest). Treatment is almost always urgent operative repair. Traumatic dislocations of the hip are rare in the pediatric population and tend to occur only in older children/adolescents. Hip dislocations are most often posterior and result from a significant trauma. Treatment for pediatric hip dislocations is urgent closed reduction. Immediate orthopedic consultation is indicated, as any significant delay in reduction is associated with a higher incidence of complications including sciatic nerve injury.

Femoral shaft

The most common mechanisms of injury are falls, pedestrian versus automobile incidents, motor vehicle collisions, and sports-related injuries. Although significant force is usually required to fracture the femoral shaft, in young healthy ambulatory children from 1 to 4 years, femur fractures can occur with low-velocity injuries such as a short fall or twisting/stumbling injury.[46] Nevertheless, it is important to consider child abuse in a child with a femur fracture who is not yet walking.[47]

The clinical findings of a femur fracture are usually obvious. There is typically tenderness and swelling over the fracture site. The child may hold the leg externally rotated and will likely refuse to bear weight. The leg may be shortened. Given the high degree of force typically needed to fracture the femur, perform a thorough evaluation for multisystem trauma. Hypotension is usually not related to an isolated femur fracture in a young child and practitioners are encouraged to look for other injuries.[47] All femoral shaft fractures require immediate orthopedic consultation.[48]

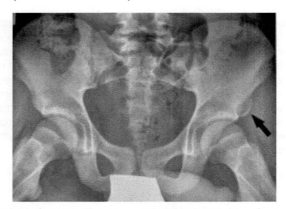

Fig. 15. Pelvic avulsion fracture. The arrow points to the avulsion fracture located at the anterior inferior iliac spine. (*Courtesy of* K. Boutis, MD, Toronto, ON.)

Slipped capital femoral epiphysis

This is characterized by slipping of the femoral epiphysis of the hip and is the most common cause of hip disability in adolescents. The etiology is multifactorial, and any child may develop slipped capital femoral epiphysis (SCFE) during a growth spurt; however, most affected children are obese adolescents whose hips are exposed to repetitive minimal trauma. Boys with SCFE present at an average age of 14 to 16 years. Girls typically present earlier, at approximately 11 to 13 years. The slippage may be chronic, acute, or acute-on-chronic. Acute SCFE are rare but quite dramatic. The child cannot bear weight, and surgery for reduction and fixation is done on an urgent basis. Acute worsening of mild chronic displacement may occur after minimal or no trauma. In cases of chronic slip, clinically, the child may develop hip (groin) pain, or pain is referred to the thigh or, much more commonly, the knee. The pain may be vague and chronic in nature. Obtain bilateral hip radiographs in any adolescent with chronic pain in the groin, hip, thigh, or knee to evaluate for SCFE because delay in diagnosis can lead to significant disability. Adequate radiographs include both anteroposterior and lateral hip views (ie, Lowenstein view). Both hips should be imaged given the high incidence of bilateral disease. The use of frog leg views is controversial given the potential for further epiphyseal displacement in this position. Radiographically, epiphyseal slippage may be detected by examining the anatomic relationship of the femoral neck to the femoral head (**Fig. 16**).

Obtain orthopedic consultation for any child with pain suspicious for SCFE in the ED. Once the diagnosis is made, the goal of treatment is to prevent further slippage: management includes strict non–weight-bearing and definitive operative management. Complications include avascular necrosis of the hip and premature closure of the physis.

Knee

Evaluation typically includes 2 radiographic views (anteroposterior and lateral) of the knee. The Ottawa Knee Rules have been validated for children older than 5 years and can help determine the need for radiographs.[49]

Fractures through the distal femoral physis

These injuries are uncommon but are at high risk of developing significant complications. The popliteal artery lies close to the distal femoral metaphysis and may be

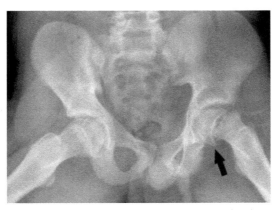

Fig. 16. Slipped Capital Femoral Epiphysis. The arrow points to the slipped epiphysis on the femoral head. (*Courtesy of* K. Boutis, MD, Toronto, ON.)

injured along with the peroneal nerve. Growth arrest may also occur secondary to permanent physeal damage. Although Salter-Harris Type I injuries may not be appreciated on plain radiographs, any child suspected of having a significant injury should receive orthopedic follow-up. Any displaced distal femoral physeal disruption needs immediate orthopedic evaluation for reduction.

Patellar dislocations

The typical mechanism of this injury is one of pivoting the knee on a fixed lower leg. There is often a history of the "knee popping out of place." If the patient remains dislocated in the ED, the displaced patella usually sits laterally, and the knee is held in flexion. Reduction need not be delayed for radiographs and is easily accomplished by gently extending the knee while another provider helps "lift" the patella into place. Obtain radiographs after the reduction to assess for fractures, which are most typically seen at either the lateral femoral condyle or the medial margin of the patella. Place the child in a knee immobilizer and arrange follow-up with orthopedics within 1 to 2 weeks.

Patellar fractures

These fractures are uncommon in children and usually occur from a direct blunt force. The "sleeve" fracture of the patella, in which the distal patellar "sleeve" is avulsed from the body of the patella, is a patellar fracture unique to children. The typical mechanism of an avulsion "sleeve" fracture is a forceful contraction of the quadriceps against a fixed lower leg. Consultation with an orthopedist is advised to determine the appropriate treatment.

Fractures of the tibial spine

From a mechanical viewpoint, an avulsion fracture of the tibial spine is the equivalent of an anterior cruciate ligament rupture in an adult. The anterior cruciate ligament inserts on the tibial eminence, also known as the anterior tibial spine, and this ligament and its insertion are much stronger than the epiphyseal bone in children. Nondisplaced fractures may be managed conservatively with immobilization in extension and orthopedic follow-up (**Fig. 17**). However, any displaced fractures need reduction and immediate orthopedic consultation.

Tibial tuberosity fractures

These are typically avulsion fractures and occur most commonly from strong contraction of the quadriceps against a fixed leg. These injuries typically occur during sports. Displaced injuries need reduction and fixation and require immediate orthopedic consultation.

Tibia and Fibula

Proximal tibial physis and metaphysis fractures

Fractures of the proximal tibial physis are relatively uncommon. The most common potential significant complication is a vascular injury to the popliteal artery, so assessment and documentation of intact pulses and an ankle brachial index is important. In proximal tibial metaphyseal fractures, there is a high risk of drift through healing and growth into a valgus deformity of the knee (Cozen phenomenon), even with proper alignment and immobilization. Orthopedic follow-up for these fractures is therefore essential.

Fractures of the tibia and fibula diaphyses

Fractures of the shaft of tibia and fibula are common in children, and one of the most common fractures in younger children is the toddler's fracture.[50] This is an isolated minimally displaced (<2 mm) spiral/oblique fracture of the distal tibia in a child

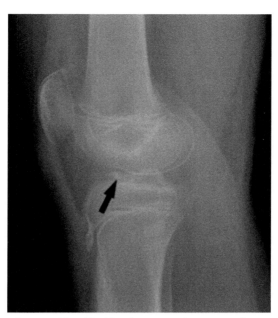

Fig. 17. Tibial spine fracture identified by the arrow. (*Courtesy of* K. Boutis, MD, Toronto, ON.)

9 months to 4 years.[51] Parents report that the child is limping or refusing to bear weight for no apparent reason or after seemingly insignificant trauma. The specific mechanism is often external rotation of the foot with the knee flexed. Clinically, there is usually pain with palpation and rotation of the distal tibia, although swelling or tenderness may be minimal or absent. Obtain radiographs of the tibia and fibula in the limping toddler, even in the absence of physical examination findings. Radiographically, a fracture line may be noticed at the distal third of the tibial shaft (**Fig. 18**). At times, initial standard plain radiographs may be normal. In these cases, oblique views may show a fracture line when standard views are negative. If a toddler's fracture is clinically suspected and initial radiographs are negative, splint immobilization and no immobilization are both management options with follow-up in one week for repeat radiographs.[52–54] If radiographs are negative, and there is also the absence of a traumatic history, clinicians are encouraged to rule out other possible diagnoses that could lead to difficulty weight bearing in a young child. For radiologically evident fractures, there is currently a wide practice variation on the need for immobilization. Options include immobilization of the injured leg in a long leg splint, removable prefabricated device or above/below knee cast.[52,54] The most commonly applied standard is a long leg splint in the ED followed by an above or below knee cast placed in the orthopedics clinic.[52,54]

In older children, if the fracture is minimally displaced and there is no evidence of compartment syndrome, immobilize in a long leg posterior splint and arrange orthopedic follow-up. However, if there is >10° of angulation in any plane, orthopedic consultation and reduction may be indicated. Where there is a high-energy injury, if the limb was in highly metabolic state at the time of injury (eg, taking part in sports), or if there is any element of a crush injury, then there is a risk of compartment syndrome, and the patient may need to be admitted for several examinations.

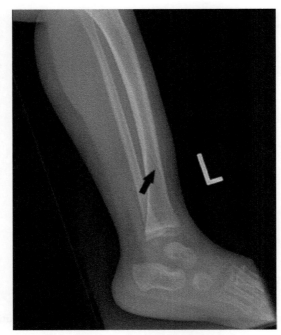

Fig. 18. Spiral fracture of the distal tibia. The arrow points to the lucency in the distal third of the tibial. (*Courtesy of* K. Boutis, MD, Toronto, ON.)

Ankle

Pediatric ankle injuries are common, but only approximately 12% of ankle injuries result in ankle fractures.[55] To avoid unnecessary radiographs in children with ankle injuries, clinical decision rules may be applied to determine which children's injuries benefit from radiographs. In a multicenter analysis, implementation of the Low-Risk Ankle Rule (**Fig. 19**)[55] safely reduced radiographs by 22% and demonstrated significant health care cost savings.[56,57] The Ottawa Ankle Rules have also been validated in children.[58–60] However, although these rules are highly sensitive, they only reduce radiographs by approximately 10%.[56] Once plain radiographs are considered necessary, standard views include anteroposterior, lateral, and oblique views. Distal tibia growth plate fractures may be at higher risk of complications, and as such additional imaging techniques such as CT and MRI can be used to help define the degree of displacement.

Distal fibula ankle fractures

These are the most common lower extremity injuries in children older than 5 years. The key fractures to consider in this location are Salter-Harris I, II, and fibular avulsion fractures. Children who present with lateral ankle injuries and no radiographic evidence of a fracture are commonly diagnosed with a distal fibular Salter-Harris I physeal fracture. However, in a recent study that included 135 skeletally immature children with this clinical scenario, MRI demonstrated that only 4 (3%) of these children had Salter-Harris I fractures of the distal fibula, 2 of which were partial injuries, and all children had ligamentous injuries or bony contusions.[61] Thus, radiograph-negative lateral ankle injuries in children are more appropriately diagnosed with ligamentous injuries and managed with a removable ankle brace and self-regulated return to activities.[62,63]

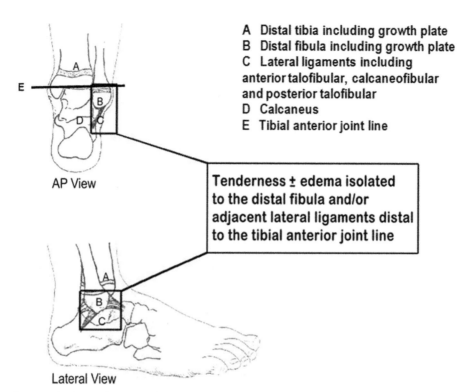

A Distal tibia including growth plate
B Distal fibula including growth plate
C Lateral ligaments including anterior talofibular, calcaneofibular and posterior talofibular
D Calcaneus
E Tibial anterior joint line

AP View

Tenderness ± edema isolated to the distal fibula and/or adjacent lateral ligaments distal to the tibial anterior joint line

Lateral View

Fig. 19. The low-risk ankle rule. AP, anteroposterior. (*Modified from* Hoppenfeld S, Hutton R, Thomas H (Eds.). Physical examination of the foot and ankle: physical examination of the spine and extremities. Appleton-Century-Crofts: New York; pp. 217-222.)

As such, routine orthopedic follow-up is not necessary for these cases and can be reserved for cases not recovering as expected.

Salter-Harris Type II (**Fig. 20**) and distal fibular avulsion fractures occur with an inversion injury. In general, when there is no significant displacement, these fractures may be managed by immobilization in a weight-bearing cast or commercial immobilizer, and orthopedic follow-up is usually not necessary.[62,63] In isolation, distal fibular Salter-Harris III-V fractures are very rare. If suspected, consult orthopedics for management.

Distal tibia ankle fractures

Salter-Harris I and II fractures of the distal tibia are the most common fractures of the distal tibia. They can be managed with immobilization and follow-up in an orthopedic clinic, but displaced fractures may require closed reduction. Salter-Harris III fractures account for approximately 25% of distal tibia fractures and may need open reduction if there is any significant displacement. Tillaux fracture is a Salter-Harris Type III fracture of the anterolateral portion of the distal tibia (see **Fig. 3**). Treatment is surgical reduction in most cases that demonstrate displacement, and thus, urgent orthopedic consultation is indicated. Salter-Harris IV fractures (see **Fig. 4**) include the triplane fracture, which involves fractures in the sagittal, coronal, and transverse planes, resulting in multiple fracture fragments. CT helps delineate the extent of the joint

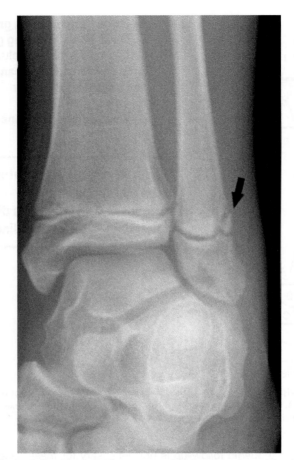

Fig. 20. Distal fibular Salter-Harris II. The arrow points to metaphyseal fracture that extends into the growth plate. (*Courtesy of* K. Boutis, MD, Toronto, ON.)

surface injury in both Salter-Harris Type III and IV ankle fractures. The management is often urgent surgical reduction.

Foot and Toe

The lack of ossification of the foot bones in younger children makes fractures in this area rare. As ossification increases with age, fractures become more common, but significant injuries are still unusual. Fractures of the mid- and hindfoot are rare, and usually result from a fall. They can often be managed with a splint and orthopedic follow-up. Fractures of the metatarsals and phalanges are relatively common in children and typically result from a direct blow from a falling object. Most nondisplaced fractures of the metatarsals and phalanges can be managed by immobilization in a posterior short-leg splint and orthopedic follow-up. Significantly displaced fractures of the metatarsals and phalanges, as well as those of the great toe that have intra-articular involvement, may require fixation, although this can typically be done on an outpatient basis. Fractures of the base of the fifth metatarsal are common with inversion injuries of the ankle, and thus the evaluation of ankle injuries should, therefore, include radiographs of the foot when there is tenderness over the fifth metatarsal. The immature skeleton consists of an ossification center lateral to the base of the fifth metatarsal (**Fig. 21**) to which the peroneus brevis tendon attaches. This ossification center may be confused with a fracture, although an avulsion fracture at this site can also occur and presents with point tenderness and displacement of the ossification center. Immobilization and orthopedic follow-up are recommended. Crush injuries to the foot may cause vascular compromise and compartment syndrome, and thus urgent orthopedic consultation is indicated.

MISSING PEDIATRIC FRACTURES IN THE EMERGENCY DEPARTMENT

One factor that may lead to missing a fracture is the extent of the history and physical examination obtained. In children, getting detailed mechanisms to help elucidate the type of injury is often not possible; further, younger children are often challenging to examine. Thus, in cases in which history or physical examination is limited, we encourage physicians to have a very low threshold to obtain radiographs. If an older child is cooperative and able to localize pain, validated clinician decision rules can be used to determine the need for imaging.[31,49,56] However, these rules are only to be used after a comprehensive physical examination is completed and are not meant to replace the physical examination. Using a rule-based physical examination can lead to missing important pathology. Other factors that may lead to missing a fracture in the ED are related to cognitive biases that impact how we process information and make clinical decisions.[64] A low clinical suspicion of a fracture on history and physical can bias the physician such that their ability to see the fracture on the radiograph may be compromised. The classic example is a subtle Tillaux fracture. On physical

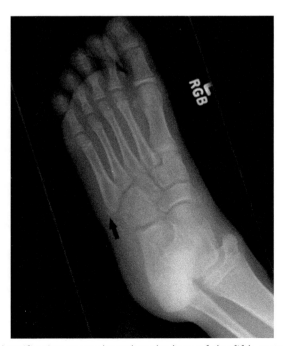

Fig. 21. A normal ossification center lateral to the base of the fifth metatarsal. The arrow points to the ossification center. (*Courtesy of* K. Boutis, MD, Toronto, ON.)

examination, the ankle demonstrates soft tissue swelling predominantly over the distal fibula: a clinical presentation similar to an ankle sprain, especially because this fracture typically occurs in older children (12–14 years). As such, the clinician reviews the radiograph with a low suspicion for a fracture and misses the more subtle radiographic presentations of this fracture. Careful examination of the anterior joint line, in this case, would demonstrate significant tenderness, cueing the physician to examine this area of the radiograph more carefully.

Another common cognitive bias is search satisficing[64]; heed the saying, "the most commonly missed fracture is the second fracture." As we reviewed previously, this can occur in Monteggia fractures where the clinician identifies the ulnar fracture and then misses the more serious radial head dislocation (see **Fig. 13**). This can also result in underestimating the seriousness of a fracture. For example, the distal radius Salter-Harris II fracture is often misdiagnosed as a distal radius buckle fracture in the ED. In this case, clinicians note the buckling of the cortex and fail to continue examining the radiograph, missing the extension of the fracture into the growth plate or any associated displacement (**Fig. 22**).

It is important for clinicians to remember that pediatric fractures are not always evident on the initial radiographs. Thus, in cases of high clinical suspicion for a fracture, even in the absence of a radiograph-visible fracture, the child should be immobilized and referred for orthopedic follow-up. Nevertheless, the most common reason for missing a fracture is due to deficiencies in physician interpretation skill of pediatric musculoskeletal images, and error rates have been reported to occur in

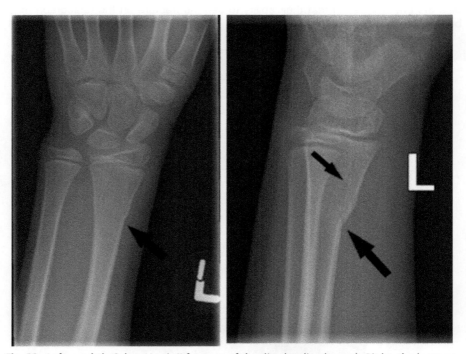

Fig. 22. Left, a subtle Salter-Harris II fracture of the distal radius (*arrow*). Right, the large arrow points to the buckling of the cortex and clinicians may stop looking and miss the more subtle extension into the growth plate indicated by the smaller arrow. (*Courtesy of* K. Boutis, MD, Toronto, ON.)

3% to 15% of pediatric musculoskeletal images.[65] Although most imaging over-reads by a radiologist may identify errors, errors are often not reported until after the patient has left the ED, which can lead to other unnecessary visits for the patient and health care system and medico-legal complaints.[66] In this scenario, it would be optimal to increase physician skill via education. Although there are many electronic resources that cover the approach to pediatric musculoskeletal images, there is currently only one that allows the deliberate active practice of cases. ImageSim (www.imagesim. com) is an evidence-based on-line learning platform that includes a course in pediatric musculoskeletal radiograph interpretation where the clinician can practice on as many as 2100 cases and receive feedback with every case completed.[65,67–69] As an additional measure, hospital-based quality assurance programs that include imaging over-reads by radiologists within 48 hours is highly recommended.

SUMMARY

Fractures are a common presenting complaint to the ED. However, relative to adults, the unique healing abilities of children allow for a lower rate of long-term fracture-related complications such as malunion, disability, arthritis. The ED management strategy of a specific pediatric fractures considers several factors. These include (but are not limited to) the age of the patient, open or closed fracture, radiographic features (location and degree of displacement/angulation of the fracture), risk of growth arrest, and/or concerns about neurovascular compromise or compartment syndrome. Minimal intervention strategies that focus on symptom relief and patient-guided return to activities are appropriate for uncomplicated mid-clavicular fractures, distal radius buckle fractures, undisplaced distal fibular Salter-Harris I, II and avulsion fractures. Nevertheless, before committing to a management strategy, it is essential that ED physicians create individual and system-level conditions to correctly diagnose the injury on the radiograph. These can include being aware of cognitive biases that lead to radiograph interpretation error, individual physician education, and radiology quality assurance of ED radiograph interpretations within 48 hours.

REFERENCES

1. Salter RB, Harris WR. Injuries involving the epiphyseal plate. J Bone Joint Surg 1963;45(3):587–622.
2. Bachman D, Santora S. Orthopedic trauma. In: Fleisher GL, Henretig F, Ruddy R, et al, editors. Textbook of pediatric emergency medicine. 4th edition. Philadelphia: Lippincott Williams & Wilkins; 2000. p. 1435–77.
3. Wilkins KE. Principles of fracture remodeling in children. Injury 2005;36(Suppl 1): A3–11.
4. Adamich J, Howard A, Camp M. Do all clavicle fractures in children need to be managed by orthopedic surgeons? Pediatr Emerg Care 2018;34(10):706–10.
5. Vander Have KL, Perdue AM, Caird MS, et al. Operative versus nonoperative treatment of midshaft clavicle fractures in adolescents. J Pediatr Orthop 2010; 30(4):307–12.
6. Shah RR, Kinder J, Peelman J, et al. Pediatric clavicle and acromioclavicular injuries. J Pediatr Orthop 2010;30:S69–72.
7. Gladstein AZ, Schade AT, Howard AW, et al. Reducing resource utilization during non-operative treatment of pediatric proximal humerus fractures. Orthop Traumatol Surg Res 2017;103(1):115–8.

8. Chaus GW, Carry PM, Pishkenari AK, et al. Operative versus nonoperative treatment of displaced proximal humeral physeal fractures: a matched cohort. J Pediatr Orthop 2015;35(3):234–9.

9. Popkin CA, Levine WN, Ahmad CS. Evaluation and management of pediatric proximal humerus fractures. J Am Acad Orthop Surg 2015;23(2):77–86.

10. Caviglia H, Garrido CP, Palazzi FF, et al. Pediatric fractures of the humerus. Clin Orthop Relat Res 2005;(432):49–56.

11. Shaw BA, Murphy KM, Shaw A, et al. Humerus shaft fractures in young children: accident or abuse? J Pediatr Orthop 1997;17(3):293–7.

12. Thomas SA, Rosenfield NS, Leventhal JM, et al. Long-bone fractures in young children: distinguishing accidental injuries from child abuse. Pediatrics 1991; 88(3):471–6.

13. Jacoby SM, Herman MJ, Morrison WB, et al. Pediatric elbow trauma: an orthopaedic perspective on the importance of radiographic interpretation. Semin Musculoskelet Radiol 2007;11(1):48–56.

14. Shrader MW, Campbell MD, Jacofsky DJ. Accuracy of emergency room physicians' interpretation of elbow fractures in children. Orthopedics 2008;31(12) [pii:orthosupersite.com/view.asp?rID=34697].

15. Dowling S, Farion K, Clifford T. Comparison views to diagnose elbow injuries in children: a survey of Canadian non-pediatric emergency physicians. CJEM 2005;7(4):237–40.

16. Ballal MS, Garg NK, Bass A, et al. Comparison between collar and cuffs and above elbow back slabs in the initial treatment of Gartland type I supracondylar humerus fractures. J Pediatr Orthop B 2008;17(2):57–60.

17. Oakley E, Barnett P, Babl FE. Backslab versus nonbackslab for immobilization of undisplaced supracondylar fractures: a randomized trial. Pediatr Emerg Care 2009;25(7):452–6.

18. Hwang RW, Bae DS, Waters PM. Brachial plexus palsy following proximal humerus fracture in patients who are skeletally immature. J Orthop Trauma 2008;22(4): 286–90.

19. Wu J, Perron AD, Miller MD, et al. Orthopedic pitfalls in the ED: pediatric supracondylar humerus fractures. Am J Emerg Med 2002;20(6):544–50.

20. Ladenhauf HN, Schaffert M, Bauer J. The displaced supracondylar humerus fracture: indications for surgery and surgical options: a 2014 update. Curr Opin Pediatr 2014;26(1):64–9.

21. Bast SC, Hoffer MM, Aval S. Nonoperative treatment for minimally and nondisplaced lateral humeral condyle fractures in children. J Pediatr Orthop 1998; 18(4):448–50.

22. Knapik DM, Gilmore A, Liu RW. Conservative management of minimally displaced (</=2 mm) fractures of the lateral humeral condyle in pediatric patients: a systematic review. J Pediatr Orthop 2017;37(2):e83–7.

23. Beaty JH JR, K. The elbow: physeal fractures, apophyseal injuries of the distal humerus, avascular necrosis of the trochlea, and T-condylar fractures. In: Rockwood CA, Wilkins KE, Beaty JH, et al, editors. Rockwood and Wilkins' fractures in children. 5th edition. Philadelphia: Lippincott Williams & Wilkins; 2001. p. 625.

24. Tarallo L, Mugnai R, Fiacchi F, et al. Pediatric medial epicondyle fractures with intra-articular elbow incarceration. J Orthop Traumatol 2015;16(2):117–23.

25. Dodds SD, Flanagin BA, Bohl DD, et al. Incarcerated medial epicondyle fracture following pediatric elbow dislocation: 11 cases. J Hand Surg Am 2014;39(9): 1739–45.

26. Caterini R, Farsetti P, D'Arrigo C, et al. Fractures of the olecranon in children. Long-term follow-up of 39 cases. J Pediatr Orthop B 2002;11(4):320–8.
27. Zimmerman RM, Kalish LA, Hresko MT, et al. Surgical management of pediatric radial neck fractures. J Bone Joint Surg Am 2013;95(20):1825–32.
28. Krul M, van der Wouden JC, Kruithof EJ, et al. Manipulative interventions for reducing pulled elbow in young children. Cochrane Database Syst Rev 2017;(7):CD007759.
29. Bexkens R, Washburn FJ, Eygendaal D, et al. Effectiveness of reduction maneuvers in the treatment of nursemaid's elbow: a systematic review and meta-analysis. Am J Emerg Med 2017;35(1):159–63.
30. Hedstrom EM, Svensson O, Bergstrom U, et al. Epidemiology of fractures in children and adolescents. Acta Orthop 2010;81(1):148–53.
31. Mulders MAM, Walenkamp MMJ, Slaar A, et al. Implementation of the Amsterdam pediatric wrist rules. Pediatr Radiol 2018;48(11):1612–20.
32. Mehlman C, Wall E. Injuries to the shafts of the radius and ulna. In: Beaty JH, Kasser JR, Rockwood CA, et al, editors. Rockwood and Wilkins' fractures in children. 6th ediiton. Philadelphia: Lippincott Williams & Wilkins; 2006. p. 400.
33. Mabrey JD, Fitch RD. Plastic deformation in pediatric fractures: mechanism and treatment. J Pediatr Orthop 1989;9(3):310–4.
34. Boutis K, Willan A, Babyn P, et al. Cast versus splint in children with minimally angulated fractures of the distal radius: a randomized controlled trial. CMAJ 2010; 182(14):1507–12.
35. Al-Ansari K, Howard A, Seeto B, et al. Minimally angulated pediatric wrist fractures: is immobilization without manipulation enough? CJEM 2007;9(1):9–15.
36. Koelink E, Schuh S, Howard A, et al. Primary care physician follow-up of distal radius buckle fractures. Pediatrics 2016;137(1). https://doi.org/10.1542/peds. 2015-2262.
37. Jiang N, Cao ZH, Ma YF, et al. Management of pediatric forearm torus fractures: a systematic review and meta-analysis. Pediatr Emerg Care 2016;32(11):773–8.
38. Ben-Yakov M, Boutis K. Buckle fractures of the distal radius in children. CMAJ 2016;188(7):527.
39. Mehlman CT. Home removal of a backslab 3 weeks after buckle fracture of the distal radius was as safe as removal at a fracture clinic. J Bone Joint Surg 2002;84(5):883.
40. Symons S, Rowsell M, Bhowal B, et al. Hospital versus home management of children with buckle fractures of the distal radius. A prospective, randomised trial. J Bone Joint Surg Br 2001;83(4):556–60.
41. Hamilton TW, Hutchings L, Alsousou J, et al. The treatment of stable paediatric forearm fractures using a cast that may be removed at home: comparison with traditional management in a randomised controlled trial. Bone Joint J 2013; 95-B(12):1714–20.
42. Jauregui JJ, Seger EW, Hesham K, et al. Operative management for pediatric and adolescent scaphoid nonunions: a meta-analysis. J Pediatr Orthop 2019; 39(2):e130–3.
43. Shaterian A, Santos PJF, Lee CJ, et al. Management modalities and outcomes following acute scaphoid fractures in children: a quantitative review and meta-analysis. Hand (N Y) 2019;14(3):305–10.
44. Lankachandra M, Wells CR, Cheng CJ, et al. Complications of distal phalanx fractures in children. J Hand Surg Am 2017;42(7):574.e1–6.
45. Grisoni N, Connor S, Marsh E, et al. Pelvic fractures in a pediatric level I trauma center. J Orthop Trauma 2002;16(7):458–63.

46. Capra L, Levin AV, Howard A, et al. Characteristics of femur fractures in ambulatory young children. Emerg Med J 2013;30(9):749–53.
47. Wood JN, Fakeye O, Mondestin V, et al. Prevalence of abuse among young children with femur fractures: a systematic review. BMC Pediatr 2014;14:169.
48. Lieber J, Schmittenbecher P. Developments in the treatment of pediatric long bone shaft fractures. Eur J Pediatr Surg 2013;23(6):427–33.
49. Vijayasankar D, Boyle AA, Atkinson P. Can the Ottawa knee rule be applied to children? A systematic review and meta-analysis of observational studies. Emerg Med J 2009;26(4):250–3.
50. Adamich JS, Camp MW. Do toddler's fractures of the tibia require evaluation and management by an orthopaedic surgeon routinely? Eur J Emerg Med 2018;25(6): 423–8.
51. Dunbar JS, Owen HF, Nogrady MB, et al. Obscure tibial fracture of infants–the Toddler's fracture. J Can Assoc Radiol 1964;15:136–44.
52. Seguin J, Brody D, Li P. Nationwide survey on current management strategies of toddler's fractures. CJEM 2018;20(5):739–45.
53. Bauer JM, Lovejoy SA. Toddler's fractures: time to weight-bear with regard to immobilization type and radiographic monitoring. J Pediatr Orthop 2019;39(6): 314–7.
54. Schuh AM, Whitlock KB, Klein EJ. Management of Toddler's fractures in the pediatric emergency department. Pediatr Emerg Care 2016;32(7):452–4.
55. Boutis K, Komar L, Jaramillo D, et al. Sensitivity of a clinical examination to predict need for radiography in children with ankle injuries: a prospective study. Lancet 2001;358(9299):2118–21.
56. Boutis K, Grootendorst P, Willan A, et al. Effect of the Low Risk Ankle Rule on the frequency of radiography in children with ankle injuries. CMAJ 2013;185(15): E731–8.
57. Boutis K, von Keyserlingk C, Willan A, et al. Cost consequence analysis of implementing the low risk ankle rule in emergency departments. Ann Emerg Med 2015; 66(5):455–63.e4.
58. Dowling S, Spooner CH, Liang Y, et al. Accuracy of Ottawa Ankle Rules to exclude fractures of the ankle and midfoot in children: a meta-analysis. Acad Emerg Med 2009;16(1):1–11.
59. Gravel J, Hedrei P, Grimard G, et al. Prospective validation and head-to-head comparison of 3 ankle rules in a pediatric population. Ann Emerg Med 2009; 54(4):534–40.
60. Plint AC, Bulloch B, Osmond MH, et al. Validation of the Ottawa Ankle Rules in children with ankle injuries. Acad Emerg Med 1999;6(10):1005–9.
61. Boutis K, Plint A, Stimec J, et al. Radiograph-negative lateral ankle injuries in children: occult growth plate fracture or sprain? JAMA Pediatr 2016;170(1):e154114.
62. Barnett PL, Lee MH, Oh L, et al. Functional outcome after air-stirrup ankle brace or fiberglass backslab for pediatric low-risk ankle fractures: a randomized observer-blinded controlled trial. Pediatr Emerg Care 2012;28(8):745–9.
63. Boutis K, Willan AR, Babyn P, et al. A randomized, controlled trial of a removable brace versus casting in children with low-risk ankle fractures. Pediatrics 2007; 119(6):e1256–63.
64. Daniel M, Khandelwal S, Santen SA, et al. Cognitive debiasing strategies for the emergency department. AEM Educ Train 2017;1(1):41–2.
65. Lee MS, Pusic M, Carriere B, et al. Building emergency medicine trainee competency in pediatric musculoskeletal radiograph interpretation: a multicenter prospective cohort study. AEM Educ Train 2019;3(3):269–79.

66. Selbst SM, Friedman MJ, Singh SB. Epidemiology and etiology of malpractice lawsuits involving children in US emergency departments and urgent care centers. Pediatr Emerg Care 2005;21(3):165–9.

67. Boutis K, Pecaric M, Pusic M. Using signal detection theory to model changes in serial learning of radiological image interpretation. Adv Health Sci Educ Theory Pract 2010;15:647–58.

68. Pusic M, Pecaric M, Boutis K. How much practice is enough? Using learning curves to assess the deliberate practice of radiograph interpretation. Acad Med 2011;86(6):731–6.

69. Pusic MV, Andrews JS, Kessler DO, et al. Determining the optimal case mix of abnormals to normals for learning radiograph interpretation: a randomized control trial. Med Educ 2012;46(3):289–98.

The Emergent Evaluation and Treatment of Hand and Wrist Injuries: An Update

Mark Sanderson, BSc, MD[a],
Bruce Mohr, BSc, MD, CCFP-EM, Diploma of Sports Medicine, FRRMS[b],
Michael K. Abraham, MD, MS[c],*

KEYWORDS

- Orthopedics • Wrist injury • Phalanx • Distal radius • Carpal bones • Fracture
- Dislocation

KEY POINTS

- There is no such thing as a simple wrist sprain; consider occult Salter-Harris fractures in pediatric injuries and occult ligamentous or cartilaginous injury in the adult population.
- For hand and wrist injuries, appropriate emergent treatment is necessary to prevent associated soft tissue injury, including compartment syndrome.
- Perform and document a detailed neurovascular examination of the injured extremity before local, regional, or procedural anesthesia, and after reduction.
- Look for specific clinical and radiographic signs of commonly missed injuries.
- Appropriate follow-up and referral are essential for optimal functional healing.

INTRODUCTION

Injury patterns of the hand and wrist can be complex and challenging for the emergency physician (EP) to diagnose and treat. The ability of the hand to perform delicate maneuvers requires a very intricate interplay of bones, ligaments, and tendons. Unfortunately, due to the omnipresence of the hand, the hand and wrist are commonly injured. These injuries can be debilitating if not managed correctly, and can be both time-consuming and fraught with medicolegal risk. This article provides the necessary

Disclosure Statement: No disclosures.
[a] Department of Emergency Medicine, University of British Columbia, Diamond Health Care Centre 2775 Laurel Street 11th floor, Vancouver, British Columbia V5Z 1M9, Canada; [b] Department of Emergency Medicine, Whistler Health Care Centre, University of British Columbia, 4380 Lorimer Road, Whistler, British Columbia V8E 1A7, Canada; [c] Department of Emergency Medicine, University of Maryland School of Medicine, UM Upper Chesapeake Health System, 500 Upper Chesapeake Drive, Bel Air, MD 21014, USA
* Corresponding author.
E-mail address: mabraham@som.umaryland.edu

knowledge to diagnose and treat common hand and wrist injuries encountered in the emergency department (ED).

EPIDEMIOLOGY OF WRIST INJURIES

Injuries of the wrist are a common ED presentation, accounting for up to 2.5% of visits to the ED in some studies.[1] The most commonly fractured bone in adult patients is the distal radius, accounting for 17.5% of all fractures. Fractures of the carpal bones account for 2.7% of adult fractures, of which the scaphoid is the most commonly fractured.[2–6]

ANATOMY

The wrist consists of the distal radius, ulna, and the carpal bones, including their articulations with the metacarpals. The bony anatomy of the wrist on radiographic imaging in the posteroanterior (PA) view can be described as having 3 lines of alignment, the *lines of Gilula* (**Fig. 1**). Knowledge of the anatomic landmarks of the wrist will lead to a more accurate diagnosis (**Fig. 2**).

CLINICAL EXAMINATION

The clinical examination of the wrist begins with a thorough history focused on the mechanism of injury (MOI). The MOI provides the clinician important information on how to focus their physical examination and provides clues toward the possible presence of wrist pathology (**Table 1**). Past history of injury or surgery and existing medical

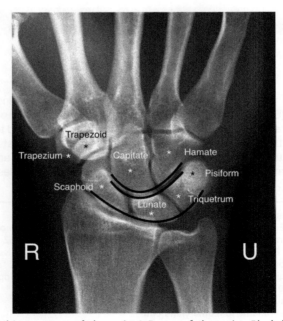

Fig. 1. Radiographic anatomy of the wrist.* Bones of the wrist. Black lines, proximal to distal = first, second, and third lines of Gilula; R, radial; U, ulnar. (*Courtesy of* B. Mohr, MD, Whistler, BC.)

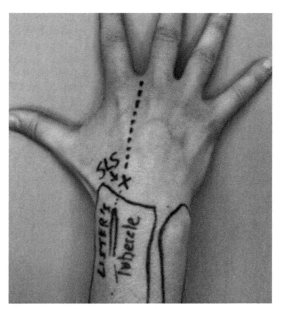

Fig. 2. Physical examination landmarks of the wrist. SLS, scapholunate space. (*Courtesy of* B. Mohr, MD, Whistler, BC.)

conditions such as osteoporosis, malignancy, and corticosteroid use will also guide your investigation.

Physical examination of the wrist is oriented by specific anatomic landmarks (see **Fig. 2**) and should proceed in an organized fashion to ensure completeness.[7] The Lister tubercle is palpable just lateral of midline on the distal radius and orients the examiner to the scapholunate space (SLS).[8] If the Lister tubercle is not palpable, a line drawn from the second web space leads directly to the SLS. Once oriented, the examiner can carefully palpate the carpal bones and adjoining ligaments in sequence. The anatomic snuffbox is a radial structure distal to the radial styloid consisting of the

Table 1	
Mechanism of injury and associated fracture or dislocation patterns	
Mechanism of Injury	**Associated Injuries**
Fall on outstretched hand (FOOSH)	• Colles fracture • Scaphoid fracture • Lunate dislocation • Perilunate dislocation • Radial head fracture[a] • Radial neck fracture[a]
Fall on volar-flexed wrist	• Smith fracture
Dorsiflexion combined with longitudinal impact on closed hand	• Carpus fractures • Metacarpal fractures[a] • Carpometacarpal subluxation
Torsional force	• Triangular fibrocartilage complex injury

[a] Outside the wrist joint.

dorsal boundary of extensor pollicus longus (EPL) and volarly by extensor pollicus bre-vis. The floor of the anatomic snuffbox is the waist of the scaphoid.[8,9] A careful neuro-vascular examination is an important part of the initial physical examination. It must be repeated after reduction. The screening motor and sensory examination include motor and sensory assessments of the radial, ulnar, and median nerves (**Table 2**). Capillary refill should be assessed (normal ≤2 seconds), as should the palpability of the radial artery.

DISTAL RADIUS FRACTURES

The distal radius is the most common fracture site in adults, accounting for up to 17% of acute fractures.[2] Common distal radius fractures and their eponyms, MOI, and best radiographic view to view the fracture are shown in **Table 3**. The most common MOI is a fall on an outstretched hand (FOOSH). Patients with distal radius fracture will typi-cally complain of radial wrist pain. This may be associated with swelling or hematoma. Tenderness over the distal radius and a mechanism consistent with distal radius frac-ture should prompt radiographic investigation (**Fig. 3**).

TREATMENT

Neurovascular compromise or presence of an open fracture is an indication for emer-gent closed reduction and orthopedic consultation. Severely displaced injuries require emergent reduction with procedural sedation and analgesia (PSA). Medical imaging should not delay emergent treatment. However, if a C-arm is present in the ED, it can be used to obtain images before reduction (**Fig. 4**).

Radiographic evidence of displacement or shortening are indications for a closed reduction before splinting (**Fig. 5**).[10] There are 4 anatomic features to attempt to restore in the reduction of a displaced distal radius fracture (**Table 4**).

Follow-up with weekly radiographs for 3 weeks or specialist referral is essential to ensure the stability of fracture reduction. Occult fractures may be indicated by convex displacement of the volar fat pad on the lateral radiograph (**Fig. 6**).

Suspected occult (or Salter 1) fractures can be treated by splinting or casting ac-cording to the patient's functional needs. It is crucial to scrutinize the lateral radio-graph for any degree of dorsal tilt that may require reduction in an otherwise nondisplaced appearing injury on anteroposterior (AP) films (**Fig. 7**).

In some populations, it may be acceptable to proceed with splinting or casting with less than anatomic reduction. In children younger than 9 there is significant remodeling yet to occur, and fracture reductions that would be unacceptable in adult patients may have acceptable or even excellent outcomes in pediatric patients.[13] Theoretically, one can accept up to 30° of dorsal angulation, although it is important to discuss the risks

| Table 2 |||||
| Screening neurologic examination of the hand and wrist |||||
Nerve	Motor	Muscle	Sensory
Radial	First digit interphalangeal (IP) extension	Extensor pollicus longus (EPL)	First dorsal web space
Median	Second digit distal interphalangeal (DIP) flexion	Flexor digitorum profundus (FDP)	Second digit volar pulp
Ulnar	Abduction of digits	Dorsal and palmar interossei	Fifth digit volar pulp

Table 3
Summary of eponymous distal radius fractures

Eponym	Fracture	Mechanism of Injury	Radiographic View Best Observed in
Colles fracture	Distal radius metaphyseal fracture with dorsal displacement; extra-articular	Low energy; FOOSH	Lateral
Smith fracture	Distal radius metaphyseal fracture with volar displacement; extra-articular	Low energy; fall on flexed wrist or direct blow to the dorsal wrist	Lateral
Barton fracture	Fracture dislocation of the distal radius and radiocarpal joint; intra-articular; volar or dorsal displacement	Low energy; FOOSH	Lateral
Die-punch fracture	Lunate facet fracture; intra-articular	Axial loading of the wrist	AP
Chauffer fracture or Hutchinson fracture	Radial styloid fracture	Low energy; FOOSH, scaphoid impaction on radial styloid, direct blow	AP

Abbreviations: AP, anteroposterior; FOOSH, fall on outstretched hand.

and benefits of leaving a fracture slightly displaced compared with performing a reduction. Most, in the authors' experience, will make the informed choice of having it reduced. An alternative, especially for minimally displaced fractures, is to perform a gentle but "firm mold" (perhaps under analgesia) so that further dorsal angulation does not occur. Timely follow-up or referral in 7 to 10 days is important before fracture healing takes place. In the elderly or those with reduced functional demands, 10° of dorsal angulation may be acceptable.

LOCAL, REGIONAL, AND PROCEDURAL ANESTHESIA

A key consideration in the management of wrist pathology requiring reduction is pain management. There are several options available to the EP, including hematoma block, Bier block, and procedural sedation. The selection of the type of anesthesia used will be dictated by the age and medical comorbidities of the patient. One must also consider the potential difficulty of reduction, time required, and provider's experience with the anesthetic technique.

Intravenous (IV) regional anesthesia (Bier block) is a safe and effective method of obtaining anesthesia for the reduction of wrist fractures.[14,15] It involves the instillation of local anesthetic into the venous system of the affected limb while isolated from the proximal circulation using a special tourniquet. At the Whistler Health Care Centre, we find that the combination of a bedside mini-C-arm and intravenous regional anesthesia create optimal conditions for obtaining an anatomic reduction of most wrist fractures and for resident teaching.

PSA involves the use of analgesics and sedatives during painful procedures. Commonly used agents include fentanyl, midazolam, ketamine, etomidate, and propofol. PSA can be combined with an IV regional block when lighter PSA is desired (eg, comorbid illness or the elderly) or when an IV regional block may not suffice

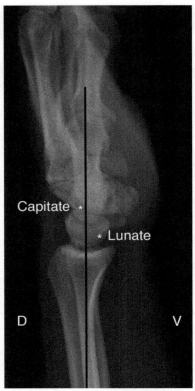

Fig. 3. Normal lateral radiograph of the wrist. There is collinearity of the radius, capitate and third metacarpal. D, dorsal; V, volar. (*Courtesy of* B. Mohr, MD, Whistler, BC.)

(eg, children or adults who are anxious or who will require significant manipulation for reduction); for example, Bayonet-type fractures (**Fig. 8**).

SPLINTING OR CASTING AND FOLLOW-UP

In general, it is safer and easier to apply a splint when treating acute fractures in the ED because of the risks associated with swelling in a circumferential cast. If you are

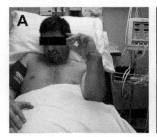
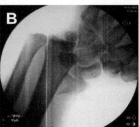
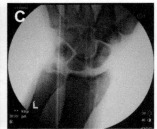

Fig. 4. Intraprocedural C-arm radiographs of a radiocarpal fracture dislocation requiring emergent reduction under PSA. (*A*) Clinical Appearance. (*B*) C-ARM Pre reduction. (*C*) C ARM Past reduction. (*Courtesy of* B. Mohr, MD, Whistler, BC.)

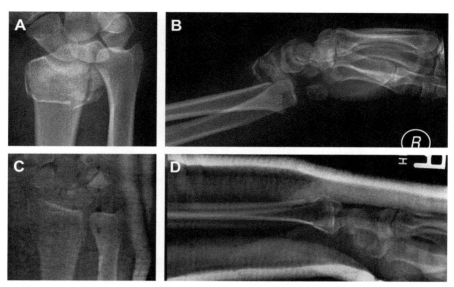

Fig. 5. Distal radius fracture and reduction. (*A*) PA radiograph of distal radius; (*B*), lateral radiograph of distal radius; (*C*), PA radiograph of distal radius postreduction; (*D*), lateral radiograph of distal radius postreduction. (*Courtesy of* B. Mohr, MD, Whistler, BC.)

performing a "soft tissue reduction," which will require subsequent surgery, always apply a splint rather than a cast. Patients who will be flying within 48 hours of their injury must be splinted or their cast must be bivalved, as per most airline regulations. If the reduction is expected to be the definitive treatment, and there are no other contraindications to cast application, you may choose to apply a carefully molded cast and give the patient explicit instructions to return for cast bivalve in the event of excessive swelling. For nondisplaced fractures at low risk for significant subsequent swelling, a splint or cast may be applied according to the functional needs of the patient and at the discretion of the EP.

We define "emergent referral" as those injuries requiring admission to hospital and consultation with an orthopedic surgeon. Urgent referral applies to fractures requiring orthopedic consultation for consideration of surgery within 7 to 10 days, and operative treatment within 10 to 14 days before the native healing process complicates surgical

Table 4
Anatomic and acceptable postreduction radiographic features of distal radius anatomy in healthy adult patients

Anatomic Feature	Normal	Acceptable Postreduction
Radial height	13 mm	<5 mm shortening
Radial inclination	22°	<5° flattening
Ulnar variance	0 mm–Neutral	Up to 4 mm positive
Volar tilt	0°–11°	From 11° volar to 5° dorsal

Data from Refs.[9,11,12]

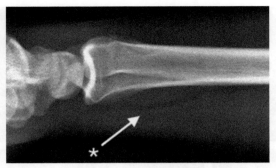

Fig. 6. Lateral radiograph of subtle nondisplaced distal radius fracture. *, Volar fat pad displacement. (*Courtesy of* B. Mohr, MD, Whistler, BC.)

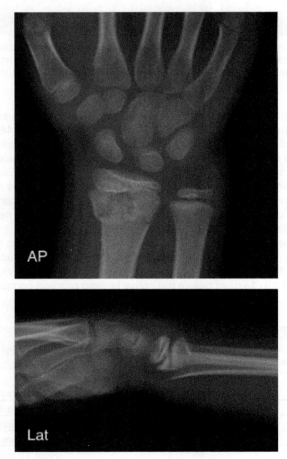

Fig. 7. Nine-year-old patient who sustained a FOOSH-type injury resulting in a distal radius fracture.

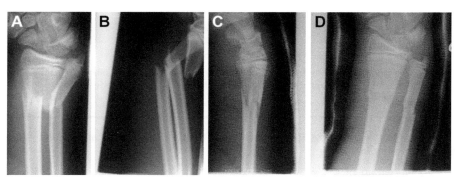

Fig. 8. Bayonet fracture. (*A*) PA - Pre reduction. (*B*) Lateral Pre reduction. (*C*) Lateral Post reduction. (*D*) PA post reduction. (*Courtesy of* Bruce Mohr, MD, Whistler, BC.)

intervention. Simple nondisplaced fractures may be appropriately followed up by primary care physicians in 1 to 2 weeks, depending on the referral patterns and level of comfort in your area.

Orthopedic injuries requiring emergent referral include the following:

- Compartment syndrome
- Neurovascular compromise (**Fig. 9**)
- Open fractures
- Concomitant trauma requiring hospital admission
- Patients with comorbidities at risk of decompensation or inability to manage at home

SCAPHOID FRACTURES

The scaphoid is the most commonly fractured carpal bone and is the second most frequently fractured bone in the wrist after the distal radius.[3] The scaphoid is most commonly fractured at its waist (approximately 70%), but also can be fractured at the distal pole, proximal pole, and the scaphoid tubercle. The location of the fracture is important in predicting the future risk of avascular necrosis (AVN) with the most proximal fractures being at significantly increased risk for AVN and nonunion.

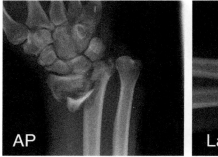
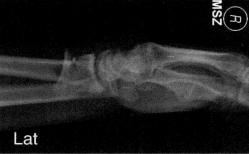

Fig. 9. Trans-scaphoid intra-articular distal radius fracture with neurovascular compromise requiring emergent open reduction internal fixation. (*Courtesy of* B. Mohr, MD, Whistler, BC.)

Box 1
Features of scaphoid fractures

- Mechanism of injury: dorsal hyperflexion; fall on outstretched hand
- Physical examination findings: pain with palpation of the anatomic snuffbox; pain with palpation of the volar scaphoid tubercle; pain with axial loading of the first digit
- Radiographic investigation: anteroposterior, lateral, scaphoid views

---

Classic features suggestive of a scaphoid fracture on history and examination (**Box 1**)[3] are the following:

- Axial loading of the wrist while extended and radially deviated (FOOSH-type mechanism)
- Pain with flexion and radial deviation of the wrist
- Tenderness over the anatomic snuffbox, the distal tubercle, and pain with axial loading of the thumb

If radiographs demonstrate no fracture, but there is strong clinical suspicion of a fracture, a computed tomography (CT) scan or MRI of the wrist may be obtained. However, it is equally reasonable in the case of a highly suspicious injury with negative radiographic findings to proceed with management as though the scaphoid has sustained an nondisplaced fracture and obtain repeat imaging in 10 to 14 days.[3] The ED management of nondisplaced acute scaphoid fractures consists of immobilization with a thumb spica (scaphoid) splint or scaphoid cast.[16] Any displaced scaphoid fractures or proximal pole fractures should be referred for surgical fixation because of the high risk of nonunion.[3]

CARPAL BONE FRACTURES EXCLUDING THE SCAPHOID

The scaphoid accounts for approximately 70% of all carpal bone fractures.[5,6,17] The remaining 30% of carpal bone fractures are heterogeneous in mechanism and outcome depending on which of the other carpal bones is affected.

Carpal bone fractures present with focal pain or tenderness, and the diagnosis requires a high index of suspicion. Plain films have limited sensitivity, and definitive diagnosis often requires a CT.[18] Patients with undisplaced carpal bone fractures should have

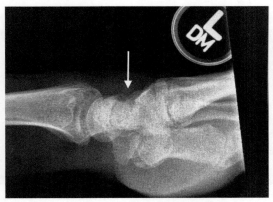

Fig. 10. Triquetral chip fracture. Often seen only on lateral views. Arrow = dorsal triquetral chip fracture. (*Courtesy of* B. Mohr, MD, Whistler, BC.)

the wrist immobilized with a volar or volar/dorsal splint, and referred for urgent orthopedic follow-up. Displaced fractures always should be referred to orthopedic surgery.

- The triquetrum is the second most commonly fractured carpal bone (15%) (**Fig. 10**).[17,18]
- Fractures of the proximal row of the carpus are more common than the distal row.[6]
- Imaging with CT may be required for definitive diagnosis.[18]
- Application of volar or volar/dorsal splint, or short arm cast, according to functional needs, with or without thumb immobilization, is indicated for simple, undisplaced carpal bone fractures.[6,18]

CARPAL BONE INSTABILITY

The most common form of ligamentous injury to the wrist is scapholunate ligament (SL) injury. The SL is an important structure in maintaining wrist biomechanics, and its disruption can lead to progressive collapse, chronic pain and disability, and ultimately degenerative arthrosis and scapholunate advanced collapse. The SL ligament is commonly injured or disrupted in conjunction with distal radius fractures, and the MOI of SL injury is a FOOSH-type mechanism.[19,20] Point tenderness, instability, or radiographic findings indicative of SL injury after an acute injury necessitate splinting of the wrist and outpatient orthopedic follow-up.

- *Terry Thomas sign*: Widening of the SLS greater than 2 mm. Typically the space between the carpal bones is uniform (**Fig. 11**).[21]

CARPAL DISLOCATIONS

Progressive wrist instability or a high-energy mechanism such as motor vehicle collisions or falls from height can result in a perilunate dislocation, lunate dislocation, or complete radiocarpal dislocation.[22] The MOI is typically wrist hyperextension in ulnar deviation, and these injuries will often present with median nerve pathology.[23]

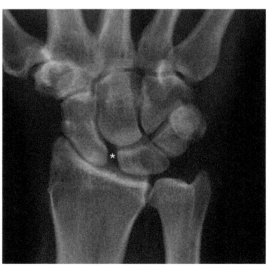

Fig. 11. Scapholunate widening, the Terry Thomas sign. *, Scapho-lunate space. (*Courtesy of* B. Mohr, MD, Whistler, BC.)

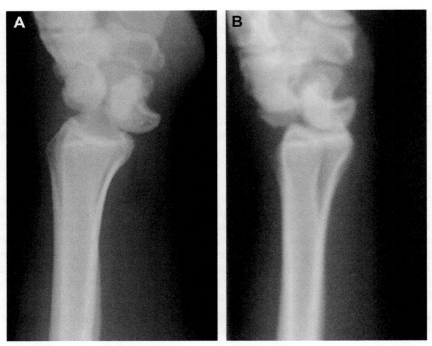

Fig. 12. Lateral radiographs of (*A*) lunate dislocation; (*B*) perilunate dislocation. (*Courtesy of* B. Mohr, MD, Whistler, BC.)

- *Perilunate dislocation*: The lunate remains in anatomic position as the carpus dislocates dorsally.[23] May present with the *Piece of Pie sign* on PA radiographs (**Fig. 12**).[24]
- *Lunate dislocation*: The lunate dislocates volarly creating the classical *Spilled cup* radiographic finding on lateral radiographs. May also present with the *Piece of P sign* on PA radiographs.[24]
- *Radiocarpal dislocation*: The entire carpus dislocates. A rare injury requiring emergent closed reduction and subsequent open repair to improve stability (**Fig. 13**).[22]

Emergent reduction and splinting should be performed for all acute injuries.[23] Reduction is usually accomplished under IV PSA or Bier block. Tips for successful reduction include using traction and dorsal angulation to open the joint space, volar pressure over the lunate if it is dislocated, followed by palmar flexion to reduce the displaced carpal bone(s). The reverse manipulation is applied to volar-type dislocations, though they are less common. Urgent referral is appropriate. Emergent surgical consultation is indicated for irreducible injuries.[22] The importance of prereduction and postreduction neurovascular examination cannot be overemphasized.

ASSOCIATED INJURIES

The distal radioulnar joint (DRUJ) and triangular fibrocartilaginous complex (TFCC) are injured with a FOOSH-type MOI plus rotational component. The TFCC is clinically tender in the foveal area just distal to the ulnar styloid and painful with TFCC compression (a combination of ulnar deviation and axial compression while performing repetitive

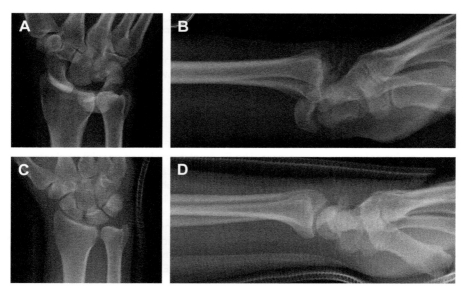

Fig. 13. Volar radiocarpal dislocation. The patient presented with median nerve sensory abnormalities that resolved with prompt ED closed reduction. (*A/B*) Pre reduction. (*C/D*) Post reduction. (*Courtesy of* B. Mohr, MD, Whistler, BC.)

flexion and extension). With DRUJ instability, the ulnar head is more pronounced, and there may be decreased supination. When the radius is stabilized, the ulna will have increased volar dorsal motion ("ballotable") compared with the uninjured side. It is important to be aware of the feeling of joint instability when performing reduction maneuvers in the wrist. You may notice DRUJ instability during or after reduction. Radiograph findings suggestive of DRUJ are a ulnar styloid fracture, positive ulnar variance, widened DRUJ on AP view, and dorsal displacement on the lateral view. Management of suspected DRUJ includes radiographs of the elbow and treating in an above elbow splint in supination. Orthopedic referral for further imaging and surgical consultation is essential for optimal functional outcomes.

HAND INJURIES
Metacarpals

The metacarpal bones connect the bones of the wrist to the phalanges. The hand does not have a large amount of soft tissue to protect the boney structures, and therefore, the metacarpals are injured in a variety of mechanisms. Axial direct force, as in a punch, or crush injuries are some of the more common mechanisms that cause injuries. Not all metacarpals are created equally, and the first digit metacarpals have injury patterns that are not seen with other metacarpal bones. The thumb is estimated to account for nearly 1 million ED visits per year.[25] Due to the dexterity and importance of the thumb for daily functions, injuries to the first metacarpal need to be accurately identified and treated. Fortunately, for the EP diagnosis of most metacarpal fractures can be done with plain radiographs.

Fractures of the First Metacarpal

Bennett fracture was first described in 1882 and is the most common fracture of the thumb. These injuries are commonly a result of a closed fist injury. Bennett fractures are an intra-articular fracture at base of carpometacarpal (CMC) joint of the thumb.[26] As a result, the attached abducens pollicis longus (APL) pulls the metacarpal and causes dorsal displacement of the metacarpal bone.

Rolando fracture, described in 1910, has a fracture pattern similar to the Bennett. Similar to Bennett, this is an intra-articular fracture; however, the fracture has a "T" or "Y" shape. As in the Bennett fracture, the pull of the APL causes dorsal displacement of the metacarpal.

Treatment
Both the Rolando and Bennett are inherently unstable, and will usually require operative fixation for definitive management. The ED treatment should consist of placement of a splint, usually a thumb spica or modified thumb spica, and discussion with a hand specialist. Pain control in these patients can be difficult as regional and hematoma blocks both have significant drawbacks and can complicate surgical planning.

The other clinically important first metacarpal fracture is an avulsion injury at the base first metacarpal from forced abduction of the thumb. This may be due to a chronic repetitive motion (ie, gamekeeper's thumb) or more commonly athletic injuries (ie, skier's thumb) (**Fig. 14**). On examination, there is laxity of the thumb joint. It is helpful to know the acuity of the symptoms; however, in the ED, the treatment will likely be

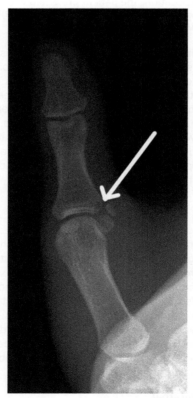

Fig. 14. Example of a gamekeeper's or skier's thumb injury (*arrow*). The insertion of the ulnar collateral ligament causes an avulsion injury. (*Courtesy of* M. Abraham, MD, Bel Air, MD.)

unchanged.[27] These injuries require diagnosis with plain radiographs, and then application of a thumb spica splint, with close follow-up. The patients will also often need operative repair for definitive management.

Fractures of the Second Through Fifth Metacarpal

Approximately 30% of hand fractures are due to the remaining metacarpals.[25] Like the thumb, these can also be from direct axial load or crush injuries, with most coming from a closed fist or falls. Once again, a physical examination can elicit the area of pain, and plain radiographs are usually diagnostic. Detailed physical examination is crucial, as open fractures with tendinous involvement can be very subtle. If missed, however, these injuries can lead to devastating infections and permanent disability. One key difference between the first and the remainder of the metacarpals is the determination of rotational deformity and angulation. In short, angulation is a radiographic term, whereas rotational deformity is a physical examination finding. To determine rotational deformity, there are 3 simple findings on clinical examination. First, have the patient clasp his or her hand so that the finger pads rest on the thenar eminence (**Fig. 15**). If there is no rotational deformity, then all of the phalanges should point to the scaphoid, with no overlap and the nails should all lie in the same plane.[28] Any rotational deformity should prompt an immediate reduction of the fractured

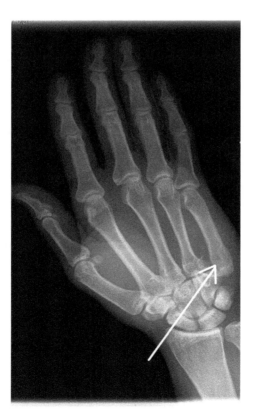

Fig. 15. Base of fifth metacarpal fracture with dislocation (*arrow*). (*Courtesy of* M. Abraham, MD, Bel Air, MD.)

metacarpal. Angulation is allowable within certain constraints. The second and third metacarpals are allowed much less angular deformity when compared with the fourth and fifth metacarpals and should be reduced if there is 5° to 10° of angulation, respectively. Fractures of the fourth and fifth metacarpals are known as a "Boxers" fracture and are the most commonly fractured metacarpal. Current literature recommends reduction if the fracture of the neck exceeds 35° to 40° of angulation.[29] One simplified algorithm is to allow 5°, 10°, 20°, and 30° of angulation for the index, middle, ring, and small fingers and perform reduction if angulation exceeds these limits.

Treatment

Although many metacarpal injuries will require surgical repair, there is some conflicting data on the best treatment.[29] Surgical outcomes have complication rates, but nonoperative repair with splinting, and even buddy-taping can have satisfactory results.[30,31] Regardless of the ultimate treatment, the ED course should consist of a radial or ulnar gutter splint for second and third fractures versus Boxers fractures, respectively.

Phalanges

The phalanges may be the least protected bones in the entire body. Their exposure, coupled with the myriad of tasks we use our hands for daily, makes for the perfect storm for injuries, and the phalanges are among the most commonly fractured bones in the body and the most common fractures in the hand.[32] Because of the complex interplay of ligaments and tendons necessary to perform the functions of the digits, there are several injury patterns that can be present. The physical examination of suspected phalanx injuries should begin with a motor examination, followed by a detailed neurovascular examination. After this has been completed, local or regional anesthesia, likely with a digital block, can be performed to assist with the remainder of the examination and treatment.

Phalanx Fractures

Damage to the proximal or middle phalanx, especially the dorsal aspect, can be important because these can lead to a Boutonniere deformity. This deformity is described as a flexion at the proximal interphalangeal (PIP) joint with hyperextension at the distal interphalangeal (DIP) joint.[33] Like avascular necrosis can develop in the posttraumatic, setting so can the Boutonniere deformity. The extensor mechanism of the digit is complex and works in close conjunction with the flexor mechanism. The flexor digitorum profundus inserts on the distal phalanx and the flexor digitorum superficialis on the middle phalanx. As a Boutonniere deformity develops, the extensor and flexor mechanisms over the dorsal PIP joint are altered due to the injury. As the extensor tendon mechanism moves down toward the volar surface of the phalanx, the pull of the extensor tendon causes extension of the DIP joint. The flexor tendon is unopposed at the PIP joint and gives the characteristic findings.[34]

If the proximal and middle phalanges are fractured, they should be immobilized with a gutter splint similar to the metacarpals as this will allow for the remainder of the uninjured digits to have functionality.

Distal Phalanx Fractures

These fractures have both bony and soft tissue implications in their management. These injuries are usually caused by a crushing force; for example, a car door or hammer. Distal tuft injuries can present with injury to the nail and nail bed. The treatment of the fracture depends on the injury patterns and the status of the nail. If there is a subungual hematoma, but the nail is intact, then the hematoma can be drained. If, however, the nail is damaged, then it should be removed, and the nail bed can be repaired. If the nail is not injured, but there is an open fracture, then depending on the circumstances, the patients may require copious irrigation, antibiotics, and possible referral to a hand specialist.[35]

Perhaps the most concerning fracture to the distal phalanx is an avulsion fracture at the base of the distal phalanx. This can lead to a mallet deformity, in which the patient cannot extend the distal phalanx. If this injury is not identified and proper treatment initiated, then a swan neck deformity may occur.[36] The swan neck deformity is characterized by extension at the PIP with flexion of the DIP, due to the unopposed action of the flexor digitorum profundus.[33] Fractures of the distal phalanx, not including tuft fractures, should be splinted in full extension for 8 weeks. This can prevent the swan neck deformity in the event the avulsion fracture is overlooked.

Ligament and Tendon Injuries

As discussed earlier in the section, there are many ligament and tendon juries that are associated with avulsion fracture, for example, skier's thumb and mallet finger. One of the most common injuries is damage to the flexor mechanism. The pulley tendons can be damaged in sports such as rock climbing, and the actual flexor insertion can be damaged as in a "jersey finger." Both of these injuries are incapacitating, as the finger cannot flex. Jersey finger has to be rapidly identified and can be done using clinical examination, but confirmation can be done with ultrasound or MRI. Jersey finger should be repaired in 7 to 10 days for optimal outcomes.[37]

SUMMARY

The hand and wrist are commonly injured. The sheer number of bones, ligaments, tendons and vascular structures with minimal overlying soft tissue for protection, make the area ripe for injury. Hand and wrist injuries should have a detailed neurovascular examination before any reduction. Plain radiographs when combined with a detailed physical examination are usually sufficient for an accurate diagnosis, although CT/MRI may be necessary for surgical planning or complex cases. Regional or procedural sedation should be used to assist in reduction and splinting when needed. Prompt and specific follow-up with the appropriate specialist should be arranged before the patient leaves the ED.

REFERENCES

1. Larsen CF, Lauritsen J. Epidemiology of acute wrist trauma. Int J Epidemiol 1993; 22(5):911–6.
2. Court-Brown CM, Caesar B. Epidemiology of adult fractures: a review. Injury 2006;37(8):691–7.
3. Sendher R, Ladd AL. The scaphoid. Orthop Clin North Am 2013;44(1):107–20.
4. Papp S. Carpal bone fractures. Hand Clin 2007;26(1):119–27.
5. Shah MA, Viegas SF. Fractures of the carpal bones excluding the scaphoid. J Am Soc Surg Hand 2002;2(3):129–40.
6. Vigler M, Aviles A, Lee SK. Carpal fractures excluding the scaphoid. Hand Clin 2006;22(4):501–16.
7. Young D, Papp S, Giachino A. Physical examination of the wrist. Hand Clin 2010; 26(1):21–36.
8. Eathorne SW. The wrist: clinical anatomy and physical examination - an update. Prim Care 2005;32(1):17–33.

9. Wulf CA, Ackerman DB, Rizzo M. Contemporary evaluation and treatment of distal radius fractures. Hand Clin 2007;23(2):209–26.

10. Fernandez DL. Closed manipulation and casting of distal radius fractures. Hand Clin 2005;21(3):307–16.

11. Medoff RJ. Essential radiographic evaluation for distal radius fractures. Hand Clin 2005;21(3):279–88.

12. Dario P, Matteo G, Carolina C, et al. Is it really necessary to restore radial anatomic parameters after distal radius fractures? Injury 2014;45(S6):S21–6.

13. Noonan KJ, Price CT. Forearm and distal radius fractures in children. J Am Acad Orthop Surg 1998;6(3):146–56.

14. Brown EM, McGriff JT, Malinowski RW. Intravenous regional anaesthesia (Bier block): review of 20 years' experience. Can J Anaesth 1989;36(3):307–10.

15. Mohr B. Safety and effectiveness of intravenous regional anesthesia (Bier block) for outpatient management of forearm trauma. (Advances) (Medical condition overview) (Clinical report). CJEM 2006;8(4):247.

16. Ram AN, Chung KC. Evidence-based management of acute nondisplaced scaphoid waist fractures. J Hand Surg Am 2009;34(4):735–8.

17. Papp S. Carpal bone fractures. Hand Clin 2010;26(1):119–27.

18. Suh N, Ek E, Wolfe S. Carpal fractures. J Hand Surg Am 2013;39(4):785–91.

19. Chinchalkar SJ, Pipicelli JG. Wrist instabilities. 2nd edition. Elsevier Inc; 2013. https://doi.org/10.1016/B978-0-323-09104-6.00026-2.

20. Caggiano N, Matullo KS. Carpal instability of the wrist. Orthop Clin North Am 2014;45(1):129–40.

21. Frankel V. The Terry-Thomas sign. Clin Orthop Relat Res 1978 Sep;135:311–2.

22. Grabow R, Catalano L. Carpal dislocations. Hand Clin 2007;21(4):288–97.

23. Budoff JE. Treatment of acute lunate and perilunate dislocations. J Hand Surg Am 2008;33(8):1424–32.

24. Newberry JA, Garmel GM. Image diagnosis: perilunate and lunate dislocations. Perm J 2012;16(1):70–1.

25. Karl JW, Olson PR, Rosenwasser MP. The epidemiology of upper extremity fractures in the United States, 2009. J Orthop Trauma 2015;29(8):242–4. Available at: https://journals.lww.com/jorthotrauma/Fulltext/2015/08000/The_Epidemiology_of_Upper_Extremity_Fractures_in.10.aspx.

26. Caldwell RA, Shorten PL, Morrell NT. Common upper extremity fracture eponyms: a look into what they really mean. J Hand Surg Am 2018;44(4):331–4.

27. Brotzman SB. Injuries to the ulnar collateral ligament of the thumb metacarpophalangeal joint (Gamekeeper's Thumb). Clin Orthop Rehabil A Team Approach 2017;29.

28. Bond M, Perron A, Abraham M. Orthopedic emergencies. 2013. Available at: https://books.google.com/books?hl=en&lr=&id=LUMIAQAAQBAJ&oi=fnd&pg=PR6&ots=3qPib9qgzz&sig=luBKG8Yh2QKwCUkCEucPGFKVZpk. Accessed April 1, 2019.

29. Padegimas EM, Warrender WJ, Jones CM, et al. Metacarpal neck fractures: a review of surgical indications and techniques. Arch Trauma Res 2016;5(3):e32933.

30. van Aaken J, Fusetti C, Luchina S, et al. Fifth metacarpal neck fractures treated with soft wrap/buddy taping compared to reduction and casting: results of a prospective, multicenter, randomized trial. Arch Orthop Trauma Surg 2016;136(1):135–42.

31. Giddins GEB. The non-operative management of hand fractures. J Hand Surg Eur Vol 2015;40(1):33–41.

32. Day CS, Stern PJ. Chapter 8. Fractures of the metacarpals and phalanges. Green's Oper Hand Surg, 2015 1:239–90.
33. McKeon K, Academy DL-J-J of the A, 2015 undefined. Posttraumatic boutonniere and swan neck deformities. Available at: https://journals.lww.com/jaaos/subjects/Trauma/Fulltext/2015/10000/Posttraumatic_Boutonni_re_and_Swan_Neck.5.aspx. Accessed April 1, 2019.
34. Grau L, Baydoun H, Chen K, SS-TJ of hand. Biomechanics of the acute Boutonniere deformity. Elsevier; 2018. Available at: https://www.sciencedirect.com/science/article/pii/S0363502317312042. Accessed April 1, 2019.
35. Carpenter S, Rohde RS. Treatment of phalangeal fractures. Hand Clin 2013;29(4): 519–34.
36. Alla SR, Deal ND, Dempsey IJ. Current concepts: mallet finger. Hand (N Y) 2014; 9(2):138–44.
37. Freilich AM. Evaluation and treatment of jersey finger and pulley injuries in athletes. Clin Sports Med 2015;34(1):151–66.

The Emergent Evaluation and Treatment of Elbow and Forearm Injuries

Dennis P. Hanlon, MD[a],*, Vasilios Mavrophilipos, MD[b]

KEYWORDS

- Elbow injury • Elbow dislocation • Radial head fractures • Olecranon fractures
- Monteggia • Galeazzi • Essex-lopresti • Tendon ruptures

KEY POINTS

- All elbow and forearm injuries require a precise neurovascular examination.
- Any injury to the paired bones of the forearm requires a careful examination, both physical and radiographic, of the joint above and below the level of injury.
- Elbow dislocations should be reduced in a timely fashion.
- Radiographic analysis of the fat pads and alignment criteria will prevent missed injuries.
- Displaced fractures of the elbow and forearm require orthopedic consultation.

INTRODUCTION

Elbow and forearm injuries are frequently seen in the emergency department (ED). The most common mechanism of injuries to the elbow and forearm results from falls from standing or as a result of sports accidents. Elbow and forearm injuries range from an equal distribution between sexes to a 2-time predominance in men compared with women.[1,2] On average, men are usually younger than women when they suffer similar injuries to the elbow.[3] Injuries around the elbow account for approximately 5% to 10% of all fractures. The most common elbow fracture involves the radial head.[4] Elbow dislocations account for the second most dislocated large joint in adults.[2] The goal of evaluation and treatment is to achieve excellent functional results and anatomic

Disclosure Statement: Neither author has a financial conflict of interest with this article or any of the content within the article. Neither received any funding for their participation in this project or in any research related to the content of the article.

[a] Department of Emergency Medicine, Allegheny General Hospital, 320 E. North Avenue, Pittsburgh, PA 15212, USA; [b] Department of Emergency Medicine, Inova Fairfax Hospital, 3300 Gallows Road, Falls Church, VA 22042, USA
* Corresponding author. Department of Emergency Medicine, Allegheny General Hospital, 320 E. North Avenue, Pittsburgh, PA 15212, USA
E-mail address: dennis.hanlon@ahn.org

Emerg Med Clin N Am 38 (2020) 81–102
https://doi.org/10.1016/j.emc.2019.09.005
0733-8627/20/© 2019 Elsevier Inc. All rights reserved.

emed.theclinics.com

reduction of any fracture or dislocation. This article highlights the early recognition of the most important adult elbow and forearm injuries evaluated in the ED.

ANATOMY

The elbow is a highly congruent, complex hinge-and-pivot joint with a high degree of inherent stability. It is composed of 3 articulations: the ulnohumeral, radiocapitellar, and proximal radioulnar joint. The ulnohumeral joint is the primary stabilizer of the elbow. The ulnohumeral and radiocapitellar are hinge joints, and the proximal radial ulnar joint is a pivot joint.[5] In addition to its stability, the elbow has a significant range of motion (ROM) with 0° in full extension and 150° of full flexion. It also has 80° of both supination and pronation. The ulnohumeral joint affords flexion and extension, whereas the proximal radioulnar joint allows forearm pronation and supination. The humeroradial joint moves in both rotation and flexion-extension. The bony articulation of the ulnohumeral consists of the trochlea and the trochlear notch of the proximal ulna. The radiocapitellar joint is formed by the articulation of the radial head with the capitellum. The coronoid process prevents the ulna from translating posteriorly on the humerus and is also an anchor to both the lateral ulnar collateral ligament (LCL) and the anterior band of the medial collateral ligament (MCL).[6] This structure is a keystone to elbow stability. The posterior olecranon process resists anterior translation of the humerus. The medial epicondyle is the origin of all the forearm flexors and contains a groove for the ulnar nerve that can be easily palpated or contused. The lateral epicondyle is the origin for the supinator muscles, extensor muscles, and the anconeus. In addition, the elbow is stabilized by the adjacent capsule and ligaments. The anterior joint capsule provides resistance to varus and valgus stress in extension but not flexion. The MCL complex is the main constraint to valgus stress, and it originates on the anterior inferior medial epicondyle and then inserts on the body of the coronoid process. The LCL complex is the main constraint to varus stress, and it originates on the lateral epicondyle and then inserts on the annular ligament on the supinator crest of the ulna. There is also dynamic stabilization provided by the muscles that cross the elbow joint.

The elbow has multiple important nerve and vascular structures that traverse the elbow joint. The brachial artery bifurcates into the radial and ulnar arteries at the level of the radial neck. The median nerve is in close proximity to the brachial artery so injury to one should prompt evaluation of the other structure. The ulnar nerve is frequently injured at the level of the medial epicondyle. The posterior interosseous nerve, a distal branch of radial nerve with pure motor function, is at risk because it courses around the lateral neck of the radial head.[7]

The integrity of the forearm structures is necessary for both elbow and hand movements. The radius and ulna are connected both proximally and distally through the radioulnar joints as well as longitudinally through the interosseous membrane (IOM). The IOM also divides the forearm into the flexor and extensor muscle compartments. The proximal radioulnar joint is supported by the annular, oblique, and quadrant ligaments. The distal radial ulnar joint (DRUJ) is supported by the superficial and deep radioulnar ligaments and the triangular fibrocartilage complex.[8] Because of the extensive attachments, the clinician must maintain a high index of suspicion for related injuries when there is an injury to one of the forearm bones. The ulna is the larger, more immobile of the 2 forearm bones so fractures of the ulna can compromise strength and require near anatomic alignment with reduction. During pronation and supination, the ulna remains relatively fixed, and the anatomic curve of the radius provides the arc of motion of the radius around the ulna. The restoration and maintenance of anatomic alignment are the key principles in managing elbow and forearm fractures and dislocations.

IMAGING

The initial step in imaging is deciding when it is clinically necessary to exclude a fracture, dislocation, or bony malalignment. There are no universally agreed upon clinical guidelines for the necessity of ordering radiographs for acute elbow injuries. If the adult patient has full ROM in all 4 movements of the elbow, this patient may be safely evaluated without radiographs.[9] The full 4-way ROM includes pronation, supination, extension, and flexion. Other investigators have assessed the inability to fully extend the elbow in the acutely injured as an indication for radiographs; they advise against this test as a single clinical decision rule for the determinant of imaging.[10] For patients who do undergo radiographs of the elbow for acute elbow trauma, the anteroposterior (AP) view and a lateral view are the standard views obtained. Some elbow series also include an oblique or radial head view.

In the AP view, the elbow is positioned extended with the forearm supinated. If the elbow cannot be fully extended owing to injury, swelling, or pain, then there may be superimposition of the radial head and capitellum causing inadequate visualization.

The lateral view elbow is performed in 90° of flexion. Alignment can be evaluated by the anterior humeral line and radial capitellar line. The anterior humeral line is drawn down the anterior aspect of the humerus and should intersect the middle third of the capitellum (**Fig. 1**). The radial capitellar line is drawn along the longitudinal axis of the radius and should bisect the capitellum (**Fig. 2**). These lines are useful in adults and pediatrics.

Analysis of the fat pads can detect occult fractures. The anterior fat pad is normally visible on the lateral view as a radiolucent stripe lying close to the coronoid fossa.

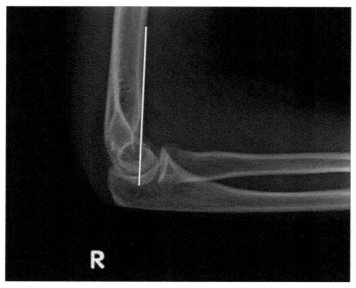

Fig. 1. Lateral elbow with an anterior humeral line, which intersects middle third of capitellum. (*Courtesy of* D. Hanlon, MD, Pittsburgh, PA.)

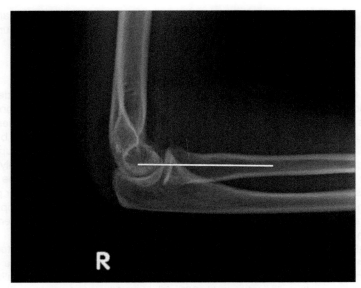

Fig. 2. Lateral elbow with a radiocapitellar line, which bisects the capitellum. (*Courtesy of* D. Hanlon, MD, Pittsburgh, PA.)

The posterior fat pad is not normally visualized, and when present, is always pathologic. A joint effusion, which is blood in the setting of trauma, will displace and elevate the anterior fat pad to produce the sail sign. Similarly, the posterior fat pad will be elevated out of the olecranon fossa and now visualized with a joint effusion (**Fig. 3**).

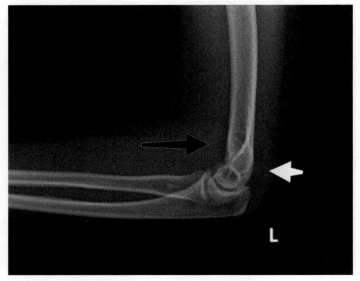

Fig. 3. Lateral elbow demonstrates a displaced anterior fat pad, "sail sign" (*black arrow*) and a posterior fat pad (*white arrow*). (*Courtesy of* D. Hanlon, MD, Pittsburgh, PA.)

Oblique view/radial head view the x-ray beam is angled at 45° to minimize overlap of the radial head with other osseous structures, primarily the coronoid process. Forearm radiographs are indicated in forearm injuries. Wrist radiographs are needed to assess the integrity of the distal radioulnar joint.

Computed tomography (CT) successfully identifies occult elbow fractures with a positive elbow extension test in patients with nondiagnostic plain radiographs.[11] Whether the detection of occult fractures by CT changes management can certainly be questioned. In any case, routine use of CT is not required with most elbow fractures. Orthopedic colleagues may request a CT of the elbow with complex fractures or fracture dislocations for further evaluation and operative planning.

Point-of-care ultrasound (POCUS) is readily available in many EDs, does not involve radiation, and can be performed at the bedside. Similar to radiographs, lipohemarthrosis can be noted on sonogram providing a sonographic fat pad sign, which has a high sensitivity for the detection of elbow fractures.[12] In cadaver studies, POCUS detected as little as 1 to 3 mL of joint fluid versus 5 to 10 mL of joint fluid that is thought to be required for detection on plain radiographs.[13] POCUS has also compared favorably to plain radiography in the detection of fractures with a degree of stepoffs and angulation and reasonably close to the performance of CT.[14] Although POCUS is not used for this purpose in most EDs, its use may increase in the future.

MRI may be necessary to follow up on complex or difficult-to-diagnose injuries, but it is not indicated in the ED for the acute management of elbow injuries.

ELBOW DISLOCATIONS

Elbow dislocations are the second most common large joint to be dislocated in the adult patient.[2] These injuries generally occur with a fall on outstretched hand (FOOSH) mechanism with an extended elbow having valgus stress. Elbow dislocations affect men more frequently than women and are most common in the 30-year-old age group.[15] In addition, most typically occur on the nondominant arm.[15] These injuries most commonly occur from falls, sports activities, assaults, and motor vehicle collisions (MVC) in that order.[15]

The initial injury of a posterior dislocation involves the disruption of the LCL. Then there is subluxation of the coronoid process over the trochlea, and finally, there is damage to the MCL, which results in complete dislocation of the radius and ulna.[2,16,17] These injuries are classified according to the displaced direction of the ulna relative to the distal humerus. Ninety percent of these dislocations are posterolateral.[16] Only 1% to 2% is dislocated anteriorly and usually occurs in combination with fractures.[5] For an anterior dislocation, the mechanisms are a blow to the posterior portion of a flexed elbow or forceful forearm extension.

Elbow dislocations are also classified as simple if not associated with a fracture, or complex if there is an associated fracture.[18] Elbow dislocations are associated with fractures in one-third of cases. Special attention should be made to exclude fractures of the radial head, coronoid process, or distal ulna. Elbow dislocations associated with both a radial head fracture and coronoid process fracture are known as the terrible triad injury, which has a high incidence of chronic instability.[19] A precise neurovascular examination is essential because of the potential for nerve or vascular injuries. Ulnar nerve injury occurs in 8% to 21% of patients with a posterior elbow dislocation.[20] Median nerve entrapment may also occur with a posterior dislocation. Median nerve deficits should raise concern for an arterial injury. Injury to the brachial artery is rare with posterior dislocations, but occurs more commonly with anterior dislocations.[20]

Patients generally arrive in the ED with the elbow flexed at 45° with pain, swelling, shortening of the forearm, and decreased ROM. There is also posterior displacement of the olecranon. With an anterior dislocation, the elbow is fully extended and the fore-arm is supinated.[18] In either case, the patient has a swollen elbow, painful decreased ROM, and an obvious deformity. Elbow dislocations are diagnosed clinically and confirmed with radiographs (**Fig. 4**). AP and lateral views of the elbow should be obtained. The films should be analyzed closely to rule out associated fracture with particular attention to the radial head and coronoid process.

The treatment of posterior elbow dislocation is closed reduction using procedural sedation. Emergent orthopedic consultation is recommended for the following: open dislocations, complex dislocations, anterior dislocations, and dislocations with persis-tent neurovascular compromise.[14] There are multiple techniques to reduce a posterior elbow dislocation. The most commonly used technique is traction-countertraction.[5] The traction-countertraction method usually requires 2 people. Before the reduction attempt, the forearm is supinated with the elbow in flexion at 30° to disengage the coronoid process and relax the biceps tendon.[5] One provider stabilizes the humerus while the second provider applies a slow continuous longitudinal traction with gradual flexion to the forearm, which should reduce the elbow. The second provider can also provide downward pressure on the forearm or pressure over the olecranon if needed (**Fig. 5**).

The leverage technique only requires a single provider. The patient is supine with the elbow flexed, the forearm supinated, and the shoulder abducted. The provider places his elbow onto the patient's distal biceps and uses his hand to interlock the patient's fingers and gradually flexes the patient's wrist using the provider's elbow as a fulcrum. The provider can use the other hand to apply medial or lateral pressure to the olec-ranon as needed (**Fig. 6**).[5,21]

Another single-provider method is the Kumar technique. The physician stands on the contralateral side of the patient's injured elbow. The patient is supine with the arm positioned across the chest with the olecranon pointing upward.[5,22] With one hand, the patient's forearm is grasped. With the other hand, the elbow is grasped and the thumb is placed over the patient's olecranon and the fingers placed over the forearm. Gentle traction is applied while the elbow is gradually flexed to disengage the coronoid process from the lower humerus. Simultaneously, the olecranon is pushed into position with the thumb.[5,22]

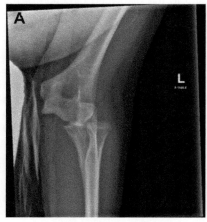 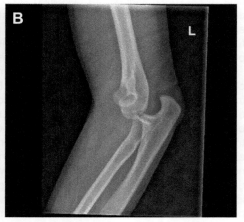

Fig. 4. (*A*) AP and (*B*) lateral elbow demonstrating a posterolateral elbow dislocation. (*Courtesy of* D. Hanlon, MD, Pittsburgh, PA.)

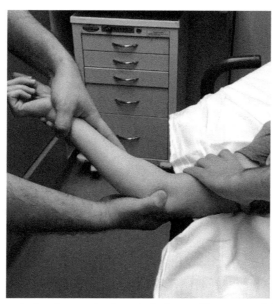

Fig. 5. Traction-countertraction reduction technique. (*Courtesy of* V. Mavrophilipos, MD,Fairfax, VA .)

Another reduction technique is the modified Stimson technique. The patient is placed prone with the shoulder abducted and the injured elbow at the edge of the stretcher with the forearm pointing down. The provider applies longitudinal traction to the forearm while manipulating the olecranon process with their other hand.[5] Alternatively, a weight can be attached to the wrist instead of downward traction. The prone position in a sedated patient is a disadvantage of this technique should the patient develop any airway emergencies.

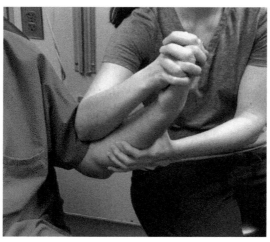

Fig. 6. Leverage technique for reduction of a dislocated elbow. (*Courtesy of* V. Mavrophilipos, MD, Fairfax, VA.)

Regardless of the reduction technique applied, a neurovascular examination must be performed before and after any reduction attempt. Neuropraxia, typically ulnar nerve, occurs in approximately 20% of cases and is usually managed conservatively.[14] Any abnormality of this examination will require orthopedic consultation. The reduced elbow should be moved through its full ROM to assess stability. Postreduction radiographs should be obtained. The elbow can be immobilized with a long-arm posterior splint and sling. After reduction, the patient should be observed for a few hours for delayed signs of vascular injury or any evolving compartment syndrome.[18,20] If there are no neurovascular complications, fractures, or joint instability, the patient may be discharged. All patients must follow up with orthopedics. The elbow should have limited use initially, in the short term, one week of immobilization, followed by early ROM with a goal of full ROM by 5 to 7 days. Immobilization greater than 3 weeks results in poor outcomes.[20] Ninety-five percent of patients can return to their previous job in functional status. Unlike shoulders, recurrent dislocations are uncommon. If joint instability is noted, the patient should be placed in a supervised rehabilitation program.

If closed reduction was unsuccessful, redislocation occurs with 50° to 60° of flexion, or if unstable fractures are present, surgery is indicated. Avulsion fractures of the coronoid process usually reduce with reduction of the dislocation. Radial head fractures and larger coronoid fractures usually require operative repair following initial closed reduction.[18,20] An unsuccessful reduction may be due to the interposition of an osteochondral fragment, most commonly a medial epicondyle fragment, and orthopedic consultation is necessary.[18,20] Recurrent instability in a simple elbow dislocation is seen in only 1% to 2% of cases.[5,20]

Anterior dislocations tend to have more ligamentous and bony instability to the joint. On examination, the arm appears to be shortened, and the forearm is elongated and held in supination. The elbow is usually held in full extension. The olecranon is palpable anteriorly.[20] These patients should be splinted in a long arm splint, and neurovascular status should be reassessed. Orthopedics should be consulted emergently. If necessary, anterior dislocations can be reduced with distal traction on the wrist, downward pressure on the forearm while an assistant provides countertraction by grasping the humerus with both hands. Gradual flexion along with the downward pressure on the forearm may be performed if needed.[5] After reduction, a neurovascular reassessment should be performed and documented. Many anterior dislocations are open, and vascular damage is quite common. Complete avulsion of the triceps mechanism is also associated with this injury.

Complications of dislocations are not uncommon. Nerve injuries are seen in up to 20% of patients and usually involve the ulnar and median nerves. The radial and anterior interosseous nerves can also be affected. These nerve injuries usually resolve with conservative management.[18,20]

Although arterial injuries are the most feared complication, there is not clear consensus on the actual incidence of such injuries because most are associated with anterior or open dislocations.[23] Closed dislocations without associated fractures are rarely associated with vascular injuries.[2,23] Posttraumatic joint stiffness with loss of the last 15° of terminal extension of the elbow is common. Heterotopic ossification occurs in greater than 75% of patients but limits motion in less than 5% of patients.[18]

RADIAL HEAD FRACTURES

Radial head fractures represent approximately one-third of all elbow fractures. Radial head fractures have a bimodal distribution of incidence with men in their late thirties to forties and women in their fifties.[3,20,24,25] Radial head fractures are most commonly caused by a FOOSH with pronation of the forearm.[20] The patients present to the ED with tenderness over the radial head and inability to fully extend their arm. Movement of the forearm can exacerbate the pain.[21] The radial head is a key aspect to the articulation of the elbow. The radial head is well vascularized, which may lead to a hemarthrosis with an injury. Ligamentous injury, including to the MCL, is also commonly associated with these fractures.[20] Special consideration should be made to fully range the elbow in active and passive movements to determine if there are any mechanical obstructions. Multiple sources suggest that drainage of the hemarthrosis and local anesthetic injection into the joint should be completed to be able to range the elbow completely.[26] However, this does not appear to translate into clinical practice because most providers do not perform such drainage. Occult fractures of the radial head may not appear on radiographs. In addition to physical examination, evidence of a posterior fat pad or a displaced anterior fat pad on imaging should prompt suspicion of a radial head fracture (**Fig. 7**).[27] POCUS can be useful for imaging such injuries.[28,29] Radial head fractures are characterized by the Mason classifications,[30–32] as seen in **Table 1** (**Fig. 8**).

Type 1 fractures are the most common (62%) and are managed with a splint or splint for comfort followed by early ROM within 2 days of injury.[20] The other types of fractures generally require surgical intervention. Most patients can be discharged from the ED with a long arm splint and close orthopedic follow-up. Various approaches to surgical repair are possible depending on the injury.[33,34] A prompt orthopedic consultation should be obtained with injuries that have evidence of a mechanical

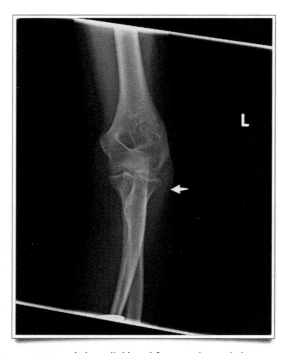

Fig. 7. AP view demonstrates subtle radial head fracture (*arrow*) that was suggested by positive fat pads on the lateral view (seen previously **Fig. 3**). (*Courtesy of* D. Hanlon, MD, Pittsburgh, PA.)

| Table 1 | |
| Mason classification | |
Type	Description
Type 1	Nondisplaced fractures (≤2 mm) without mechanical obstruction
Type 2	Displaced fractures (>2 mm)
Type 3	Comminuted fractures
Type 4	Fractures with elbow dislocation

From Mason MI. Some observations on fractures of the head of the radius with a review of one hundred cases. Br J Surg 1954; 42:123 – 132; with permission.

obstruction, open fracture, unstable elbow joint, or neurovascular deficits. Patients usually tolerate these injuries well; however, limited ROM, osteoarthritis, nerve deficits, and avascular necrosis can occur.[35] The most commonly associated nerve injury is the posterior interosseous nerve, usually with displaced fractures, and these patients cannot extend their fingers.[18,20]

CORONOID PROCESS FRACTURES

The coronoid provides critical stability and integrity to the elbow joint as part of the ulnohumeral joint.[36] It is also a site of attachment for the MCL and a portion of the anterior capsule. Coronoid process fractures are caused by axial compression on the coronoid process by the trochlear.[37] Examination reveals tenderness and swelling over the antecubital fossa. These fractures are usually associated with other injuries, particularly elbow dislocations, and rarely isolated. These injuries are visualized best on the lateral radiograph of the elbow. A medial oblique film (lateral film with forearm pronated 45°) may be required to remove the overlap of the radial head on the coronoid process. If identified, a coronoid fracture requires a careful look for other injuries to the joint. Although not necessarily needed in the ED, CT is recommended to identify the exact location of the fracture and enhances the recognition of instability patterns.[38] If associated with dislocation, reduction dislocation usually reduces the fracture. Any significant fracture of the coronoid process produces instability and will require open reduction internal fixation of the fracture.

Tables 2 and **3** highlight the types of coronoid fractures. A higher type is associated with a worse prognosis.[39] Type 1 fractures should be treated conservatively. Type 2 and 3 fractures require surgical repair. There is another classification system that is

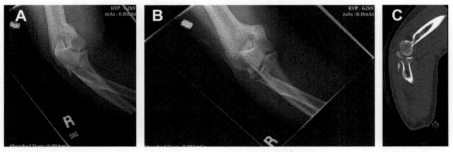

Fig. 8. (*A*) Lateral view with inappropriate degree of flexion but obvious fracture. (*B*) AP view of displaced fracture. (*C*) CT scan demonstrates comminuted, displaced fracture more clearly, Mason type 3. (*Courtesy of* D. Hanlon, MD, Pittsburgh, PA.)

Table 2
Regan and Morrey classification system

Type	Description
Type 1	Avulsion fracture of the tip
Type 2	Fracture involving <50%
Type 3	Fracture involving >50%

Data from Regan W, Morrey B. Fractures of the coronoid process of the ulna. J Bone Joint Surg Am 1989; 71: 1348 – 1354.

gaining popularity among orthopedic surgeons, the O'Driscoll System, which is anatomic based but also requires a CT.[6] From an emergency medicine perspective regardless of the classification system, the essential concept is that any fracture beyond an avulsion fracture of the coronoid process requires surgery.[6] Displaced coronoid process fractures require emergent orthopedic consultation, especially if greater than 50% of the coronoid process is fractured or the elbow is unstable.[6,18] For stable fractures, the elbow is placed in a posterior splint at 90° flexion with the forearm in supination. Early orthopedic follow-up for surgical repair should be arranged. These injuries are associated with arthritis.

OLECRANON FRACTURES

Fractures of the olecranon account for 10% of elbow fractures.[40] These fractures are often comminuted when due to a direct fall on the elbow, but usually are a transverse or oblique noncomminuted fracture if owing to a FOOSH mechanism.[40] The fracture pattern and site are determined by the degree of flexion of the elbow at the time of injury.[37] The triceps brachii inserts on the posterior third of the olecranon and may displace the fracture. These fractures occur more frequently in adults than children because the pediatric olecranon is short, thick, and relatively stronger than the distal humerus.[40] Pain and tenderness will be noted over the olecranon. Inability to fully extend the elbow against force is suggestive of an olecranon injury.[41] Particular attention should be paid to the ulnar nerve when evaluating the patient. Although olecranon fractures are usually isolated injuries, they can be associated with elbow dislocations and fractures of the radial head, radial shaft, and distal humerus.[40] Excluding avulsion fractures, olecranon fractures are intraarticular, and as such, strict anatomic alignment of the residual contour of the articular surface is critical to maintaining joint integrity.[42]

AP and lateral radiographs of the elbow should be obtained. The lateral view should be evaluated for any bony disruption, the degree of comminution, and the degree of displacement (**Fig. 9**). If there is no fracture displacement in 90° of flexion on the lateral

Table 3
Mayo classification system

Type	Description
Type 1	Stable, nondisplaced (≤2 mm) with or without comminution
Type 2	Stable, displaced >2 mm with or without comminution
Type 3	Highly unstable, displaced fractures with dislocation with or without comminution

Data from Newman SD, Mauffrey C, Krikler S. Olecranon Fractures. Injury 2009; 40: 575 – 581 and Tamaoki MJ, Matsunaga FT, Silveria JD, et al. Reproducibility of classifications for olecranon fractures. Injury 2014; 45S 5: S18 – S20.

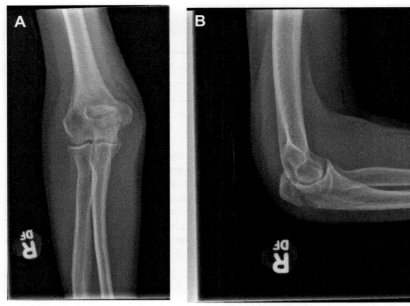

Fig. 9. Displaced olecranon fracture. (*A*) AP view. (*B*) Lateral view. (*Courtesy of* D. Hanlon, MD, Pittsburgh, PA.)

radiograph, then the triceps aponeurosis is likely intact.[12] There are multiple classification syndromes, but the Mayo Classification System is most widely used.[40]

Type 1 fractures can be treated nonoperatively; type 2 and 3 require surgical repair. Nonoperative treatment of type 1 fractures consists of long arm splint at 45° to 90° of flexion and follow-up in 5 to 7 days. Immobilization continues for up to one month followed by protective ROM. Type 2 and 3 fractures can be subdivided according to whether they are noncomminuted (type A) or comminuted (type B). Mayo type 3 fractures have poor functional outcomes.[40,43]

If there is greater than 2 mm of displacement, an orthopedic consultation should be obtained for possible surgical repair. Geriatric patients may be the exception to this displacement rule because this group does well with displacement up to 5 mm with nonoperative management.[44]

Displaced fractures or fractures associated with an elbow dislocation/fracture will need orthopedic consultation for eventual surgical repair, but the initial management can be the same as a nondisplaced fracture. Complications include arthritis, decreased ROM, and nonunion (5%).[18,40]

DISTAL HUMERUS FRACTURES

Distal humerus fractures account for approximately 2% of all fractures in the adult population.[45] Humeral fractures are usually associated with a high energy impact; however, in the osteoporotic, geriatric population, low-energy events, such as falls, have a higher incidence. Because the distal humerus contains insertion sites for extension and flexion of the elbow, injury to this area usually leads to a significant decrease in ROM and swelling. With transcondylar fractures, the fracture line extends through both condyles just proximal to the articular surface of the elbow within the joint capsule. With intercondylar fractures, 2 types ("T" or "Y") occur depending on the fracture line pattern. Independent of the type, the distal fracture line enters the intra-articular surface of the distal humerus. A fracture with a fracture line passing equally through both condyles defines a T-type fracture, which bisects the distal humeral segment. The Y-type fracture occurs when the lateral or medial segment passes through just the lateral condyle. Regardless of whether it is a transcondylar or intra-condylar fracture, ulnar nerve injuries are common, and a comprehensive neurovascu-lar examination of the upper extremity should be completed.[46]

Standard radiographs of the shoulder, humerus, and elbow should be obtained. Good-quality radiographs may be difficult to obtain because of patient discomfort. For the distal humerus, the AP view is taken with the elbow flexed to 40°, rather than fully extended, to facilitate olecranon disengagement from the fossa, allowing for better visualization of the distal humerus (**Fig. 10**).[45]

Multiple classifications systems exist to characterize these fractures. The most common one is the Orthopedic Trauma Association classification, as seen in **Table 4**. Type A fractures associated with supracondylar fractures occur commonly in children, whereas transcondylar fractures occur more often in adults.

Surgical intervention is required for most of these fractures and is superior to nonoperative management.[46,47] Conservative management is usually reserved for cases with nondisplaced fractures and high-risk surgical candidates.[48] There are multiple surgical approaches for repair. The goal is to maintain full mobility and sta-bility of the elbow. Type A fractures can be placed in a splint for comfort with early ROM of the joint and follow-up with orthopedics. Orthopedics should be consulted for type B and C fractures, and in cases with open fractures or neurovascular compromise. Complications include loss of elbow function secondary to prolonged immobilization, arthritis, ulnar nerve impingement, nonunion, and valgus or varus deformity.

NIGHTSTICK FRACTURES

Isolated diaphyseal fractures to the ulna are nightstick fractures. These injuries usually occur with a direct blow to the ulna, such as in assaults, MVCs, and occasionally, falls.[49] The presentation includes localized pain and tenderness. One should evaluate closely for open fractures and ensure a complete neurovascular examination is completed. Radiographs of the wrist and elbow should be obtained in addition to

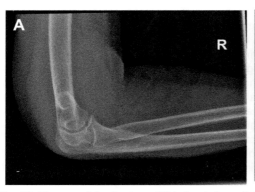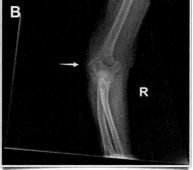

Fig. 10. Transcondylar fracture. (*A*) Lateral view, distorted distal humerus. (*B*) AP view, easily seen displaced fracture (arrow). (*Courtesy of* D. Hanlon, MD, Pittsburgh, PA.)

Table 4	
Orthopedic Trauma Association classification	
Type	**Description**
Type A	Extraarticular fractures
Type B	Partial articular fracture (single column)
Type C	Complete articular fracture (both columns)

Data from Meinberg E, Agel J, Roberts C, et al. Fracture and Dislocation Classification Compendium–2018, Journal of Orthopaedic Trauma. Volume 32: Number 1; Supplement, January 2018.

the forearm to rule out further injuries, especially disruptions to the distal and proximal radioulnar joints.

Most injuries can be reduced and placed in a sugar-tong or long arm splint. Close follow-up with orthopedic surgery should be arranged. The elbow should be flexed at 90° with the forearm in a neutral position. Immediate orthopedic consultation should be obtained for surgical repair in fractures with more than 10° to 15° of angulation or more than 50% displacement.

Potential complications include limited ROM, pain, and nonunion.[50] Fractures involving the middle and proximal thirds of the ulna shaft have an increased risk for malunion and other complications.[20] Also, higher rates of complications are associated with increased angulation and displacement.[51] Early mobilization may lead to better outcomes with lower rates of morbidity.[52,53]

MONTEGGIA FRACTURE

A fracture of the proximal third of the ulnar shaft in conjunction with a radial head dislocation is a Monteggia fracture. These injuries usually result as a consequence of a direct blow to the forearm, in either high-impact or low-impact injuries, such as a FOOSH with the forearm in pronation. Energy from the ulnar fracture leads to injury to the quadrate and annular ligaments that destabilizes the radiocapitellar joint, leading to the associated radial head dislocation.[54] Patients present forearm deformities, point tenderness, limited ROM of the elbow, especially with pronation and supination, and neurovascular deficits. Clinical tenderness to palpation of the proximal radioulnar joint in the presence of a proximal ulnar fracture should raise suspicion for this injury. The posterior interosseous nerve is the most commonly injured nerve in such injuries and can present with limited extension of the fingers. Injuries to the radial and median nerves also occur, although less commonly.

Imaging studies should include the elbow, forearm, and wrist. Although the ulnar fracture is usually readily seen, identifying a subtle radial head dislocation may be difficult. Under normal alignment, drawing a straight line through the axis of the radius should intersect the middle third of the capitellum (**Fig. 11**).[55,56] Any deviation from the radiocapitellar line suggests a radial head dislocation. These injuries are reportedly missed in 20% to 50% of cases on the initial evaluation.[55,56]

Monteggia fractures are classified into 4 different types under the BADO classification system that is based on the direction of the radial head dislocation (**Table 5**).[57] Type I injuries are associated with an anterior dislocation of the radial head, most commonly seen in children. Type II injuries are associated with a posterior radial head dislocation, most commonly seen in adults. Type III injuries are associated with a lateral dislocation, and type IV injuries are associated with anterior dislocations in combination with both proximal ulnar and radial shaft fractures.

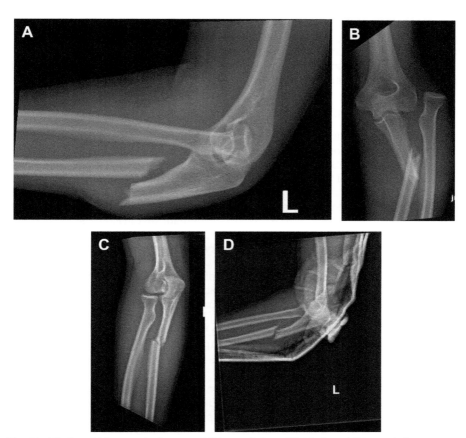

Fig. 11. Displaced Monteggia fracture. (*A*) Lateral view. (*B*) AP view. (*C*) Lateral view postreduction. (*D*) AP view postreduction. Surgery will still be required. (*Courtesy of* V. Mavrophilipos, MD, Fairfax, VA.)

Pediatric injuries are commonly treated with reduction and placement in a long arm splint. ED management of adult Monteggia fractures includes immediate placement in a long arm splint for comfort, analgesia, and urgent orthopedic consultation for surgical repair. All cases should be discussed with orthopedics. If orthopedics is not

Table 5
Bado classification: Monteggia fractures

Type	Injury
I	Ulnar diaphysis + anterior RHD
II	Ulnar diaphysis + posterior RHD
III	Ulnar diaphysis + lateral RHD
IV	Both bone fractures proximal 1/3 + RHD

Abbreviation: RHD, radial head dislocation.
From Waters PM. Monteggia fracture-dislocation in children. In Rockwood and Wilkins' Fractures in Children, 7th Ed. Beaty JH, Kasser JR (Eds). Lippincott Williams & Wilkins: Philadelphia; 2010. p.446-74.

available for bedside consult, reduce the fracture, place the patient in a sugar-tong splint, and arrange for close follow-up for operative repair. Missed radial head dislocations become irreducible after 2 to 3 weeks, except by surgical intervention.[58] Mistreated injuries can lead to significant mobility limitations, neurologic deficits, and osteoarthritis.[59,60] Malunion rates occur in 2% to 10% of all repairs.[59]

GALEAZZI FRACTURE-DISLOCATION

The Galeazzi fracture-dislocation is a fracture of the middle to distal third of the radius with a concomitant dislocation of the distal ulna or instability of the DRUJ. The mechanism is usually a FOOSH with the forearm in pronation.[61] The patient is tender and has pain over the site of the radius fracture and tenderness over the DRUJ. Ulnar styloid palpation leads to suspicion of this injury during examination because an overly prominent styloid process suggests a dorsal dislocation, and the loss of prominence suggests a palmar dislocation. The DRUJ ballottement test involves stabilizing the distal radius and trying to move the distal ulna volarly or dorsally comparing any laxity with the uninjured extremity.[61,62] Peripheral nerve injuries are relatively rare.

The initial assessment includes radiographs of the wrist, forearm, and elbow. The Galeazzi fracture may seem to be a simple radius fracture on plain imaging; careful analysis of the DRUJ is necessary to pick up subtle changes (**Fig. 12**). DRUJ dislocations are often missed because of subtle physical and radiographic findings. AP films may show a relatively shortened radius (>5 mm) and a widened interspace (>1–2 mm) between the radioulnar articulation at the DRUJ.[62] These findings coincide with a lack of overlap of the ulnar head on the radius on AP films.[62] An associated ulnar styloid fracture may be a marker for DRUJ instability because the radioulnar ligament attaches to the base of the ulnar styloid.[62]

Successful treatment depends on recognition of the lesion because, generally, the treatment is surgical repair in adults. Orthopedics should be consulted in the acute setting. Some investigators think that the proposed radiographic criteria for DRUJ instability are only moderately accurate, and they recommend an orthopedist perform an intraoperative assessment of the DRUJ after fixation of the radial fracture.[8,62] Rarely, children may be managed conservatively with closed reduction and splinting. Complications of an unrecognized DRUJ disruption include chronic pain and weakness associated with diminished supination and pronation.[18]

ESSEX-LOPRESTI INJURIES

The Essex-Lopresti injury is a rare complex injury that is a combination of fractured radial head, disruption of the DRUJ, and a torn IOM of the forearm.[63]

The mechanism is a violent, longitudinal compression of high-impact FOOSH. The impaction of the radial head on the capitellum causes fracture of the radial head, disruption of IOM, and disruption of the DRUJ.[18]

In addition to tenderness over the radial head and wrist, the patient may have ecchymosis along the path of the IOM disruption. In a patient with a radial head fracture, pain on compression of the wrist is an early indication that an Essex-Lopresti injury is present.[64]

The initial assessment includes radiologic evaluation of the wrist, forearm, and elbow. With the right mechanism and only a radial head fracture seen on plain radiographs, the diagnosis should still be pursued, particularly if there is wrist pain. If not diagnosed in the acute setting, the ruptured IOM allows the radius to migrate proximally, producing chronic instability of the forearm.[8,64]

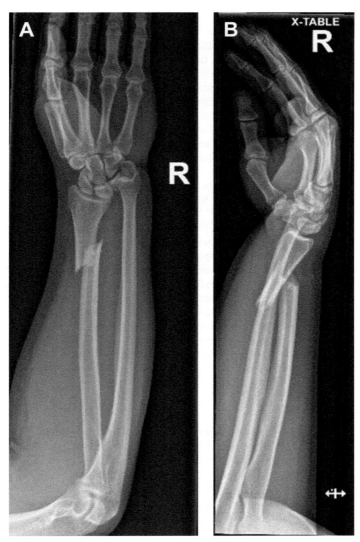

Fig. 12. Galeazzi fracture-dislocation. (*A*) AP view. Obvious radial shortening, loss of distal radial ulnar overlap. (*B*) Lateral view. (*Courtesy of* D. Hanlon, MD, Pittsburgh, PA.)

Initial treatment is a well-padded long posterior splint, analgesia, and emergent orthopedic consultation. Early diagnosis is essential because this injury needs to be managed operatively to realign both the radial capitellum joint and the DRUJ. Delayed diagnosis and treatment can lead to proximal migration of the radius, and chronic instability at the DRUJ, which is difficult to treat surgically.[8,65] One should be sure to evaluate for compartment syndrome and posterior interosseous nerve injury.

DISTAL BICEPS TENDON RUPTURE

Distal biceps tendon rupture is a relatively uncommon injury and only accounts for 3% of all biceps tendon ruptures.[66] Typically, it affects the dominant arm of men in the fourth to– fifth decade of life.[66] The mechanism is a sudden injury from an eccentric force on the forearm while the elbow is attempting to flex. Patients often report a sharp, tearing sensation in antecubital fossa associated with a pop.[67] The sharp pain will often subside to a dull ache, but they will continue to have weak supination and flexion. There may be a visible deformity of the muscle belly; however, it may be obscured by swelling, obesity, or sometimes an intact brachioradialis muscle.[67]

Partial tears are more difficult to diagnose because they will not have the apparent deformity and have more subtle clinical findings.

The hook test is very sensitive for diagnosing a complete biceps tendon rupture.[68] The patient actively flexes his forearm to 90°, and then the examiner attempts to place his finger behind the distal biceps tendon from the lateral aspect of the antecubital fossa.[68] The examiner will be unable to hook the tendon with a complete rupture. The squeeze test is performed with the forearm slightly pronated and resting on the patient's leg; the examiner squeezes the biceps and should notice slight supination of the forearm if the tendon is intact.[69] Two additional physical examination adjuncts are the supination-pronation test and the biceps crease interval. The supination pronation test is negative if the biceps moves toward the shoulder with supination and toward the elbow with pronation, and signifies the tendon is intact.[70] The biceps crease interval is positive if the distance between the antecubital crease and the distal biceps muscle is measured to be greater than 6 cm or 20% longer on the affected arm.[70] Imaging is not required acutely if the diagnosis can be made clinically. POCUS may be diagnostic and can confirm the diagnosis if readily available. MRI is diagnostic, although not indicated in the ED, and will usually be done in follow-up.

These injuries should be referred early to an orthopedist. Acute complete ruptured distal biceps tendon often requires an early surgical reattachment. Partial tears are treated conservatively with mobilization, and surgical repair is only done for refractory dysfunction.[66]

TRICEPS TENDON RUPTURE

Triceps tendon rupture is the most uncommon of major tendon injuries.[7] This injury primarily occurs in men in the third to fifth decade of life.[71] Geriatric patients with underlying systemic diseases are another major group to suffer this injury. Associated risk factors include renal failure, endocrine disorders, metabolic bone disease, olecranon bursitis, local steroid injections, and anabolic steroid use.[7,71] The mechanism is usually a FOOSH because the triceps is contracted.[7,71] The site of rupture is at the insertion of the tendon on the olecranon.[7]

Patients will have posterior elbow swelling and tenderness with limited ability to extend the elbow against gravity or resistance. Squeezing the triceps tendon normally results in some elbow extension; this is not seen if the tendon is ruptured.[7] A defect may be palpated unless it is obscured by swelling. The injury can be associated with an avulsion fracture olecranon, which can be seen as a bony flake on the lateral elbow.[7,71] The diagnosis is often made clinically, although POCUS may be diagnostic. MRI is definitively diagnostic and usually obtained as an outpatient for preoperative planning.[72]

Initial treatment is splinting at 30° of flexion. Urgent orthopedic consultation is recommended. Most patients require early surgical repair.[72]

SUMMARY

Emergency physicians must be proficient in the management of acute elbow and forearm injuries. Most are initially evaluated in the ED and require imaging studies, adequate limb immobilization, rest, ice, and analgesia. A thorough neurovascular examination is necessary to appropriately evaluate such injuries. Most nondisplaced fractures without neurovascular involvement can be treated nonoperatively in consultation with an orthopedist. A subset of injuries, such as elbow dislocations, complex forearm fracture-dislocations, and displaced supracondylar fracture, is potential limb-threatening injuries that require immediate identification as well as timely intervention to avoid neurovascular complications and chronic dysfunction. In addition, early recognition of unstable injuries can help avoid chronic instability and corrective surgeries.

REFERENCES

1. Kaas L, van Riet RP, Vroemen JP, et al. The epidemiology of radial head fractures. J Shoulder Elbow Surg 2010;19:520–3.
2. Kuhn MA, Ross G. Acute elbow dislocations. Orthop Clin North Am 2008;39: 155–61.
3. Duckworth AD, Clement ND, Jenkins PJ, et al. The epidemiology of radial head and neck fractures. J Hand Surg 2012;37A:112–9.
4. Karl JW, Olson PR, Rosenwasser MP. The epidemiology of upper extremity fractures in the United States, 2009. J Orthop Trauma 2015;29:242–4.
5. Gottlieb M, Schiebout J. Elbow dislocations in the emergency department: a review of reduction techniques. J Emerg Med 2018;54:849–54.
6. Manikadis N, Sperelakis I, Hackney R, et al. Fractures of the ulnar coronoid process. Injury 2012;43:989–98.
7. Kokkalis ZT, Ballas EG, Mavrogenis, et al. Distal biceps and triceps ruptures. Injury 2013;44:318–22.
8. Omokawu S, Iida A, Fujitani R, et al. Radiographic predictors of DRUJ instability with distal radial fracture. J Wrist Surg 2014;3:2–6.
9. Vinson DR, Kann GS, Gaona GS, et al. Performance of the 4-way range of motion test for radiographic injuries after blunt elbow trauma. Am J Emerg Med 2016;34: 235–9.
10. Appelbaum A, Reuben AD, Benger JR, et al. Elbow extension test to rule out elbow fracture: multicentre, prospective validation and observational study of diagnostic accuracy in adults and children. BMJ 2008;337:a2428.
11. Acar K, Aksay E, Oray D, et al. Utility of computed tomography in elbow trauma patients with normal x-ray study and positive elbow extension test. J Emerg Med 2016;50:444–8.
12. Rabiner JE, Khine H, Avner JR, et al. Accuracy of point of care ultrasonography for diagnosis of elbow fractures in children. Ann Emerg Med 2013;61:9–17.
13. De Maessner M, Jacobson JA, Jaovisidha S, et al. Elbow effusions: distribution of joint fluid with flexion and extension and imaging implications. Invest Radiol 1998; 33:117–25.
14. Avci M, Kozai N, Beydilli I, et al. The comparison the bedside point of care ultrasound and computed tomography in the elbow injuries. Am J Emerg Med 2016; 34:2186–90.
15. Stonebeck JW, Owens BD, Syckes J, et al. Incidence of elbow dislocations in the United States population. J Bone Joint Surg Am 2012;94:240–5.
16. McCabe MP, Savoie FH. Simple elbow dislocations: evaluation, management, and outcomes. Phys Sportsmed 2012;40:62–71.
17. Hobgood ER, Khan SO, Field LD. Acute dislocations of the adult elbow. Hand Clin 2008;24:1–7.

18. Falcon-Chevre JL, Mathew D, Cabanas JG, et al. Management and treatment of the elbow and forearm injuries. Emerg Med Clin North Am 2010;28:765–88.
19. Giannicola G, Calella P, Piccioli A, et al. Terrible triad of the elbow: is it still a troublesome injury? Injury 2015;46:S68–76.
20. Goldham K. Evaluation and treatment of the elbow and forearm injuries in the emergency department. Emerg Med Clin North Am 2015;33:409–21.
21. Skelley NW, Chamberlain A. A novel reduction technique for elbow dislocations. Orthopedics 2015;38:42–4.
22. Kumar A, Ahmed M. Closed reduction of posterior dislocation of the elbow: a simple technique. J Orthop Trauma 1999;13:58–9.
23. Cadie SJ, Germann CA, Darcus AA, et al. Orthopedic pitfalls in the ED: neurovascular injury associated with posterior elbow dislocations. Am J Emerg Med 2010; 28:960–5.
24. Burkhart KJ, Wegmann K, Muller LP, et al. Fractures of the radial head. Hand Clin 2015;31:533–46.
25. Black WS, Becker JA. Common forearm fractures in adults. Am Fam Physician 2009;80:1096–102.
26. Rosenblatt Y, Athwal G, Faber K. Current recommendations for the treatment of radial head fractures. Orthop Clin North Am 2008;39:173–85.
27. Pappas N, Bernstein J. Fractures in brief, radial head fractures. Clin Orthop Relat Res 2010;468:914–6.
28. Malahias M, Manolopoulos P, Kadu V, et al. Bedside ultrasonography for early diagnosis of occult radial head fractures in emergency room: a CT-comparative diagnostic study. Arch Bone Jt Surg 2018;6:539–46.
29. Pavic R, Margetic P, Hnatesen D. Diagnosis of occult radial head and neck fractures in adults. Injury 2015;46S:S119–24.
30. Mason MI. Some observations on fractures of the head of the radius with a review of one hundred cases. Br J Surg 1954;42:123–32.
31. Johnston GW. A follow-up of one hundred cases of fracture of the head of the radius with a review of the literature. Fracture and orthopaedic service. Ulster Med J 1962;31:51–6.
32. Hotchkiss RN. Displaced fractures of the radial head: internal fixation or excision? J Am Acad Orthrop Surg 1997;5:1–10.
33. Duparc F, Merlet M. Prevention and management of early treatment failures in elbow injuries. Orthop Traumatol Surg Res 2019;105:S75–87.
34. Vannabouathong C, Akhter A, Athwal GS, et al. Interventions for displaced radial fractures: network meta-analysis of randomized trials. J Shoulder Elbow Surg 2018;12:2232–41.
35. Jordan RW, Jones AD. Radial head fractures. Open Orthop J 2017;11:1405–16.
36. Matzon JL, Widmer BJ, Draganich LF, et al. Anatomy of the coronoid process. J Hand Surg Am 2006;31:1272–8.
37. Amis AA, Miller JH. The mechanisms of elbow fractures: an investigation using impact tests in vitro. Injury 1995;26:163–8.
38. Lindenhovius A, Karanicolas PJ, Bhandari M, et al. Interobserver reliability of coronoid fracture classification: two-dimensional versus three-dimensional computed tomography. J Hand Surg Am 2009;34:1640–6.
39. Regan W, Morrey B. Fractures of the coronoid process of the ulna. J Bone Joint Surg Am 1989;71:1348–54.
40. Newman SD, Mauffrey C, Krikler S. Olecranon fractures. Injury 2009;40:575–81.
41. Rommens PM, Kuchle R, Schneider RU, et al. Olecranon fractures in adults: factors influencing outcome. Injury 2004;35:1149–57.

42. Lavigne G, Baratz M. Fractures of the olecranon. J Am Soc Surg Hand 2004;4: 94–102.
43. Tamaoki MJ, Matsunaga FT, Silveria JD, et al. Reproducibility of classifications for olecranon fractures. Injury 2014;45S 5:S18–20.
44. Veras Del Monte L, Sirera Vercher M, Busquets Net R, et al. Conservative treatment of displaced fractures of the olecranon in the elderly. Injury 1999;30:105–10.
45. Beazley JC, Baraza N, Jordon R, et al. Distal humeral fractures–current concepts. Open Orthop J 2017;11:1353–63.
46. Nauth A, McKee MD, Ristevski B, et al. Distal humeral fractures in adults. J Bone Joint Surg Am 2011;93:686–700.
47. Srinivasan K, Agarwal M, Matthews S, et al. Fractures of the distal humerus in the elderly: is internal fixation the treatment choice? Clin Orthop Relat Res 2005;434: 222–30.
48. Amir S, Jannis S, Daniel R. Distal humerus fractures: a review of current therapy concepts. Curr Rev Musculoskelet Med 2016;9:199–206.
49. Williams A, Friedrich J. Retrospective analysis demonstrates no advantage to operative management of distal ulna fractures. Hand 2011;6:378–83.
50. McAuliffe JA. Isolated diaphyseal fractures of the ulna. J Hand Surg Am 2012;37: 145–7.
51. Coulibaly MO, Jones CB, Siestsema DL, et al. Results of 70 consecutive ulnar nightstick fractures. Injury 2015;46:1359–66.
52. Cai X-Z, Yan S-G, Giddins G. A systemic review of the non-operative treatment of nightstick fractures of the ulna. Bone Joint J 2013;95-B:52–9.
53. Pollock FH, Pankovich AM, Prieto JJ, et al. The isolated fracture of the ulnar shaft. Treatment without immobilization. J Bone Joint Surg Am 1983;65:339–42.
54. Beutel BG. Monteggia fractures in pediatric and adult populations. Orthopedics 2012;35:138–44.
55. Perron AD, Hersh RE, Brady WJ, et al. Orthopedic pitfalls in the ED: Galeazzi and Monteggia fracture-dislocation. Am J Emerg Med 2001;19:225–8.
56. Storen G. Traumatic dislocation of the radial head as an isolated lesion in children; report of one case with special regard to roentgen diagnosis. Acta Chir Scand 1959;116:114–47.
57. Bado JL. The Monteggia lesion. Clin Orthop Relat Res 1967;50:71–86.
58. Delpont M, Louahem D, Cottalorda J. Monteggia injuries. Orthop Traumatol Surg Res 2018;104:S113–20.
59. Wong JC, Getz CL, Abboud JA. Adult Monteggia and olecranon fracture dislocations of the elbow. Hand Clin 2015;31:565–80.
60. Hamaker M, Zheng A, Eglseder A, et al. The adult Monteggia fracture: patterns and incidence of annular ligament incarceration among 121 cases at a single institution over 19 years. J Hand Surg 2018;43:85.e1-6.
61. George AV, Lawton JN. Management of complications of forearm fractures. Hand Clin 2015;31:217–33.
62. Tsismenakis T, Tornetta P. Galeazzi fractures: is DRUJ instability predicted by current guidelines? Injury 2016;47:1472–7.
63. Jungbluth P, Frangen TM, Arens S, et al. The undiagnosed Essex-Lopresti injury. Hand Clin 2008;24:125–37.
64. Grassmann JP, Hakimi M, Gehrmann SV, et al. The treatment of the acute Essex-Lopresti injury. Bone Joint J 2014;96-B:1385–91.
65. Schnetzke M, Porschke F, Hoppe K, et al. Outcome of early and late diagnosed Essex-Lopresti injury. J Bone Joint Surg Am 2017;99:1043–50.

66. Sarda P, Qaddori A, Nauschutz F, et al. Distal biceps tendon rupture: current concepts. Injury 2013;44:417–20.
67. Pflederer N, Zitterkopf Z, Saxena S. Bye bye biceps: case report describing presentation, physical examination, diagnostic workup, and treatment of acute distal biceps brachii tendon rupture. J Emerg Med 2018;55:702–6.
68. O'Driscoll SW, Goncalves LBJ, Dietz P. The hook test for distal biceps tendon avulsion. Am J Sports Med 2007;35:1865–9.
69. Ruland RT, Dunbar RP, Bowen JD. The biceps squeeze test for diagnosis of distal biceps tendon ruptures. Clin Orthop Relat Res 2005;437:128–31.
70. Sherman SC, Afifi N. Distal biceps tendon rupture. J Emerg Med 2012;43: e469–70.
71. Tom JA, Kumar NS, Cerynik DL, et al. Diagnosis and treatment of triceps tendon injuries: a review of the literature. Clin J Sport Med 2014;24:197–204.
72. Balazs GC, Brelin AM, Dworak TC, et al. Outcomes and complications of triceps tendon repair following acute rupture in American military personnel. Injury 2016; 47:2247–51.

The Emergent Evaluation and Treatment of Shoulder, Clavicle, and Humerus Injuries

Jacob Stelter, MD[a],*, Sanjeev Malik, MD[a],
George Chiampas, DO[a,b]

KEYWORDS

- Shoulder emergencies • Proximal humerus fracture • Acromioclavicular separation
- Shoulder dislocations • Septic arthritis • Clavicle fractures • Rotator cuff tears
- Shoulder labral injury

KEY POINTS

- The shoulder is the most mobile joint in the body and is prone to injuries that are often evaluated in the emergency department.
- Emergency providers need to be facile in evaluating and treating common shoulder injuries, including dislocations, rotator cuff tears and labral injuries.
- Clavicle fractures and proximal humerus fractures are also commonly seen as causes of shoulder pain and need thorough evaluation in the emergency department.
- The emergency department must be familiar with what diagnoses need immediate treatment in the emergency department and which need primarily outpatient treatment.

INTRODUCTION

The shoulder joint serves many functions and is very mobile. In exchange for enhanced mobility, the shoulder also has inherent instability, placing it at an increased risk of injury. Shoulder injuries are frequent causes of seeking medical attention, accounting for 8% to 13% of athletic injuries.[1] Expertise in the acute diagnosis, stabilization, and management of these injuries is an essential part of the skill set of an emergency provider (EP).

EVALUATION

When evaluating a patient with shoulder pain, the EP should complete an accurate history and physical examination, considering infectious, bony, and soft tissue injuries.

Disclosure Statement: The authors have no financial interest to disclose.
[a] Department of Emergency Medicine, Feinberg School of Medicine, Northwestern University, 211 East Ontario Street, Suite 200, Chicago, IL 60611, USA; [b] United States Soccer Federation
* Corresponding author.
E-mail address: jacobqstelter@gmail.com

Emerg Med Clin N Am 38 (2020) 103–124
https://doi.org/10.1016/j.emc.2019.09.006
0733-8627/20/© 2019 Elsevier Inc. All rights reserved.

emed.theclinics.com

Table 1, although not exhaustive, provides reference to musculoskeletal differential diagnoses stratified by historical features. In addition to these, emergent diagnoses can present as shoulder pain and should be considered (eg, biliary disease, diaphragmatic irritation, myocardial ischemia, and cervical injuries).

During the physical examination, the EP should examine the shoulder, clavicle, and humerus, ensuring to carefully inspect and palpate the area, test passive and active range of motion (ROM), assess neurovascular status, test strength, and perform indicated provocative tests that may help to establish a diagnosis. It is essential that the joints proximal, cervical spine, and distal, elbow, be examined as well.

Palpation of the sternoclavicular (SC) joint, clavicle, acromioclavicular (AC) joint, and proximal humerus should be performed to assess for crepitus and tenderness. External rotation of the shoulder allows the long head of the biceps to track in the intertubercular groove and can be palpated here. Passive ROM of the shoulder can normally be performed to 170° abduction, 150° to 170° forward flexion, 90° external rotation, and internal rotation to the level of the T7 spinous process.[5,6] Diagnoses of adhesive capsulitis, osteoarthritis, fracture, or dislocation will limit passive ROM, whereas most other injuries have preserved passive ROM.[2] After an evaluation of passive ROM, the EP should evaluate the patient's ability to actively range the shoulder, which may be limited by pain or functional deficits.

It is critical that the EP assesses for any signs of neurovascular deficits in any musculoskeletal injury. Fracture dislocations, old age, hematoma, and inferior dislocations are associated with increased risk of neurovascular injury, with the most

Table 1
Suggested differential diagnoses with certain historical features

Historical Feature	Differential Diagnoses to Consider
Age <40 y	Glenohumeral instability/dislocation, labral tears, acromioclavicular separations
Age >40 y	Rotator cuff tears, proximal humeral fractures, impingement syndrome, adhesive capsulitis
Duration–acute	Glenohumeral dislocations, acromioclavicular separations, shoulder contusions, rotator cuff tear, biceps/pectoralis rupture
Duration–chronic	Impingement syndrome, biceps tendinosis
Mechanism–traumatic	Glenohumeral dislocations, acromioclavicular separations, proximal humerus fractures
Mechanism–atraumatic or repetitive microtrauma	Impingement syndrome, labral tears, glenohumeral instability, osteoarthritis
History of diabetes	Adhesive capsulitis, septic arthritis
Limitations in passive range of motion	Glenohumeral dislocations, proximal humerus fracture, adhesive capsulitis
Mechanical symptoms	Labral tear, osteoarthritis, intra-articular loose body
Muscle weakness	Rotator cuff tear, brachial plexus injury
Prior instability or dislocation	Glenohumeral instability or dislocation, impingement syndrome, labral tears, biceps tendinosis
Fever	Septic arthritis, rheumatologic disorder

Data from Refs.[2–4]

commonly injured nerves being axillary (37%), suprascapular (29%) and radial (22%).[7,8] It is essential that immediate reduction of fracture fragments or dislocations be performed in the setting of acute neurovascular compromise in the emergency department (ED) and that an orthopedic surgeon is promptly involved.[8]

After neurovascular testing, the EP should next evaluate the shoulder joint for any injuries that may involve the rotator cuff, which consists of the subscapularis, supraspinatus, teres minor, and infraspinatus muscles. **Table 2** describes the rotator cuff muscles and their specific diagnostic tests in more detail.

A positive test is defined as the presence of weakness in the affected shoulder when compared with the normal, uninjured contralateral side. Objective weakness is highly specific to detect a partial or complete rotator cuff tear, whereas the presence of pain without weakness may suggest rotator cuff impingement.[2] Refer to **Fig. 1** for demonstrations of rotator cuff muscle testing. **Fig. 2** demonstrates both the Neer[13] and Hawkins[14] tests, which are useful in the diagnosis of rotator cuff impingement syndrome.

Two highly sensitive and specific tests that may be performed to assess for instability in patients with suspected subluxation, recent dislocation, or instability are the apprehension test and the relocation test.[2] To perform the apprehension test, the patient is placed in the supine position with the affected arm abducted 90° and flexed 90° at the elbow.[15] The EP should then apply an external rotational force to the arm. If the patient develops discomfort and a sensation of impending dislocation, the test is suggestive of anterior glenohumeral instability. If the apprehension test is positive, the relocation test may also be performed with the EP applying a posteriorly directed force to the humeral head. A decrease in patient discomfort with the relocation test further suggests anterior instability.[2,3]

The cross-arm adduction test (sensitivity of 0.77) can be used to evaluate suspected AC injuries.[16,17] The arm is flexed forward to 90° and adducted across the body toward the contralateral arm, providing a compressive force at the AC joint. Pain localized at this joint suggests AC pathology. If biceps tendon pathology is suspected, the EP may perform the Speed test (sensitivity of 0.54 and specificity of 0.81) by resisting forward flexion with the arm extended at the elbow and the forearm supinated.[18] Palpable subluxation or pain localized in the intertubercular groove is suggestive of biceps tendon involvement.[19]

Plain radiographs consisting of anteroposterior (AP) view and lateral views is the initial imaging modality to perform in the ED. A true lateral view should take the form of a scapular Y-view. An axillary view can be obtained as well to assess for dislocations or subtle fractures of the glenohumeral joint. However, this view may be difficult to obtain owing to pain.[20] An AP view and 45° cephalic tilt view is recommended for evaluation of a suspected clavicle fracture. A serendipity view (40° cephalic tilt centered on the manubrium) may be performed for better assessment of medial clavicle fractures and SC joint injuries, whereas a Zanca view (10°–15° cephalic tilt)

Table 2 Muscles of the rotator cuff				
Muscle	**Action**	**Test**	**Sensitivity**	**Specificity**
Supraspinatus	Abduction	Empty can test	0.50–0.89	0.50–0.98
Infraspinatus	External Rotation	External rotation test	0.51	0.84
Teres Minor	External rotation	External rotation test	0.51	0.84
Subscapularis	Internal rotation	Liftoff test	0.17–0.92	0.60–0.92

Data from Refs.[9–12]

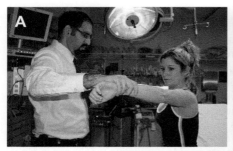
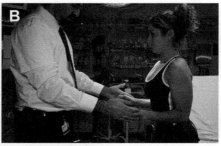
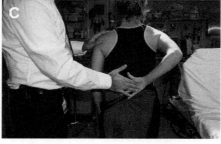

Fig. 1. Rotator cuff strength testing. (*A*) Empty can test.[10] The examiner isolates the supraspinatus by placing the patient's arm in 90° abduction and 30° forward flexion with the elbow in full extension and the arm in internal rotation with the thumb pointed downward. The examiner than places downward pressure on the arm while the patient resists. (*B*) External rotation test. The examiner resists active external rotation by the patient with the arm adducted at the side and the elbow flexed at 90°. (*C*) Liftoff test.[12] The patient places the affected arm behind his or her back with the dorsum of his or her hand against the lumbar spine. The patient then attempts to actively lift the hand away from the spine against resistance provided by the examiner. (*Reproduced with permission* of the Department of Emergency Medicine, Feinberg School of Medicine, Northwestern University.)

provides a better visualization of the distal clavicle and AC joint.[21,22] A computed tomography (CT) scan is the test of choice in evaluating suspected SC injuries.[23,24] Magnetic Resonance Imagery (MRI), although providing an excellent assessment of the soft tissue structures, has limited value in the acute evaluation of patients in the ED setting.

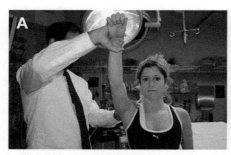
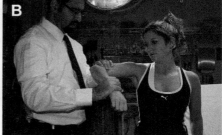

Fig. 2. Tests for impingement. (*A*) Neer[13] test. The examiner performs passive forward flexion of the arm to 180° with the arm fully pronated. Reproduction of pain above 90° suggest impingement. (*B*) Hawkins and Kennedy[14] test. The patient's arm is placed in 90° forward flexion with the elbow flexed. The examiner then forcibly internally rotates the arm. Discomfort suggest impingement.[3] (*Reproduced with permission* of the Department of Emergency Medicine, Feinberg School of Medicine, Northwestern University.)

CAUSES OF SHOULDER PAIN
Septic Arthritis

Septic arthritis of any joint is an emergency diagnosis and cannot be missed. More than 16,000 visits annually in the ED are attributed to septic arthritis.[25] It is the result of inoculation of bacteria into the joint via either hematogenous spread, direct spread from adjacent structures, or direct inoculation from trauma, surgery, or joint injections. The hip and knee are the most commonly affected joints, although the glenohumeral joint is involved in approximately 5% to 12% of cases.[26] The majority (56%) of septic arthritis is caused by Staphylococci, mostly *Staphylococcus aureus,* with methicillin-resistant *S aureus* making up 10% of all septic arthritis.[27] Streptococci species make up the next largest group, causing about 16% of septic arthritis cases, whereas gram-negative rods such as *Escherichia coli* and *Pseudomonas aeruginosa* make up 15% of septic arthritis cases.[27] In sexually active young adults, the most common cause of polyarticular septic arthritis is *Neisseria gonorrhoeae.*[28]

The diagnosis of septic arthritis can be challenging for various reasons. Children with septic arthritis often seem to be ill, have vital signs that are consistent with sepsis (eg, tachycardia, tachypnea, fever, and hypotension), and have severe pain and resist movement of the affected joint. However, in adults, the presentation may be vaguer with an indolent progression of symptoms. Risks factors that may suggest a diagnosis of septic arthritis include preexisting intrinsic joint pathology (eg, rheumatoid arthritis, gout, or lupus), recent trauma or surgery, diabetes, renal disease, and intravenous drug use.[27] The patient with septic arthritis often has localized pain and swelling to the joint. The patient often holds the joint in a position of comfort and avoids excess movement. A fever is noted in only 57% of cases.[29]

The initial ED evaluation of a patient with a concern for septic arthritis has traditionally included a white blood cell (WBC) count, erythrocyte sedimentation rate, and C-reactive protein. Although these tests can be useful, they are not at all sensitive or specific. In a recent review article, it was noted that the sensitivity of these tests varies widely.[30] These serum tests are still often obtained to help guide evaluation of the patient as data points to consider when making a medical decision and plan. Indeed, if a patient has a significant leukocytosis or highly elevated inflammatory markers, the suspicion for septic arthritis will most certainly be heightened. However, the critical point to consider is that normal or marginally elevated inflammatory markers and WBC do not exclude septic arthritis. These tests should be used as adjuncts and not as definitive diagnostics. A shoulder radiograph should be obtained to evaluate for bony erosions and to exclude a fracture as the cause of a painful swollen joint.

The gold standard evaluation to diagnose a septic shoulder is the analysis of synovial fluid, obtained by arthrocentesis. There are no absolute contraindications to an arthrocentesis, although relative contraindications include overlying cellulitis and a prosthetic joint.[28] It is advisable to attempt to discuss arthrocentesis of a prosthetic joint with an orthopedic surgeon before performing this procedure. Once the synovial fluid is obtained, it should be analyzed for cell count, crystals, Gram stain, and bacterial culture. Classically, a WBC count of 50,000/mm^3 or greater is diagnostic of septic arthritis. However, studies suggest no absolute WBC count is sensitive or specific enough to diagnosis septic arthritis.[31] It is appreciated that, as the WBC count increases, the likelihood of septic arthritis also increases, with a 90% to 99% specificity when the synovial WBC count is 100,000/mm^3 or greater.[30] However, a low WBC count does not exclude septic arthritis.

When treating septic arthritis, a few antibiotics are considered to be first line. In general, ampicillin/sulbactam or a third-generation cephalosporin such as ceftriaxone provides adequate coverage, especially if a large joint that is involved.[29] If the patient has diabetes or there is a concern for *Pseudomonas,* then piperacillin-tazobactam is the preferred choice.[29] The addition of vancomycin should be considered in any case with a reasonable suspicion for methicillin-resistant *S aureus* infection.

It is essential that an orthopedic surgeon is involved, preferably early, in the treatment course of a patient with septic shoulder arthritis. There are varying surgical methods for the treatment of septic arthritis, including serial aspiration, arthroscopy, and irrigation or open arthrotomy.[32] Up to one-third of patients who have had an arthroscopy and irrigation procedure need repeated procedures, demonstrating that this is a serious and potentially life-threatening condition.[32]

Bony Injuries

Glenohumeral dislocations

The shoulder is the most commonly dislocated joint in the body, accounting for about 50% of large joint dislocations, with about 95% being anterior, instead of the less frequent posterior and inferior dislocations.[1,33] Anterior dislocations tend to be associated with a posterior force directed against an abducted and extended arm. Posterior dislocations have a pathognomonic association with lightning injuries and seizures.

Physical examination of the anteriorly dislocated shoulder often reveals a squared-off appearance, as displacement of the humerus makes the acromion more prominent. The patient tends to hold the arm in slight abduction with anterior dislocations, versus in adduction and internal rotation with posterior dislocations.[1] As with all injuries, perform a thorough neurovascular examination with particular attention to axillary nerve function (ie, deltoid muscle innervation with sensation over the shoulder region).[8] In addition to an AP radiograph, it is critical to obtain a lateral or Y-view, because as many as 50% of posterior dislocations are missed without the lateral view.[1,33–35] Ideally, an axillary or modified axillary view can be obtained because the Y-view can be challenging to interpret. Obtaining pre-reduction and postreduction radiographs are the only reliable way to evaluate for existing fractures and provides the most complete evaluation of the patient. Iatrogenic fractures from reduction techniques are relatively rare, but still occur.[36–38]

There are multiple different methods that are commonly used to decrease glenohumeral dislocations (**Fig. 3**). A summary of these techniques is in **Table 3**. A recent study suggests that, with the sole use of oral analgesics, the Milch technique was successful during first attempt 82.8% of the time, over the Stimson technique, which was successful during first attempt only 28% of the time.[50] Analgesia is an important consideration when reducing these dislocations. Glenohumeral dislocations can be quite painful, and adequate analgesia is not only important for patient care, but also to facilitate the reduction. The use of narcotic analgesia or procedural sedation as premedication for the reduction provides excellent analgesia and has a high rate of success.[51] However, the risks of complications, including respiratory depression and aspiration, must be considered. As such, intra-articular injection with lidocaine is becoming a preferred method of analgesia. In fact, one systematic review identified 6 randomized controlled trials that concluded that there was no statistically significant difference in success rates between intra-articular lidocaine versus procedural sedation with analgesia. However, intravenous sedation was much more likely to have complications, the most concerning of which is respiratory depression and apnea.[51] Length of stay was significantly shorter in intra-articular

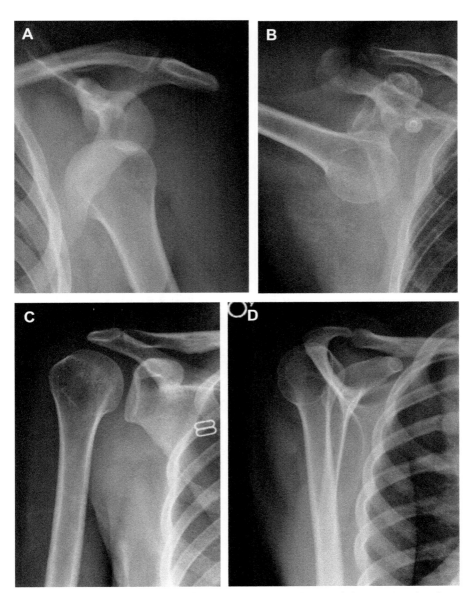

Fig. 3. Glenohumeral dislocations. (*A*) Anteroposterior (AP) view of the anterior glenohumeral dislocation. (*B*) AP view of luxatio erecta (inferior) dislocation. (*C*) AP view of posterior glenohumeral dislocation. Note that radiographic signs are subtle and easily missed. (*D*) Scapular Y-view showing humeral head migration posteriorly in the same patient as in C. (*Reproduced with permission* of the Department of Emergency Medicine, Feinberg School of Medicine, Northwestern University.)

lidocaine patients versus patients who undergo procedural sedation with analgesia.[52] Intravenous agents (ie, propofol, benzodiazepines, etomidate, and narcotics) are advantageously and widely used in both for sedation or analgesia. However, the authors advocate first to try, if able, a method with fewer complications such as

Table 3
Comparison of common glenohumeral reduction techniques

Technique	No. of Operators	Patient Position	Description	Disadvantages	Success Rate
Modified Hippocratic (traction–countertraction)	Two	Supine	One operator provides a longitudinal traction force with the arm slightly abducted. A second operator provides countertraction (typically with a bed sheet wrapped around the thorax in the axilla).	Requires significant force	86%
Kocher[39]	One	Seated	Starting position: arm should be adducted at the side with elbow flexed. Gently adduct the arm further and externally rotate the elbow. When resistance is felt, the arm is forward flexed upward and then internally rotated.	Higher incidence of fracture	72%–100%
Milch[39–41]	One	Supine	Starting position: arm fully abducted above the head with extended elbow. Apply longitudinal traction and external rotation of the arm.	None	70%–89%
Scapular manipulation[42]	Two	Prone	One operator provides downward traction to arm forward flexed 90°. A second operator attempts to adduct and medially rotate inferior border of scapula.	Difficult to monitor sedation, operator dependent	79%–90%
External rotation[43,44]	One	Supine/seated	Starting position: arm fully adducted, shoulder forward flexed 20°, and at side with elbow flexed. Perform slow, passive external rotation of arm with downward traction.	None	80%–90%
Stimson[45,46]	One	Prone	Arm hangs off stretcher in 90° forward flexion and a 5- to 10 pound weight attached to affected arm (can combine with scapular).	Equipment; difficult to monitor sedation	91%–96%
Snowbird[47]	Two	Seated	Starting position: patient seated in chair with arm adducted and flexed at elbow. Operator applies downward traction by placing foot in a loop of stockinette wrapped around the patient's forearm.	None	97%
Spaso[48,49]	One	Supine	Starting position: arm forward flexed 90° toward the ceiling. Apply longitudinal traction toward ceiling and passive external rotation.	Operator back discomfort (rare)	67%–91%

Data from Ufberg JW, Vilke GM, Chan TC, et al. Anterior shoulder dislocations: beyond traction-countertraction. J Emerg Med 2004;27(3):301-6.

intra-articular lidocaine. **Fig. 4** demonstrates the lateral approach to the intra-articular injection of lidocaine.

Refer patients to an orthopedic surgeon for follow-up. Counsel patients on the risk of recurrent dislocation. Patients younger than 30 years of age have a 50% to 64% risk of recurrent dislocation and this risk decreases with age.[53] Interestingly, patients with an associated greater tuberosity fracture are at significantly lower risk of recurrence than patients who do not have fractures.[54] This recurrence is attributed to the disruption of the inferior glenohumeral ligament-labrum complex, commonly referred to as a Bankart lesion, which occurs in 97% of first-time glenohumeral dislocations.[53]

Stabilization of the Bankart lesion is thought to decrease the recurrence of dislocation. Although usual treatment uses an internal rotation sling, MRI studies have shown better anatomic reduction of the Bankart lesion with the shoulder in external rotation.[55,56] A prospective clinical trial of 198 patients in Japan showed a 38.2% relative risk reduction for recurrent dislocation at 2 years in patients immobilized in an external rotation sling for 3 weeks compared with the internal rotation sling.[57]

Proximal humerus fractures

Proximal humerus fractures account for up to 5% of all fractures that present to the ED and are the third most common fracture in older patients, with more than 70% of these fractures occurring in women older than 60 years.[58–60] The humerus is most likely to be injured from a fall at an oblique angle onto an outstretched hand, usually from a standing height.[58,61,62] Younger patients with proximal humerus fractures tend to involved in a high mechanism trauma with a direct blow to the lateral humerus or shoulder.[58]

On examination, there is often point tenderness over the proximal humerus with some degree of swelling or ecchymosis, with obvious deformity often being obscured by the surrounding musculature. Given the proximity of the axillary nerve and brachial plexus, it is essential to evaluate for neurovascular injury, which may be present in up to 36% of these patients.[63] Axillary nerve injury is more common in fracture cases that also involve glenohumeral dislocation or displacement of the fracture.[64] Fractures of the anatomic neck of the humerus place vascular structures including the axillary artery and its branches, the anterior and posterior circumflex arteries, at greater risk of injury.[63,64]

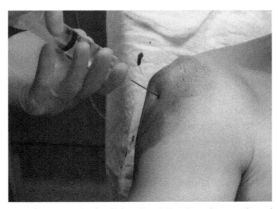

Fig. 4. Demonstration of intra-articular lidocaine injection. (*Reproduced with permission* of the Department of Emergency Medicine, Feinberg School of Medicine, Northwestern University.)

Because more than 80% of proximal humerus fractures are nondisplaced or minimally displaced, treatment consists of primarily conservative management, including a sling, application of ice to the affected area, and discharge with pain control and orthopedic follow-up.[65] In fact, even for proximal humerus fractures with displacement, surgery seems to provide little benefit when compared with immobilization and conservative management.[66] A recent systematic review also suggests that, in older patients with displaced humerus fractures, there is difference in functional outcomes of patients who were treated surgically or nonsurgically.[67] The data suggest that early ROM and physical therapy after one(1) week may result in decreased pain and improved functional outcomes.[68–70] Simple ROM exercises such as pendulum swings and wall walk-ups should be encouraged and can be quickly demonstrated in the ED. These exercises help to prevent the development of adhesive capsulitis of the shoulder.

Clavicle fractures

Clavicle fractures occur in 30 to 64 per 100,000 people per year, accounting for approximately 2.6% to 5% of all fractures, and up to 44% of all fractures of the shoulder joint.[1,23] The majority of patients with clavicular fractures are males between the ages of 15 and 30, with a second peak incidence occurring in women older than 80 years.[71,72]

The Allman system is used to classify clavicle fractures based on the location of the fracture.[73] The most common location for a clavicle fracture is the middle one-third of the clavicle (type I), which makes up 69% to 80% of all clavicle fractures. Fractures in the distal (ie, lateral, type II) one-third of the clavicle account for 21% to 28% of all fractures whereas proximal (ie, medial, type III) one-third fractures are relatively uncommon, occurring in only 2% of all clavicle fractures.[23,60] Both distal and proximal clavicle fractures are seen more commonly in the older patient, presumably owing to the weaker trabecular bone at the ends of the clavicle secondary to aging.[23,61]

Fractures of the clavicle in young people frequently require a high-impact mechanism, such as those experienced during collision sports or a motor vehicle collision. Unlike adolescents and young adults, the older population tends to fracture after a low-energy trip and fall.[23,60]

Patients with clavicle fractures typically guard and hold the affected arm close to the body. The superficial location of the clavicle allows for appreciation of tenting, palpation of step-offs or deformities, and ecchymosis. It is critical to complete a full neurovascular examination in addition to the standard musculoskeletal examination because of the proximity of the brachial plexus and subclavian vessels. Although rare, there have been reports of pneumothorax caused by displaced clavicle fractures.[74]

Clavicle fractures are managed conservatively, including ice, anti-inflammatories, short-term immobilization, physical therapy, and orthopedic referral, especially for acutely displaced mid-shaft and distal clavicle fractures. Figure-of-8 braces have been used in the past for treatment of clavicle fractures. However, there is no improvement in outcomes with these braces as compared with a traditional sling, and they have been associated with brachial plexus injuries and patient discomfort.[75,76] As a result, figure-of-8 braces are now avoided. Gentle ROM exercises should be encouraged early in nondisplaced fractures to improve functional recovery and prevent complications, such as adhesive capsulitis and muscle atrophy. Overhead activity is typically restricted until comfort allows and radiographic healing is evident.[77]

Conservative care remains the mainstay of management of nondisplaced clavicle fractures.[23,78] However, the evidence suggests that the rates of nonunion for certain types of clavicle fractures are greater than previously thought, indicating that surgery may be of benefit in certain patients. In one analysis, the overall rate of nonunion for conservatively managed clavicle fractures is 5.9% compared with 2.5% for surgically managed patients.[79] Advanced age, female sex, displacement, and comminution of the fracture have been found to be independent predictors of nonunion.[80] In particular, displaced mid-shaft clavicle fractures have a 15.1% rate of nonunion, which decreased to 2.2% with surgical fixation.[79] In addition, fractures with more than 1.5 cm of shortening are associated with increased risk of nonunion, decreased shoulder strength, and patient dissatisfaction and should be evaluated for surgical management.[78,81]

The majority of lateral clavicle fractures are nondisplaced and are managed conservatively. Displacement of lateral clavicle fractures is associated with an approximately 11% rate of nonunion.[80] Some surgeons recommend operative management, but studies suggest higher rates of complications than previously believed, and nonunion of these fractures may be relatively asymptomatic, especially in the older patient.[23,82] Medial clavicle fractures are rare and are typically managed nonoperatively.

Acromioclavicular separations

AC joints injuries are quite common and are frequently diagnosed in patients with shoulder pain. These injuries are commonly seen in contact sports and are more likely to occur in men than in women.[83] Falling onto an adducted shoulder often causes injury to one of the ligaments making up the AC joint, those being the AC and coracoclavicular ligaments.[1,84] Tenderness along the AC joint as well as pain with cross-arm adduction is suggestive of an AC injury.[16,17] Plain shoulder radiographs should be performed to evaluate for possible fracture as well as for AC joint widening. Radiographic findings that would suggest an AC separation is widening of the AC joint of more than 3 mm and a coracoclavicular distance increase of more than 13 mm.[84,85] AC joint injury severity is classified by the Rockwood system, with type I and II injuries being conservatively managed and types III to VI needing orthopedic or sports medicine evaluation.[86] **Fig. 5** demonstrates a type III AC injury. The Rockwood classification, its findings, and ED management are described in detail in **Table 4**.[87]

Emergency treatment and management of AC injuries varies based on the Rockwood type. The current recommendation for the management of type I and II AC injuries is to place the patient in a sling, use ice and anti-inflammatories as needed for 1 to 2 weeks, followed by physical therapy and strengthening activities.[88] Although most type III injuries do well when managed conservatively, there is still some controversy on conservative versus surgical management.[88] Type IV to VI injuries should have orthopedics consulted from the ED or close follow-up, because these injuries nearly always require surgical management.[4]

Sternoclavicular dislocations

SC dislocations are rare but are often serious injuries, usually associated with a high-force impact, such as in contact sports or motor vehicle collisions.[1,89,90] Anterior SC dislocations are 9 times more common than posterior dislocations and are usually benign, whereas posterior dislocations can be fatal owing to the proximity to mediastinal structures.[89,91]

The presentation of SC dislocations usually includes chest and shoulder pain, with the shoulder held in adduction with elbow flexion.[1] Patients may also note shortness of breath, paresthesias, or dysphagia. A complete physical examination is essential, with an immediate assessment of airway, breathing, and circulation. The affected shoulder may seem to be shortened, with a prominent medial clavicle in anterior

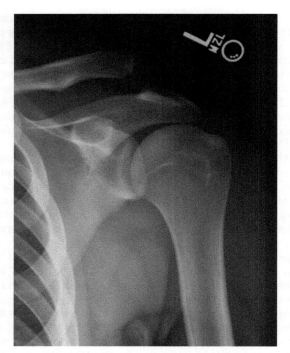

Fig. 5. Type III AC separation. Note widening of the AC joint and increased coracoclavicular distance. (*Courtesy of* Northwestern Emergency Medicine Orthopedics, Northwestern Memorial Hospital, Chicago, IL.)

dislocations.[21,89] Plain radiographs are of limited usefulness and, as such, a CT of the chest with angiography should be performed to assess for both bony abnormalities as well as possible vessel compromise.[21,91]

Anterior SC dislocations are unstable and often continue to be unstable after treatment.[1,21,89] These dislocations can be reduced in the ED. The most common technique involves placing the patient supine with a rolled towel between his or her shoulder blades. The affected shoulder is then abducted and traction is applied while an assistant applies posterior pressure to the medial clavicle.[90,92,93] After reduction, place the patient in a figure-of-8 sling or a clavicle harness for immobilization. Prompt orthopedic follow-up is essential. Patients may be managed by use of one of the slings for up to 6 weeks. Operative repair is considered if conservative management fails.[92]

Unlike anterior dislocations, posterior dislocations are usually managed operatively. Because of the location of vital mediastinal structures, all reduction techniques, whether open or closed, should be performed in consultation with an orthopedic surgeon and a cardiothoracic surgeon.[93] Closed reduction may be attempted with traction to the abducted and extended arm. If unsuccessful, a sterile towel clip may be used to pull the medial clavicle out from behind the sternum.[1] Alternatively, caudal traction can be applied to the adducted arm with posterior pressure on both shoulders.[94] If closed reduction fails or if there is delayed presentation after more than 48 hours or an associated disruption to the medial clavicular physis, open reduction is indicated.[95] Unlike anterior dislocations, posterior dislocations are usually stable

Table 4
Rockwood classification of AC injuries and associated findings

Type	Pathology	Clinical Findings	Radiographic Findings	ED Management	Definitive Management
Type I	AC sprain, CC intact	AC tenderness	Normal	Sling 7–10 d, pain control	Conservative
Type II	AC torn, CC sprain	AC tenderness	AC >3 mm	Sling 2–3 wk, pain control	Conservative
Type III	AC torn, CC torn, D and T torn	AC tenderness, deformity	AC >3 mm, CCD >13 mm, 25%–100% displacement	Sling, pain control	Controversial, nonoperative[a]
Type IV	AC torn, CC torn, D and T torn, posterior displacement of clavicle through trapezius	Prominent acromion	AC >3 mm, CCD >13 mm, Posterior displacement of clavicle on axillary lateral	Sling, pain control, neurovascular assessment	Surgical
Type V	AC torn, CC torn, D and T torn, severe superior displacement of clavicle	Deformity	AC >3 mm, CCD >13 mm, 100%–300% displacement	Sling, pain control, neurovascular assessment	Surgical
Type VI	AC torn, CC intact, inferior displacement of clavicle subcoracoid	Associated trauma	AC >3 mm, CCD decreased	Sling, pain control, neurovascular assessment	Surgical

Abbreviations: CC, coracoclavicular; CCD, coracoclavicular distance; D, deltoid attachment at clavicle; T, trapezius attachment at clavicle.
[a] Management of type III injuries is controversial. Nonoperative management is most common but surgical management may be considered in select populations.

Data from Simovitch R, Sanders B, Ozbaydar M, et al. Acromioclavicular joint injuries: diagnosis and management. J Am Acad Orthop Surg 2009;17(4):207-19; and Williams GR, Nguyen VD, Rockwood CR. Classification and radiographic analysis of acromioclavicular dislocations. Appl Radiol 1989;18:29-34.

after reduction.[93] Patients should be placed in a figure-of-8 strap for 6 to 8 weeks with orthopedic follow-up.[21,92]

Soft Tissue Injuries

Rotator cuff injuries

Rotator cuff injuries are a common cause of shoulder pain. Multiple causes can lead to rotator cuff injuries, including inflammatory and degenerative conditions that lead to impingement syndromes or acute tears of the tendons that make up the rotator cuff.

Rotator cuff injuries are usually able to be diagnosed just from a history and physical examination. Rotator cuff tears are very common, affecting 7% to 30% of older patients and may occur because of an acute traumatic injury or from the progression of impingement.[96–98] Rotator cuff pain is often localized to the lateral deltoid, is usually worse with overhead activity, and may wake patients up at night.[24] Passive ROM is preserved, but active ROM is limited owing to pain. Weakness in the affected extremity is suggestive of a rotator cuff tear, but may be clinically difficult to distinguish from weakness secondary to pain. A diagnostic injection of 10 mL of 1% lidocaine into the subacromial space may be performed to assist in the diagnosis of impingement syndrome. If pain and strength improve, this finding is suggestive of rotator cuff impingement. Meanwhile, if weakness persists, the patient likely has a rotator cuff tear.[13,99]

Impingement syndrome, which incorporates rotator cuff strains, tendonitis, and subacromial bursitis, occurs as a result of mechanical irritation of the rotator cuff tendons on the anteroinferior portion of the acromium.[99]

When a rotator cuff injury is suspected, radiographs should still be obtained to evaluate for other diagnoses. Superior migration of the humeral head toward the acromion (ie, acromiohumeral distance of <7 mm) can be suggestive of a rotator cuff tear, whereas the presence of a hooked type acromion may suggest impingement.[100,101] Rotator cuff injuries can be challenging to diagnose in the ED owing to acute pain and the insensitivity of radiographs. Outpatient follow-up is often indicated to orthopedics or sports medicine for further evaluation and possible physical therapy.

Treatment of rotator cuff pathology in the ED includes ice, analgesia typically with nonsteroidal anti-inflammatory drugs (NSAIDs), a sling for comfort, and a referral to an appropriate specialist. Conservative management and physical therapy often improve impingement and partial thickness rotator cuff tears. Full-thickness tears may require operative management.[99]

Labral tears

The shoulder labrum is commonly injured and presents as shoulder pain in ED patients. The labrum is a fibrocartilaginous structure attached to the glenoid that helps to form the glenohumeral articulation and enhances the stability of the joint.[102] In particular, repetitive overhead athletic activities, such as those performed by baseball pitchers, increase the propensity to develop a superior labrum anterior–posterior lesion. These injuries involve labral detachment posterior to the insertion point of the long head of the biceps tendon.[4] Other mechanisms that can predispose to superior labrum anterior–posterior injuries are falls on an outstretched hand and direct injury to the shoulder joint itself.[4]

Labral injuries present with pain that is often difficult for the patient to localize, often described as deep within the shoulder joint. It may also present with pain that wakes the patient up in the middle of the night. When conducting a thorough physical examination, O'Brien's active compression test can be performed. This test is often positive in the setting of a labral injury.[103]

The initial treatment for labral tears is conservative, with NSAIDs, ice, and early reha-bilitation.[102] Importantly, unlike many other injuries, shoulder immobilization is not rec-ommended for a suspected superior labrum anterior–posterior tear, because the goals of treatment are early mobilization and rehabilitation to restore ROM.[4,102] Outpatient follow-up with orthopedics or sports medicine within 1 to 2 weeks should be provided to these patients at discharge from the ED.

Shoulder impingement syndrome

Shoulder impingement syndrome (SIS) is another potential cause of shoulder pain. The pathophysiology is primarily related to the rotator cuff tendons (most commonly the supraspinatus), and subacromial bursa become compressed in between 3 struc-tures of the shoulder, being the acromion, the humeral head, and the coracoacromial ligament.[76,104] Repetitive movement of the tendons through this impinged area leads to inflammation and eventual fibrosis and predisposes to tendon tears.[76] The anatomic morphology of the shoulder, including that of the acromion, can also predis-pose to developing SIS.[105] Repetitive overhead motions tend to predispose to SIS, because this motion narrows the subacromial space and over time can lead to signif-icant functional deficits.[76,106]

The examination reveals pain over the lateral aspect of the shoulder where the actual impingement occurs. Two examination maneuvers have been shown to improve diagnostic accuracy when evaluating for SIS. Those are the Neer sign and the Hawkins-Kennedy Test. The Neer sign is performed by stabilizing the patient's scapula while forward flexing at the shoulder.[107] The Hawkins-Kennedy test is done by flexing the shoulder to 90° and then rotating it internally.[107] Both of these maneu-vers are considered positive if they reproduce the patient's pain laterally over the impingement area.

Treatment of SIS can initially be conservative with ice, NSAIDs, a sling for comfort, and a referral to orthopedics or sports medicine for physical therapy and further eval-uation. Performing a subacromial injection of steroids with or without local anesthetic may help relieve pain. However, a recent meta-analysis suggests that there is no sig-nificant evidence to support routine steroid injection use for rotator cuff pathology.[108]

Adhesive capsulitis

Adhesive capsulitis, commonly known as frozen shoulder, typically presents with an insidious onset of progressive pain, stiffness, and loss of motion.[109] The exact mech-anism for the development of adhesive capsulitis is not entirely clear, but there is a strong association with heart disease, endocrine disorders (eg, diabetes and hypothy-roidism), and most often occurs in middle-aged women.[110] There is an especially strong correlation between adhesive capsulitis and diabetes. Approximately 20% of diabetic patients suffer from adhesive capsulitis compared with 2% to 5% of the gen-eral population.[111,112] It has been noted that 52% of patients with adhesive capsulitis who do not meet criteria for diabetes do meet the criteria for prediabetes.[112] Another category of patients that develop adhesive capsulitis are patients who have been immobilized in a sling for prolonged periods of time as a treatment for another condi-tion, such as a proximal humerus fracture.

Clinical diagnosis of adhesive capsulitis involves ruling out other possible diagno-ses, such as rotator cuff tears and impingement. Patients will usually have significant limitation to ROM, including less than 100° forward flexion and at least 50% loss in external rotation.[111] Importantly, although patients with rotator cuff injuries tend to have preserved passive ROM, patients with adhesive capsulitis have limited passive ROM.[109]

When managing adhesive capsulitis in the ED, particular attention should be given to pain control with NSAIDs and local steroids, and referral to an orthopedist or sports medicine specialist.[111] Avoid systemic steroids in patients with diabetes. The cornerstone of outpatient management is physical therapy and may also include steroid injections and operative manipulation.[111] Given its association with diabetes, patients should be referred for diabetes screening.[111,112]

Bicipital tendinosis and biceps tendon rupture

Bicipital tendinosis is another diagnosis to consider in patients presenting with shoulder pain. The long head of the biceps tendon sits in the intertubercular groove of the proximal humerus and attaches proximally to the glenoid labrum. Pain associated with bicipital tendinosis tends to be anterior pain, worse with overhead motion, elbow flexion, and forearm supination. Tenderness in the intertubercular groove with the arm at 10° internal rotation and discomfort with the Speed test is suggestive of the diagnosis.[113,114] Isolated bicipital tendinosis is rare, and usually accompanies rotator cuff injuries, most notably the subscapularis tendon.[113,115] This condition is most commonly seen in older individuals aged 40 to 60 years, but may also be seen in young athletes with repetitive overhead activity.

Bicipital tendinosis predisposes to acute biceps tendon rupture, involving an isolated tear of the long head of the biceps tendon in 97% of cases.[116] Patients with biceps tendon rupture will often present to the ED with acute onset of anterior shoulder pain and weakness with elbow flexion. The classic Popeye deformity may be present on examination as the biceps muscle belly retracts distally. In addition, patients may demonstrate weakness in supination, and have pain with the Speed test.[113]

Treatment of bicipital tendinosis in the ED is also conservative, using ice, NSAIDs, and physical therapy.[117] A recent study has suggested benefit from platelet-rich plasma injection for cases with refractory symptoms.[118] Prompt referral to orthopedic surgery is indicated, especially if the patient has an acute biceps rupture. Treatment of acute biceps tendon rupture is usually surgical to preserve function, whereas partial tears may treated conservatively.[119]

SUMMARY

Shoulder injuries account for a large number of ED visits with significant morbidity for the affected patients. This article, although not a comprehensive review, focuses on providing an up-to-date review of the current state of the literature on emergent conditions of the shoulder seen in the ED and their optimal management.

REFERENCES

1. Daya M. Shoulder. In: Marx JA, Hockberger RS, Walls RM, editors. Rosen's emergency medicine. 5th edition. Philadelphia: Mosby; 2002. p. 576–606.
2. Burbank KM, Stevenson JH, Czarnecki GR, et al. Chronic shoulder pain: part I. Evaluation and diagnosis. Am Fam Physician 2008;77(4):453–60.
3. Woodward TW, Best TM. The painful shoulder: part I. Clinical evaluation. Am Fam Physician 2000;61(10):3079–88.
4. Guyer C. Shoulder. In: Waterbrook AL, editor. Sports medicine for the emergency physician. New York: Cambridge University Press; 2016. p. 2–56.
5. Boone DC, Azen SP. Normal range of motion of joints in male subjects. J Bone Joint Surg Am 1979;61(5):756–9.

6. Bay E, Strong C. Mild traumatic brain injury: a Midwest survey of discharge teaching practices of emergency department nurses. Adv Emerg Nurs J 2011;33(2):181–92.

7. de Laat EA, Visser CP, Coene LN, et al. Nerve lesions in primary shoulder dislocations and humeral neck fractures. A prospective clinical and EMG study. J Bone Joint Surg Br 1994;76(3):381–3.

8. Visser CP, Coene LN, Brand R, et al. The incidence of nerve injury in anterior dislocation of the shoulder and its influence on functional recovery. A prospective clinical and EMG study. J Bone Joint Surg Br 1999;81(4):679–85.

9. Hegedus EJ, Goode A, Campbell S, et al. Physical examination tests of the shoulder: a systematic review with meta-analysis of individual tests. Br J Sports Med 2008;42(2):80–92 [discussion: 92].

10. Jobe FW, Moynes DR. Delineation of diagnostic criteria and a rehabilitation program for rotator cuff injuries. Am J Sports Med 1982;10(6):336–9.

11. Park HB, Yokota A, Gill HS, et al. Diagnostic accuracy of clinical tests for the different degrees of subacromial impingement syndrome. J Bone Joint Surg Am 2005;87(7):1446–55.

12. Gerber C, Krushell RJ. Isolated rupture of the tendon of the subscapularis muscle. Clinical features in 16 cases. J Bone Joint Surg Br 1991;73(3):389–94.

13. Neer CS 2nd. Impingement lesions. Clin Orthop Relat Res 1983;(173):70–7.

14. Hawkins RJ, Kennedy JC. Impingement syndrome in athletes. Am J Sports Med 1980;8(3):151–8.

15. Harryman DT 2nd, Sidles JA, Clark JM, et al. Translation of the humeral head on the glenoid with passive glenohumeral motion. J Bone Joint Surg Am 1990; 72(9):1334–43.

16. Mc LH. On the frozen shoulder. Bull Hosp Joint Dis 1951;12(2):383–93.

17. Chronopoulos E, Kim TK, Park HB, et al. Diagnostic value of physical tests for isolated chronic acromioclavicular lesions. Am J Sports Med 2004;32(3): 655–61.

18. Ben Kibler W, Sciascia AD, Hester P, et al. Clinical utility of traditional and new tests in the diagnosis of biceps tendon injuries and superior labrum anterior and posterior lesions in the shoulder. Am J Sports Med 2009;37(9):1840–7.

19. Bennett WF. Specificity of the Speed's test: arthroscopic technique for evaluating the biceps tendon at the level of the bicipital groove. Arthroscopy 1998; 14(8):789–96.

20. Zhao Y, Fesharaki NJ, Liu H, et al. Using data-driven sublanguage pattern mining to induce knowledge models: application in medical image reports knowledge representation. BMC Med Inform Decis Mak 2018;18(1):61.

21. Macdonald PB, Lapointe P. Acromioclavicular and sternoclavicular joint injuries. Orthop Clin North Am 2008;39(4):535–45, viii.

22. Lovell MR, Iverson GL, Collins MW, et al. Measurement of symptoms following sports-related concussion: reliability and normative data for the post-concussion scale. Appl Neuropsychol 2006;13(3):166–74.

23. Khan LA, Bradnock TJ, Scott C, et al. Fractures of the clavicle. J Bone Joint Surg Am 2009;91(2):447–60.

24. Hanby CK, Pasque CB, Sullivan JA. Medial clavicle physis fracture with posterior displacement and vascular compromise: the value of three-dimensional computed tomography and duplex ultrasound. Orthopedics 2003;26(1):81–4.

25. Singh JA, Yu S. Septic arthritis in emergency departments in the US: a national study of health care utilization and time trends. Arthritis Care Res (Hoboken) 2018;70(2):320–6.

26. Jiang JJ, Piponov HI, Mass DP, et al. Septic arthritis of the shoulder: a comparison of treatment methods. J Am Acad Orthop Surg 2017;25(8):e175–84.
27. Ross JJ. Septic arthritis of native joints. Infect Dis Clin North Am 2017;31(2): 203–18.
28. Margaretten ME, Kohlwes J, Moore D, et al. Does this adult patient have septic arthritis? JAMA 2007;297(13):1478–88.
29. Clerc O, Prod'hom G, Greub G, et al. Adult native septic arthritis: a review of 10 years of experience and lessons for empirical antibiotic therapy. J Antimicrob Chemother 2011;66(5):1168–73.
30. Carpenter CR, Schuur JD, Everett WW, et al. Evidence-based diagnostics: adult septic arthritis. Acad Emerg Med 2011;18(8):781–96.
31. McGillicuddy DC, Shah KH, Friedberg RP, et al. How sensitive is the synovial fluid white blood cell count in diagnosing septic arthritis? Am J Emerg Med 2007;25(7):749–52.
32. Abdel MP, Perry KI, Morrey ME, et al. Arthroscopic management of native shoulder septic arthritis. J Shoulder Elbow Surg 2013;22(3):418–21.
33. Blake R, Hoffman J. Emergency department evaluation and treatment of the shoulder and humerus. Emerg Med Clin North Am 1999;17(4):859–76, vi.
34. Hawkins RJ, Neer CS 2nd, Pianta RM, et al. Locked posterior dislocation of the shoulder. J Bone Joint Surg Am 1987;69(1):9–18.
35. Clough TM, Bale RS. Bilateral posterior shoulder dislocation: the importance of the axillary radiographic view. Eur J Emerg Med 2001;8(2):161–3.
36. Hendey GW, Chally MK, Stewart VB. Selective radiography in 100 patients with suspected shoulder dislocation. J Emerg Med 2006;31(1):23–8.
37. Emond M, Le Sage N, Lavoie A, et al. Clinical factors predicting fractures associated with an anterior shoulder dislocation. Acad Emerg Med 2004;11(8): 853–8.
38. Kahn JH, Mehta SD. The role of post-reduction radiographs after shoulder dislocation. J Emerg Med 2007;33(2):169–73.
39. Beattie TF, Steedman DJ, McGowan A, et al. A comparison of the Milch and Kocher techniques for acute anterior dislocation of the shoulder. Injury 1986; 17(5):349–52.
40. Johnson G, Hulse W, McGowan A. The Milch technique for reduction of anterior shoulder dislocations in an accident and emergency department. Arch Emerg Med 1992;9(1):40–3.
41. Milch H. Treatment of dislocation of the shoulder, Surgery 1938;3:732–40.
42. Baykal B, Sener S, Turkan H. Scapular manipulation technique for reduction of traumatic anterior shoulder dislocations: experiences of an academic emergency department. Emerg Med J 2005;22(5):336–8.
43. Marinelli M, de Palma L. The external rotation method for reduction of acute anterior shoulder dislocations. J Orthop Traumatol 2009;10(1):17–20.
44. Eachempati KK, Dua A, Malhotra R, et al. The external rotation method for reduction of acute anterior dislocations and fracture-dislocations of the shoulder. J Bone Joint Surg Am 2004;86-a(11):2431–4.
45. Miller SL, Cleeman E, Auerbach J, et al. Comparison of intra-articular lidocaine and intravenous sedation for reduction of shoulder dislocations: a randomized, prospective study. J Bone Joint Surg Am 2002;84-a(12):2135–9.
46. Stimson L. An easy method of reduction dislocation of the shoulder and hip. Med Rec 1900;57:356.
47. Westin CD, Gill EA, Noyes ME, et al. Anterior shoulder dislocation. A simple and rapid method for reduction. Am J Sports Med 1995;23(3):369–71.

48. Yuen MC, Yap PG, Chan YT, et al. An easy method to reduce anterior shoulder dislocation: the Spaso technique. Emerg Med J 2001;18(5):370–2.
49. Fernandez-Valencia JA, Cune J, Casulleres JM, et al. The Spaso technique: a prospective study of 34 dislocations. Am J Emerg Med 2009;27(4):466–9.
50. Amar E, Maman E, Khashan M, et al. Milch versus Stimson technique for non-sedated reduction of anterior shoulder dislocation: a prospective randomized trial and analysis of factors affecting success. J Shoulder Elbow Surg 2012; 21(11):1443–9.
51. Fitch RW, Kuhn JE. Intraarticular lidocaine versus intravenous procedural sedation with narcotics and benzodiazepines for reduction of the dislocated shoulder: a systematic review. Acad Emerg Med 2008;15(8):703–8.
52. Waterbrook AL, Paul S. Intra-articular lidocaine injection for shoulder reductions: a clinical review. Sports Health 2011;3(6):556–9.
53. McNeil NJ. Postreduction management of first-time traumatic anterior shoulder dislocations. Ann Emerg Med 2009;53(6):811–3.
54. Hovelius L, Olofsson A, Sandstrom B, et al. Nonoperative treatment of primary anterior shoulder dislocation in patients forty years of age and younger. a prospective twenty-five-year follow-up. J Bone Joint Surg Am 2008;90(5):945–52.
55. Itoi E, Sashi R, Minagawa H, et al. Position of immobilization after dislocation of the glenohumeral joint. A study with use of magnetic resonance imaging. J Bone Joint Surg Am 2001;83-a(5):661–7.
56. Scheibel M, Kuke A, Nikulka C, et al. How long should acute anterior dislocations of the shoulder be immobilized in external rotation? Am J Sports Med 2009;37(7):1309–16.
57. Itoi E, Hatakeyama Y, Sato T, et al. Immobilization in external rotation after shoulder dislocation reduces the risk of recurrence. A randomized controlled trial. J Bone Joint Surg Am 2007;89(10):2124–31.
58. Court-Brown CM, Garg A, McQueen MM. The epidemiology of proximal humeral fractures. Acta Orthop Scand 2001;72(4):365–71.
59. Lauritzen JB, Schwarz P, Lund B, et al. Changing incidence and residual lifetime risk of common osteoporosis-related fractures. Osteoporos Int 1993;3(3): 127–32.
60. Nordqvist A, Petersson CJ. Incidence and causes of shoulder girdle injuries in an urban population. J Shoulder Elbow Surg 1995;4(2):107–12.
61. Kelsey JL, Browner WS, Seeley DG, et al. Risk factors for fractures of the distal forearm and proximal humerus. The Study of Osteoporotic Fractures Research Group. Am J Epidemiol 1992;135(5):477–89.
62. Palvanen M, Kannus P, Parkkari J, et al. The injury mechanisms of osteoporotic upper extremity fractures among older adults: a controlled study of 287 consecutive patients and their 108 controls. Osteoporos Int 2000;11(10):822–31.
63. Bahrs C, Rolauffs B, Dietz K, et al. Clinical and radiological evaluation of minimally displaced proximal humeral fractures. Arch Orthop Trauma Surg 2010; 130(5):673–9.
64. Visser CP, Coene LN, Brand R, et al. Nerve lesions in proximal humeral fractures. J Shoulder Elbow Surg 2001;10(5):421–7.
65. Skariah JM, Rasmussen C, Hollander-Rodriguez J, et al. Rural curricular guidelines based on practice scope of recent residency graduates practicing in small communities. Fam Med 2017;49(8):594–9.
66. Handoll HH, Brorson S. Interventions for treating proximal humeral fractures in adults. Cochrane Database Syst Rev 2015;(11):CD000434.

67. Rabi S, Evaniew N, Sprague SA, et al. Operative vs non-operative management of displaced proximal humeral fractures in the elderly: a systematic review and meta-analysis of randomized controlled trials. World J Orthop 2015;6(10): 838–46.
68. Lefevre-Colau MM, Babinet A, Fayad F, et al. Immediate mobilization compared with conventional immobilization for the impacted nonoperatively treated proximal humeral fracture. A randomized controlled trial. J Bone Joint Surg Am 2007;89(12):2582–90.
69. Kristiansen B, Angermann P, Larsen TK. Functional results following fractures of the proximal humerus. A controlled clinical study comparing two periods of immobilization. Arch Orthop Trauma Surg 1989;108(6):339–41.
70. Hodgson S. Proximal humerus fracture rehabilitation. Clin Orthop Relat Res 2006;442:131–8.
71. Postacchini F, Gumina S, De Santis P, et al. Epidemiology of clavicle fractures. J Shoulder Elbow Surg 2002;11(5):452–6.
72. Robinson CM. Fractures of the clavicle in the adult. Epidemiology and classification. J Bone Joint Surg Br 1998;80(3):476–84.
73. Allman FL Jr. Fractures and ligamentous injuries of the clavicle and its articulation. J Bone Joint Surg Am 1967;49(4):774–84.
74. Geraci G, Pisello F, Sciume C, et al. Clavicle fracture complicated by pneumothorax. Case report and literature review. G Chir 2007;28(8–9):330–3 [in Italian].
75. Andersen K, Jensen PO, Lauritzen J. Treatment of clavicular fractures. Figure-of-eight bandage versus a simple sling. Acta Orthop Scand 1987;58(1):71–4.
76. Hussain A, Malik S. Shoulder. In: Sherman S, editor. Simon's emergency orthopedics. 8th edition. New York: McGaw-Hill; 2019. p. 331–84.
77. Jeray KJ. Acute midshaft clavicular fracture. J Am Acad Orthop Surg 2007; 15(4):239–48.
78. Smekal V, Oberladstaetter J, Struve P, et al. Shaft fractures of the clavicle: current concepts. Arch Orthop Trauma Surg 2009;129(6):807–15.
79. Zlowodzki M, Zelle BA, Cole PA, et al. Treatment of acute midshaft clavicle fractures: systematic review of 2144 fractures: on behalf of the Evidence-Based Orthopaedic Trauma Working Group. J Orthop Trauma 2005;19(7):504–7.
80. Robinson CM, Court-Brown CM, McQueen MM, et al. Estimating the risk of nonunion following nonoperative treatment of a clavicular fracture. J Bone Joint Surg Am 2004;86-a(7):1359–65.
81. McKee MD, Pedersen EM, Jones C, et al. Deficits following nonoperative treatment of displaced midshaft clavicular fractures. J Bone Joint Surg Am 2006; 88(1):35–40.
82. Kona J, Bosse MJ, Staeheli JW, et al. Type II distal clavicle fractures: a retrospective review of surgical treatment. J Orthop Trauma 1990;4(2):115–20.
83. Bishop JY, Kaeding C. Treatment of the acute traumatic acromioclavicular separation. Sports Med Arthrosc Rev 2006;14(4):237–45.
84. Simovitch R, Sanders B, Ozbaydar M, et al. Acromioclavicular joint injuries: diagnosis and management. J Am Acad Orthop Surg 2009;17(4):207–19.
85. Rios CG, Mazzocca AD. Acromioclavicular joint problems in athletes and new methods of management. Clin Sports Med 2008;27(4):763–88.
86. Gastaud O, Raynier JL, Duparc F, et al. Reliability of radiographic measurements for acromioclavicular joint separations. Orthop Traumatol Surg Res 2015;101(8 Suppl):S291–5.
87. Willams GR, Nguyen VD, Rockwood CR. Classification and radiographic analysis of acromioclavicular dislocations. Appl Radiol 1989;18:29–34.

88. Felder JJ, Mair SD. Upper extremity: acromioclavicular joint injuries. Curr Orthop Pract 2015;26(2):113–8.

89. Ferrera PC, Wheeling HM. Sternoclavicular joint injuries. Am J Emerg Med 2000; 18(1):58–61.

90. Yeh GL, Williams GR Jr. Conservative management of sternoclavicular injuries. Orthop Clin North Am 2000;31(2):189–203.

91. Ono K, Inagawa H, Kiyota K, et al. Posterior dislocation of the sternoclavicular joint with obstruction of the innominate vein: case report. J Trauma 1998; 44(2):381–3.

92. Bicos J, Nicholson GP. Treatment and results of sternoclavicular joint injuries. Clin Sports Med 2003;22(2):359–70.

93. Robinson CM, Jenkins PJ, Markham PE, et al. Disorders of the sternoclavicular joint. J Bone Joint Surg Br 2008;90(6):685–96.

94. Buckerfield CT, Castle ME. Acute traumatic retrosternal dislocation of the clavicle. J Bone Joint Surg Am 1984;66(3):379–85.

95. Laffosse JM, Espie A, Bonnevialle N, et al. Posterior dislocation of the sternoclavicular joint and epiphyseal disruption of the medial clavicle with posterior displacement in sports participants. J Bone Joint Surg Br 2010;92(1):103–9.

96. SooHoo NF, Rosen P. Diagnosis and treatment of rotator cuff tears in the emergency department. J Emerg Med 1996;14(3):309–17.

97. Moosmayer S, Smith HJ, Tariq R, et al. Prevalence and characteristics of asymptomatic tears of the rotator cuff: an ultrasonographic and clinical study. J Bone Joint Surg Br 2009;91(2):196–200.

98. Yamamoto A, Takagishi K, Osawa T, et al. Prevalence and risk factors of a rotator cuff tear in the general population. J Shoulder Elbow Surg 2010;19(1):116–20.

99. Ahmad C, Yamaguchi K, Wolfe I. The shoulder. In: Scuderi G, McCann P, editors. Sports medicine a comprehensive approach. 2nd edition. Philadelphia: Elsevier Mosby; 2005. p. 227–48.

100. Kotzen LM. Roentgen diagnosis of rotator cuff tear. Report of 48 surgically proven cases. Am J Roentgenol Radium Ther Nucl Med 1971;112(3):507–11.

101. Moosikasuwan JB, Miller TT, Burke BJ. Rotator cuff tears: clinical, radiographic, and US findings. Radiographics 2005;25(6):1591–607.

102. Mlynarek RA, Lee S, Bedi A. Shoulder injuries in the overhead throwing athlete. Hand Clin 2017;33(1):19–34.

103. O'Brien SJ, Pagnani MJ, Fealy S, et al. The active compression test: a new and effective test for diagnosing labral tears and acromioclavicular joint abnormality. Am J Sports Med 1998;26(5):610–3.

104. Dong W, Goost H, Lin XB, et al. Treatments for shoulder impingement syndrome: a PRISMA systematic review and network meta-analysis. Medicine (Baltimore) 2015;94(10):e510.

105. Balke M, Schmidt C, Dedy N, et al. Correlation of acromial morphology with impingement syndrome and rotator cuff tears. Acta Orthop 2013;84(2):178–83.

106. Mayerhoefer ME, Breitenseher MJ, Wurnig C, et al. Shoulder impingement: relationship of clinical symptoms and imaging criteria. Clin J Sport Med 2009; 19(2):83–9.

107. Hughes P. The Neer sign and Hawkins-Kennedy test for shoulder impingement. J Physiother 2011;57(4):260.

108. Koester MC, Dunn WR, Kuhn JE, et al. The efficacy of subacromial corticosteroid injection in the treatment of rotator cuff disease: a systematic review. J Am Acad Orthop Surg 2007;15(1):3–11.

109. Kelley MJ, McClure PW, Leggin BG. Frozen shoulder: evidence and a proposed model guiding rehabilitation. J Orthop Sports Phys Ther 2009;39(2):135–48.
110. Sharma SP, Baerheim A, Moe-Nilssen R, et al. Adhesive capsulitis of the shoulder, treatment with corticosteroid, corticosteroid with distension or treatment-as-usual; a randomised controlled trial in primary care. BMC Musculoskelet Disord 2016;17:232.
111. Brue S, Valentin A, Forssblad M, et al. Idiopathic adhesive capsulitis of the shoulder: a review. Knee Surg Sports Traumatol Arthrosc 2007;15(8):1048–54.
112. Tighe CB, Oakley WS Jr. The prevalence of a diabetic condition and adhesive capsulitis of the shoulder. South Med J 2008;101(6):591–5.
113. Patton WC, McCluskey GM 3rd. Biceps tendinitis and subluxation. Clin Sports Med 2001;20(3):505–29.
114. Churgay CA. Diagnosis and treatment of biceps tendinitis and tendinosis. Am Fam Physician 2009;80(5):470–6.
115. Post M, Benca P. Primary tendinitis of the long head of the biceps. Clin Orthop Relat Res 1989;(246):117–25.
116. Mariani EM, Cofield RH, Askew LJ, et al. Rupture of the tendon of the long head of the biceps brachii. Surgical versus nonsurgical treatment. Clin Orthop Relat Res 1988;228:233–9.
117. Nho SJ, Strauss EJ, Lenart BA, et al. Long head of the biceps tendinopathy: diagnosis and management. J Am Acad Orthop Surg 2010;18(11):645–56.
118. Sanli I, Morgan B, van Tilborg F, et al. Single injection of platelet-rich plasma (PRP) for the treatment of refractory distal biceps tendonitis: long-term results of a prospective multicenter cohort study. Knee Surg Sports Traumatol Arthrosc 2016;24(7):2308–12.
119. Glass C. Upper arm. In: Sherman S, editor. Simon's emergency orthopedics. 8th edition. New York: McGraw-Hill; 2019. p. 323–30.

Traumatic Injuries of the Pelvis

Jason V. Brown, MD, MC, USAF[a],*, Sharleen Yuan, MD, PhD[b]

KEYWORDS

- Pelvic fracture • Hip fracture • REBOA • Intertrochanteric fracture • Hip dislocation

KEY POINTS

- Fascia iliaca block is a safe and effective pain control modality for patients with a hip fracture.
- High-energy trauma resulting in fractures of the pelvis are associated with multiple other traumatic injuries.
- Exsanguination is the common cause of death in the first 6 hours following a severe pelvis fracture.
- Gross hematuria is highly associated with severe pelvic fractures.
- Hip fractures can occur in the elderly with minimal trauma and result in significant morbidity and mortality.

Traumatic injuries to the pelvis and hip are common in the emergency department (ED). The ability to diagnose and manage these often-complex injuries is essential for all emergency medicine practitioners (EMPs).

Fractures of the pelvis occur in a bimodal distribution with young patients experiencing catastrophic injuries from high-energy mechanisms, whereas elderly patients tend to sustain injuries from low-energy mechanisms such as a fall from standing. Hip fractures, conversely, occur almost exclusively in patients more than 65 years of age and often from low-energy mechanisms.

This article will educate readers on the anatomy and physiology, epidemiology, diagnosis, disposition, and associated considerations related to these injuries.

INTRODUCTION

Pelvic fractures are broadly categorized as either stable or unstable. Stable pelvic fractures can often be subtle and should be suspected in the elderly presenting

Disclosure: Drs J.V. Brown and S. Yuan have no commercial interests to disclose.
[a] Emergency Medical Services, United States Air Force, 96TW/SGOE, 307 Boatner Road, Eglin AFB, FL 32542, USA; [b] Department of Emergency Medicine, University of Maryland Medical Center, 110 South Paca Street, 6th Floor, Suite 200, Baltimore, MD 21201, USA
* Corresponding author.
E-mail address: jason.v.brown8.mil@mail.mil

with a fall from standing or other minor trauma. Morbidity and mortality can be higher for this population because of comorbidities rather than the degree of trauma.[1] Unstable fractures of the bony pelvis are often a result of high-energy mechanisms and carry a high rate of morbidity and mortality. Worldwide, the overall mortality is between 6% and 35%.[2–5] Recent evidence has shown decreasing mortalities because of advances in prehospital recognition and hospital management, including advances in resuscitation, interventional radiology, and surgical techniques.[6] Pelvic ring disruptions and fractures are often associated with polytrauma and should be considered in any patient presenting with multiple traumatic injuries. Unstable ring fractures often occur concurrently with chest trauma (21.2%), head injuries (16.9%), liver and spleen injuries (8%), and multiple long-bone fractures (7.8%).[4] These concomitant injuries often lead to delayed death (>6 hours), whereas immediate death (<6 hours) is most commonly associated with uncontrolled abdominal or pelvic hemorrhage.[3] The primary predictors for immediate mortality are hemodynamic instability and findings on computed tomography (CT) suggestive of arterial bleeding.[7]

ANATOMY

A basic review of the anatomy of the pelvis can be found in reference textbooks; therefore, this article focuses on important anatomic considerations that can lead to missed injuries.

The pelvis is a semirigid structure despite having 5 internal joints. Because of the inflexibility of the ring structure, if a single fracture is identified, further investigation is needed to ensure that a second fracture is not present.

Typically, disruption of the pelvic ring is difficult because of a robust ligamentous architecture that provides mechanical stability and limited flexibility within the pelvis (**Fig. 1**). Disruption of these ligamentous structures requires enormous forces and often results in injuries to the underlying structures of both the abdomen and pelvis.

The vascular architecture of the pelvis is robust and, as such, hemorrhage within the pelvis can lead to exsanguination and death. Important points to remember are that the superior gluteal artery continues posteriorly toward the hip joint and is in close proximity to the posterior arch, whereas the obturator and internal pudendal branches course anteriorly toward the ramus. Fractures in these areas can lead to vascular injuries that can be missed on the initial examination.

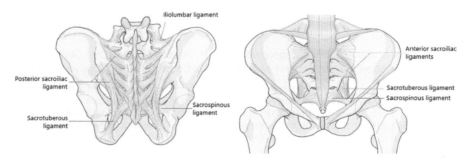

Fig. 1. Ligamentous architecture of the pelvis. (*From* Tile M, Kellam JF. Anatomy of the pelvic ring. In: Tile M, Helfet DL, Kellam JF, Vrahas M, eds. Fractures of the pelvis and Acetabulum: principles and methods of management. 4th ed. Davos Platz, Switzerland: AO Foundation; 2015; with permission. Copyright by AO Foundation, Switzerland.)

The venous vasculature largely mirrors the arterial supply, but there is a large, retroperitoneal venous plexus that collects along the pelvic wall and is susceptible to shearing forces, making it a common source of retroperitoneal and pelvic hemorrhage. Bleeding from this region can often be limited by restoring the pelvis to its native shape.

Pathophysiology

Pelvic fractures are described either mechanistically or in terms of posterior arch stability (**Fig. 2**). The Young-Burgess (YB) system is based on mechanism and has 4 subtypes:

- Anterior-posterior compression (APC)
- Lateral compression (LC)
- Vertical sheer (VS)
- Combined mechanical injury (CMI)[8]

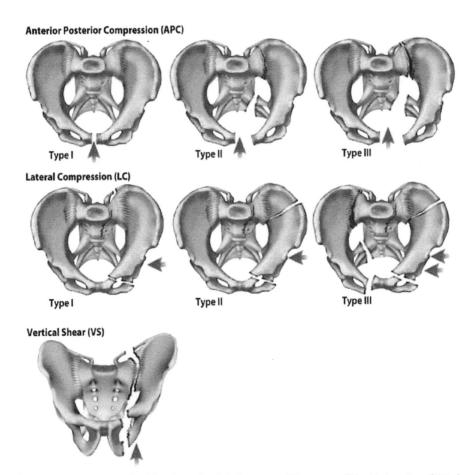

Fig. 2. Young-Burgess classification of pelvic fractures. (*Courtesy of* The University of Washington, Seatte, WA.)

The Tile classification (A–C) refers to posterior arch stability and has 3 subtypes :

A. Stable
B. Rotationally unstable, vertically stable
C. Both rotationally and vertically unstable[9]

Independent of the system used, identification of these patterns and delineation of stable from unstable fractures is important because this informs the management of the patient.[10]

The YB system is more commonly used in practice because it is more descriptive of the forces involved in creating the injury patterns. Within the YB classification, LC fractures represent roughly two-thirds of fractures[11] and generally result from a motor vehicle crash wherein the vehicle is broadsided, or T-boned. This injury creates a compression of the pelvis, resulting in fracture of the pubic symphysis at a minimum and varying instability of the posterior arch (**Fig. 3**).

APC fractures are the second most common fracture, accounting for one-fourth of unstable pelvic fractures. This injury results from an anterior-to-posterior force, such as a head-on motor vehicle crash or a motorcycle crash. This force vector causes the pelvis to open, resulting in widening of the pubic symphysis and varying damage to the posterior arch (**Fig. 4**).

VS fractures occur rarely, but should be suspected in falls from height. The force vector here disrupts the pubic rami and sacroiliac joint inferiorly to superiorly (**Fig. 5**).

In addition to the aforementioned unstable, high-energy pelvic fractures, there are a variety of single-bone and avulsion fractures that occur in the pelvis (**Figs. 6** and **7**). Although most of these are treated nonsurgically with routine orthopedic follow-up, special consideration should be given to fractures of the iliac wing and the sacrum. These fractures typically involve a significant amount of energy and should prompt further investigation for concomitant injuries. Isolated pelvic fractures occurring in the elderly, even from benign mechanisms such as a fall from ground level, can result in significant morbidity and mortality.[12]

Acetabular fractures

The acetabulum is a deep, socket-shaped structure that is formed superiorly by the ilium, inferiorly by the ischium, and medially by the pubis. Injuries occur in a bimodal distribution, with young patients sustaining high-energy mechanisms, such as a fall

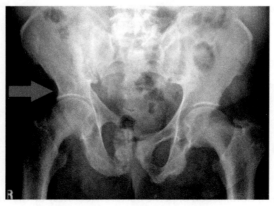

Fig. 3. A lateral compression fracture pattern (*arrow*).

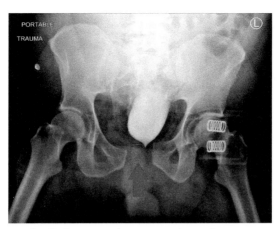

Fig. 4. An anteroposterior (AP) compression pattern (*arrow*).

from a great height or a high-speed motor vehicle crash; conversely, elderly patients can have acetabular fractures caused by osteopenia/osteoporosis from ground-level falls.[1] These injuries often exist concurrently with ipsilateral injuries of the knee (15%–25%), hip (7%), and pelvis (5%) and should prompt further work-up.[13] Most acetabular fractures involve posterior displacement of the femoral head and can result in sciatic or peroneal nerve injuries.[14]

Emergency Department Management

Seriously injured patients with a suspected pelvic fracture should be treated in accordance with Advanced Trauma Life Support (ATLS) guidelines. Initial management includes the establishment of 2 large-bore supradiaphragmatic points of intravenous access, rapid blood resuscitation, and an orderly procession through the primary and secondary surveys.

Focused assessment with sonography in trauma (FAST), an adjunct of the primary survey, is a useful tool for the immediate disposition of hemodynamically unstable

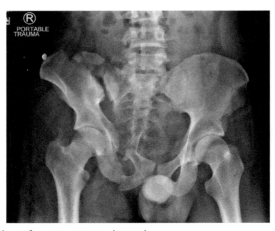

Fig. 5. A vertical shear fracture pattern (*arrow*).

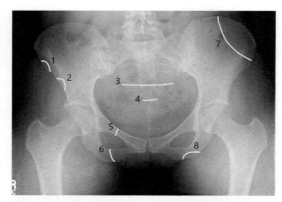

Fig. 6. Stable pelvic fractures. (1) Avulsion of anterosuperior iliac spine, (2) avulsion of anteroinferior iliac spine, (3) transverse fracture of the sacrum, (4) fracture of the coccyx, (5) fracture of superior pubic ramus, (6) fracture of inferior pubic ramus, (7) fracture of iliac wing, (8) avulsion of the ischial tuberosity. (*Courtesy of* Dr. Frank Gaillard, rID 8248, Radiopaedia. org.)

patients with trauma. Unstable patients with a positive FAST examination generally require emergent exploratory laparotomy.[15] Stable patients with a positive FAST and patients with a negative FAST likely require CT imaging to further delineate their injuries.

Examination of the pelvis, as part of the secondary survey, should include a single provider assessing the stability of the pelvis with gentle medial compression and distraction of the pelvis at the level of the anterior superior iliac spine. If movement is felt, then a pelvic binder or other pelvic stabilizing device (eg, a bed sheet) should be positioned over the greater trochanters of the femur and secured in place. This technique reduces the pelvic volume and stabilizes periosteal clots to reduce hemorrhage. Repeated manipulation of the pelvis should be avoided.

Digital rectal examination (DRE) and bimanual pelvic examination are a necessary part of the evaluation of patients with a pelvic fracture. The presence of blood or the palpation of bony fragments on DRE or bimanual examination should prompt antibiotic administration and direct visualization, including proctoscopy or speculum examination.

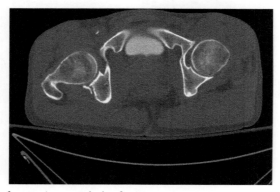

Fig. 7. CT image of posterior acetabular fracture.

Diagnostics

The use of pelvic radiographs in patients with blunt abdominal trauma has been the standard of care as an adjunct to the primary survey. However, routine use of pelvic radiographs in awake, hemodynamically stable patients may not be needed because physical examination alone is often sufficient to exclude significant pelvic fractures.[16,17] In stable patients with a suspected pelvic fractures who will undergo CT as part of their work-up, pelvic radiographs are redundant.[18] Otherwise, a standard anteroposterior (AP) pelvic radiograph can help to quickly identify severe injuries and guide therapy.

CT has long been superior to plain radiographs for the identification of pelvic fractures.[19] Plain films of the pelvis have a less than 85% sensitivity for the detection of fractures compared with CT in patients with blunt trauma.[20] In addition, CT identifies the instability of the pelvic ring more easily than plain films.[19] Therefore, patients with suspected pelvic fracture but negative plain films should undergo CT with contrast. In patients with ongoing, undifferentiated hemorrhage, the addition of CT angiography has a 100% sensitivity in ruling out a pelvic source.[21]

Interventions

Roughly 85% of hemorrhage associated with pelvic fractures is venous and can be controlled with maneuvers that reduce the pelvic volume and stabilize the pelvis.[22] These maneuvers include pelvic binding and operative external pelvic fixation. The remaining 15% is associated with an arterial source that requires either extraperitoneal pelvic packing or endovascular embolization.

Pelvic packing is a useful temporizing measure for patients requiring laparotomy for other reasons (eg, bowel perforation) or patients who are hemodynamically unstable. Transcatheter arterial embolization (TAE) has been shown to have an 81% to 100% efficacy for controlling arterial pelvic hemorrhage and is the modality of choice when available.[23] However, these patients often present with multiple injuries and the sequence of treatment modalities is often difficult to determine. When available, TAE should be accomplished as soon as possible to reduce mortality.[24] If any delay is anticipated, then extraperitoneal packing has been shown to reduce mortality while awaiting TAE.[25] Pelvic packing and TAE are not thought of as competing treatment modalities but as complementary, depending on the specific patient needs. In addition, individual facilities often have different preferences on modalities with which EMPs should be familiar.

Resuscitative endovascular balloon occlusion of the aorta (REBOA) is an emerging treatment being used to provide proximal hemorrhage control in patients with isolated subdiaphragmatic injuries instead of thoracotomy. This treatment was first described by Colonel Carl W. Hughes[26] during the Korean war and has recently reemerged in the trauma literature.[27] Numerous retrospective studies have shown mixed results,[27–30] whereas a single prospective clinical study[31] showed no difference in survival compared with open aortic occlusion via emergent resuscitative thoracotomy. REBOA is typically used to occlude the aorta in zone III, below the renal arteries and above the aortic bifurcation. This technique acts as a temporizing measure only, and the true utility of its use in the ED is still a topic of discussion. Protocols should be in place to facilitate definitive surgical repair before REBOA use in an ED.

Associated injuries

Pelvic fractures are considered compound, or open, when there is communication between the pelvis and the rectum, vagina, or skin. These open fractures have high mortalities and are often associated with urogenital and intra-abdominal injuries.[32] Careful inspection of the perineum, rectum, and vaginal vault within the trauma bay is essential to avoid a missed diagnosis. Associated rectal injuries carry an especially high mortality[33] and often require early diverting colostomy, external pelvic fixation, and serial operative washouts.[34]

Urogenital trauma is common among patients with pelvic fracture. The urethra and bladder are commonly injured, whereas ureteral and gynecologic injuries are rare among bluntly injured patients. Urethral injuries should be suspected in patients with a high-riding prostate (recently removed from ATLS 10th edition[35]), inability to urinate, perineal/genital ecchymosis, blood in the vaginal vault, or blood at the urethral meatus and should prompt retrograde urethrography for further work-up.[36] Prompt bladder drainage should be accomplished in patients with a urethral injury. Although attempts to place a Foley catheter blindly in patients with suspected urethral injury are contraindicated, current guidelines support a single, well-lubricated attempt at placement by an experienced provider.[37,38] If this is unsuccessful, then placement of a suprapubic catheter should be done.

Bladder injuries occur in 29% of patients with pelvic fracture and gross hematuria.[36] These patients require emergent CT cystography for evaluation. Intraperitoneal ruptures are caused by so-called blow-out injuries to the dome of the bladder and are unlikely to heal spontaneously by bladder drainage; therefore, they require emergent repair when appropriate. Extraperitoneal ruptures are either uncomplicated or complicated. Complicated extraperitoneal ruptures (eg, bone fragments within the bladder wall or concurrent vaginal/rectal injuries) require surgical fixation. Uncomplicated extraperitoneal ruptures are managed with bladder decompression.

Hip dislocation
Hip dislocation is a rare injury that requires emergent treatment to prevent long-term complications. Posterior dislocation (**Figs. 8** and **9**) results from an anterior-to-posterior force directed through the knee while the hip is flexed at 90°, most often when the knee impacts the dashboard during a high-speed motor vehicle crash. Patients most commonly present with a shortened internally rotated leg with slight adduction and knee flexion. Anterior dislocations occur when a posterior force is applied to an abducted and externally rotated leg. Traditionally, this was associated with a heavy weight falling on a prone person with legs splayed apart; however, high-speed motor vehicle crashes are now the most common mechanism.[39]

Initial work-up involves plain radiographs, but CT is essential in all cases of hip dislocation to better examine the acetabulum and femoral head/neck.[40] Closed reduction should be performed within 6 hours of injury in order to reduce the chance of adverse outcomes.[41]

There are many techniques described in the literature for posterior hip reductions.[42] Because many techniques require either multiple providers or place the provider at risk from climbing on the bed, this article focuses on the Captain Morgan and Whistler techniques. The Captain Morgan reduction is performed with the patient supine and the patient's pelvis fixed to the bed. The affected hip and knee are then flexed to 90° and the operator places a knee behind the patient's knee. The operator then simultaneously applies upward traction to the hip by lifting their leg and pushing downward on the patient's ankle to produce a fulcrum effect.[43] The Whistler technique involves 2 providers. The first provider flexes the unaffected leg to 90° with the foot on the bed. The second provider then flexes the affected hip to 90° and places a forearm under the patient's knee and a hand on the contralateral knee. The second operator's forearm acts as a fulcrum and allows upward traction with concurrent downward force placed on the ankle of the affected leg.[44]

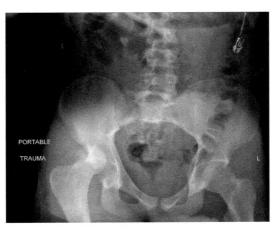

Fig. 8. AP radiograph of a posterior hip dislocation.

Anterior dislocations are typically reduced with a combination of hip extension, external rotation, in-line traction, and abduction, which can be accomplished with 2 providers using a lateral traction technique. One provider places a sheet under and around the patient's affected thigh and applies lateral traction and external rotation while the second provider provides in-line traction.

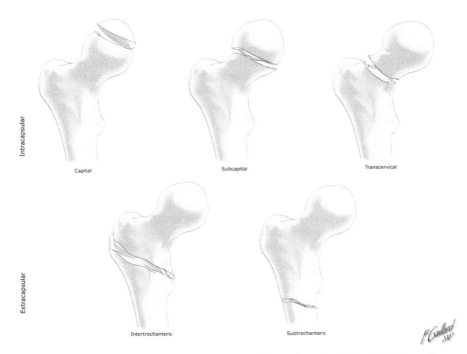

Fig. 9. Proximal femur fractures. (Case courtesy of A.Prof Frank Gaillard, Radiopaedia.org, rID: 35815.)

The most common early complications of hip dislocations are sciatic nerve and vascular injury. Approximately 10% to 20% of posterior dislocations result in damage to the sciatic nerve either from stretching of the nerve as the femoral head displaces it posteriorly or from fracture fragments causing direct damage to the nerve.[39] Damage to the superior gluteal artery is rare but, if suspected, should prompt vascular imaging because it may lead to avascular necrosis.

TRAUMATIC INJURIES OF THE HIP
Introduction

In the United States, proximal femur fractures, commonly referred to as hip fractures, are common, with more than 300,000 patients hospitalized yearly.[43] Morbidity associated with hip fractures is substantial and approximately 50% of individuals who lived independently before the hip fracture are unable to maintain their independent lifestyles.[44] This loss of independence can be debilitating for elderly individuals without social support.

Hip fractures are strongly associated with loss of bone density and commonly occur as a result of low-energy trauma.[45] Most causes of these fractures are secondary to a fall from standing height, usually reflecting an individual's decreased reflexes, increased bone loss, and reduced bone strength.[44]

The average age of patients with hip fractures is more than 70 years old, and nearly 80% are women.[2] Mortality with a hip fracture is approximately 5% to 10% after 1 month, with 33% of patients passing after 1 year, compared with a baseline of 10%. Only 33% of those who perish do so as a direct result of the fracture; the remainder die of their comorbidities.

Pathophysiology

The proximal femur is divided into 4 zones: the femoral head, the femoral neck, the intertrochanteric region, and the subtrochanteric region (**Fig. 10**). Fractures of the femoral head and neck are intracapsular, whereas intertrochanteric and subtrochanteric fractures are extracapsular. This distinction is important when considering associated injuries. Most hip fractures occur in the femoral neck and the intertrochanteric region; in total, these 2 regions account for roughly 90% of fractures.[45]

Femoral head fractures are rare and are typically associated with hip dislocations. These fractures are usually discovered on plain radiographs following closed reduction of a posteriorly dislocated hip. Femoral neck fractures occur between the distal femoral head articular cartilage and the intertrochanteric line (subcapital region). Intertrochanteric fractures include any fracture below the intertrochanteric line, but above the inferior border of the lesser trochanter.[46] Subtrochanteric fractures are any below and within 5 cm of the lesser trochanter.

The intracapsular portion of the hip is supplied by the artery of the ligamentum teres, terminal branches of the lateral femoral circumflex artery, and terminal branches of the medial femoral circumflex artery (MFCA). The lateral epiphyseal artery (a terminal branch of the MFCA) supplies most of the femoral head and is susceptible to shearing forces.[47] Displaced intracapsular fractures and posterior hip dislocations can result in damage to this tenuous blood supply and lead to avascular necrosis, heterotopic ossification, and arthrosis.[48] The incidence of these complications increases proportionally to the length of time that the joint/fracture is nonreduced, so prompt reduction is essential in minimizing these long-term complications.[49]

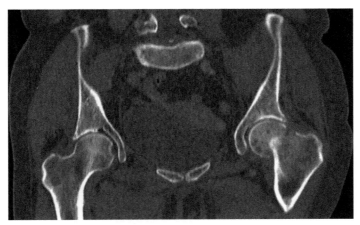

Fig. 10. CT image of a subcapital femur fracture.

The major neurologic structure at risk is the sciatic nerve as it courses posterior to the femoral head and neck. Posterior displacement of the femoral head or neck can cause compression and necrosis of the sciatic nerve, resulting in neurologic deficits in the lower leg, most commonly foot drop.

Presentation

In most cases, the patient presents with hip pain following a fall; however, the provider must obtain a thorough history because many cases of hip and groin pain have other underlying causes (eg, stones, labral tears, pelvic inflammatory disease, malignancies). In addition, pain can be described as knee, groin, or pelvic in location. Patients are often elderly and may have been immobile for a prolonged period of time. Take care to assess for associated injuries, metabolic abnormalities, and any concomitant disease processes.

The positioning of the patient's afflicted leg can be telling. External rotation, abduction, and shortening is most likely a femoral neck fracture, whereas external rotation and shortening indicates an intertrochanteric fracture.[44,50] Initial examination of the hip should consist of rolling the leg on the bed to assess pain with external and internal rotation. If this produces pain, further manipulation should be avoided. A full neurologic examination is warranted for proximal femur fractures to assess for loss of sensation. In addition, lower extremity perfusion should be evaluated by evaluating pulses, and clinicians should consider obtaining an ankle-brachial index.

Imaging

Plain radiographs are the initial imaging modality of choice for assessment using the AP pelvic view and cross-table lateral views, with the femur internally rotated as tolerated. The cross-table lateral view is important if the fracture is suspected to be in the subtrochanteric region. However, initial radiographs may be insensitive, particularly if the patient is more than 50 years old or has a history of bone density loss. MRI is favored in these situations. One 10-year retrospective study noted that 69 out of 98 patients had negative radiographs, whereas MRI was able to accurately identify their proximal femur fractures.[51] However, MRI may not be feasible in the ED. A CT without contrast of the pelvis and hips can be supplemented with radiographs for characterization and identification of nondisplaced proximal femur fractures.[43]

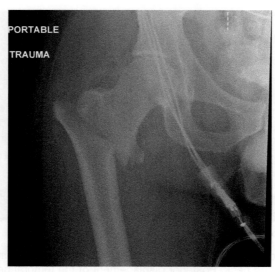

Fig. 11. Radiograph of an intertrochanteric femur fracture.

Femoral Neck Fractures

Femoral neck fractures (**Fig. 11**) are classified as either displaced or nondisplaced. They are further classified based on their location: basicervical (capital), subcapital (most common), and transcervical fractures (see **Fig. 10**). The Garden classification is the most widely used system for femoral neck fractures, especially in the elderly. It uses 4 categories of subcapital fractures based on AP radiographs, with stages I and II indicating nondisplaced fractures, whereas stages III and IV are partially or fully displaced (**Table 1**).[52,53]

Nondisplaced fractures include fractures that are truly nondisplaced and fractures that are impacted into a valgus position. Although these fractures have a lower rate of avascular necrosis and nonunion, they are still associated with significant functional impact.[54,55]

Intertrochanteric Fractures

Classifications for these fractures is not reliable, but the most commonly used is the Evans-Jensen classification system (**Table 2**). This system divides the fractures into 3 groups based on the number of bone fragments:

- Class I: nondisplaced or stable displaced 2-fragment fractures

Table 1	
Garden classification of subcapital femoral neck fractures	
Stages	**Description**
I	Incomplete and nondisplaced
II	Complete and nondisplaced
III	Complete and partially displaced
IV	Complete and fully displaced

From Garden RS. Low-angle fixation in fractures of the femoral neck. J Bone Joint Surg Br. 1961;43:647–663; with permission.

- Class II: unstable 3-fragment fractures with posterolateral (greater trochanteric) or posteromedial (less trochanteric) involvement
- Class III: unstable 4-fragment fractures[43]

Intertrochanteric fractures can be associated with other traumatic injuries, including upper extremity fractures. Therefore, a thorough assessment of all limbs, spine, and contralateral hip is required.

Subtrochanteric Fractures

Subtrochanteric fractures account for 11% of all femur fractures, with 30% to 50% of these patients presenting with ipsilateral fractures in the pelvis, other long bones, and spine (**Fig. 12**).[50] Subtrochanteric fractures are mainly seen in 2 patient populations: spiral fractures in osteoporotic patients and atypical insufficiency fractures that happen after no to low-energy trauma (eg, patients who use long-term bisphosphate therapy).[43,56] The Seinsheimer classification (**Table 3**) for subtrochanteric fractures is the most commonly used and studied.[57]

Emergency Department Management

Because hip fractures most commonly occur in elderly patients with multiple comorbidities, a thorough investigation of the precipitating event (eg, syncope, stroke) as well as potential coexisting disease processes (eg, diabetic ketoacidosis, cerebrovascular event) is essential.

Pain control is important for patient comfort. Opioids may be first-line therapy, and femoral nerve blocks may be an excellent adjunct modality to maintain patient comfort. These blocks allow quick onset of pain relief and decreased use of opioid medications. The relief can last for hours, especially if a long-acting analgesic such as bupivacaine is used.

In the ED, a fascia iliaca block can be performed as a simple and effective treatment of hip pain. After identifying the inguinal ligament and femoral artery, a 21-gauge needle can be inserted in a perpendicular fashion to the skin. Per Monzon, "the insertion should be 1 cm below the lateral and medial two-thirds of a line that joins the pubic tubercle to the anterior superior iliac spine."[58] Continue to insert the needle until a lack of resistance is felt as the fascia lata is passed. It is important to advance the needle until a second resistance loss is felt as the fascia iliaca is penetrated (2 pops may be felt). After aspiration of the syringe to ensure no blood return, injection of 0.3 mL/kg of 0.25% bupivacaine can provide excellent pain relief for the patient. This type of relief can be an effective and very safe alternative to opioid analgesics and femoral nerve blocks.[59] Fascia iliaca blocks have rapid onset and provide prolonged relief with

Table 2		
Evans-Jensen classification for intertrochanteric fractures		
Class	**Description**	
I	Nondisplaced or displaced 2-fragment stable fractures	
II	Unstable 3-fragment fractures with greater trochanteric or lesser trochanteric involvement	
III	Very unstable 4-fragment fractures	

Data from Evans EM. The treatment of trochanteric fractures of the femur. J Bone Joint Surg Br 1949; 31B: 190-203 and Jensen JS, Michaelsen M. Trochanteric femoral fractures treated with McLaughlin osteosynthesis. Acta Orthop Scand. 1975;46(5):795–803.

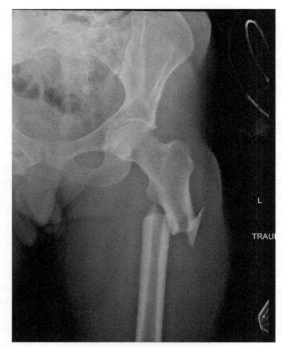

Fig. 12. Radiograph of a subtrochanteric femur fracture.

analgesic onset at roughly 15 minutes and relief for up to 8 hours, especially with concurrent use of nonsteroidal antiinflammatory drugs.[60]

Disposition

Femoral head fractures require open reduction and internal fixation (ORIF) for all fractures with residual displacement of 1 mm or more. Because these fractures are rare in isolation, they are often repaired in conjunction with their associated injuries.

Table 3 Seinsheimer classification of subtrochanteric fractures	
Grade	**Description**
I	Any fracture with <2-mm displacement
II	Two-part fractures Grade IIa: 2-part transverse fractures Grade IIb: 2-part spiral fracture, lesser trochanteric in proximal fragment Grade IIc: 2-part spiral fracture, lesser trochanteric in distal fragment
III	Three-part fractures Grade IIIa: 3-part spiral fractures in which the third fragment is the lesser trochanter Grade IIIb: 3-part fracture in which the third fragment is a butterfly fragment
IV	Composed of 4 or more parts
V	Any fracture that extends into the greater trochanter

Data from Seinsheimer F. J Subtrochanteric fractures of the femur Bone Joint Surg Am. 1978 Apr;60(3):300-6.

For femoral neck fractures, surgery depends on the fracture type and ambulatory nature of the patient. In nondisplaced femoral neck fractures, ORIF is the best modality for treatment, especially to prevent displacement because more than 46% can be displaced if not treated surgically.[52] Displaced femoral neck fractures should undergo arthroplasty because of the high failure rate of internal fixation. Total hip replacement is also an option for very active patients.

Intertrochanteric fractures are treated with ORIF through nail fixation or implants, with the sliding hip screw system being most commonly used. Arthroplasty for these fractures can be used if internal fixation has failed.[61]

Subtrochanteric fractures are typically unstable; therefore, treatment is usually intramedullary nail fixation. In such surgeries, complications include malreductions, neurovascular injury, impingement, and nail penetration into the femoral cortex.

Postoperative complications occur in 20% of patients older than 60 years. Avascular necrosis is the most often seen complication, accounting for up to 39% of cases, particularly with intracapsular fractures treated with ORIF. Other complications include hardware-related complications, malunion, discrepant leg length, hip osteoarthritis, and infection.[43,44,62–64]

SUMMARY

Traumatic injuries to the hip and pelvis are associated with significant morbidity and mortality. These injuries occur most often in either the young or old. Young patients tend to have high-energy mechanisms and often present with polytrauma. Expert trauma management by the EMP is essential to reduce both immediate and late complications. In contrast, the elderly are often injured from ground-level falls and have higher morbidity and mortality because of their comorbidities. Expert evaluation, diagnosis, and disposition of these patients is an essential skill for all EMPs.

REFERENCES

1. Rinne PP, Laitinen MK, Huttunen T, et al. The incidence and trauma mechanisms of acetabular fractures: a nationwide study in Finland between 1997 and 2014. Injury 2019;48(10):2157–61.

2. Vaidya R, Scott A, Tonnos F. Patients with pelvic fractures from blunt trauma . What is the cause of mortality and when? Am J Surg 2016;211(3):495–500.

3. Yoshihara H, Yoneoka D. Demographic epidemiology of unstable pelvic fracture Demographic epidemiology of unstable pelvic fracture in the United States from 2000 to 2009: trends and in-hospital mortality. J Trauma Acute Care Surg 2014; 76(2):8–13.

4. Giannoudis PV, Ortho EEC, Grotz MRW, et al. Prevalence of pelvic fractures , associated injuries , and mortality: the United Kingdom perspective. J Trauma 2001;63(4):875–83.

5. Hauschild O, Strohm PC, Culemann U, et al. Mortality in patients with pelvic fractures: results from the German pelvic injury register. J Trauma 2008;64(2):449–55.

6. Black SR, Sathy AK, Jo C, et al. Improved survival after pelvic fracture: 13-year experience at a single trauma center using a multidisciplinary Institutional Protocol. J Orthop Trauma 2016;30(1):22–8.

7. Tanizaki S, Maeda S, Matano H, et al. Time to pelvic embolization for hemodynamically unstable pelvic fractures may affect the survival for delays up to 60 min. Injury 2018;45(4):738–41.

8. Dalar S, Burgess A, Siegel J, et al. Pelvic fracture in multiple trauma: classification by mechanism is key to pattern of organ injury, resuscitative requirements, and outcome. J Trauma 1989;28(7):1084.

9. Tile M. Acute pelvic fractures: I . causation and classification. J Am Acad Orthop Surg 1996;4(3):143–51.

10. Eastridge B, Starr A, Minei JO, et al. The importance of fracture pattern in guiding therapeutic decision-making in patients with hemorrhagic shock and pelvic ring disruptions. J Trauma 2002;53(3):446–51.

11. Manson T, Robert V, Toole O, et al. Young-burgess classification of pelvic ring fractures: does it predict mortality, transfusion requirements, and non-orthopaedic injuries? J Orthop Trauma 2010;24(10):603–9.

12. Dodge G, Brison R. Low-impact pelvic fractures in the emergency department. CJEM 2010;12(6):509–13.

13. Kempegowda H, Maniar HH, Tawari AA, et al. Knee injury associated with acetabular fractures: a multicenter study of 1273 patients. J Orthop Trauma 2016;30(1):2013–6.

14. Fassler P, Swiontkowski M, Kilroy A, et al. Injury of the sciatic nerve associated with acetabular fracture. J Bone Joint Surg Am 1993;75(8):1157–66.

15. Ruchholtz S, Waydhas C, Lewan U, et al. Free abdominal fluid on ultrasound in unstable pelvic ring fracture: is laparotomy always necessary? J Trauma 2004; 57:278–87.

16. Gonzalez RP, Fried PQ, Bukhalo M. The utility of clinical examination in screening for pelvic fractures in blunt trauma. J Am Coll Surg 2002;7515(01):121–5.

17. Duane TM, Tan BB, Golay D, et al. Blunt trauma and the role of routine pelvic radiographs: a prospective analysis. J Trauma 2002;53(3):463–8.

18. Soto JR, Zhou C, Hu D, et al. Skip and save: utility of pelvic x-rays in the initial evaluation of blunt trauma patients. Am J Surg 2015;210(6):1076–81.

19. Berg E, Chebuhar C, Bell R. Pelvic trauma imaging: a blinded comparison of computed tomography and roentgenograms. J Trauma 1996;41(6):994–8.

20. Clement N, Court-Brown C. Elderly pelvic fractures: the incidence is increasing and patient demographics can be used to predict the outcome. Eur J Orthop Surg Traumatol 2014;24(8):1431–7.

21. Juern JS, Milia D, Codner P, et al. Clinical significance of computed tomography contrast extravasation in blunt trauma patients with a pelvic fracture. J Trauma Acute Care Surg 2017;82(1):138–40.

22. White C, Hsu J, Holcomb J. Haemodynamically unstable pelvic fractures. Injury 2009;40(10):1023–30.

23. Papakostidis C, Kanakaris N, Dimitriou R, et al. The role of arterial embolization in controlling pelvic fracture haemorrhage: a systematic review of the literature. Eur J Radiol 2018;81(5):897–904.

24. Schwartz DA, Medina M, Cotton BA, et al. Are we delivering two standards of care for pelvic and on weekends increases time to therapeutic intervention. J Trauma Acute Care Surg 2013;76(1):134–9.

25. Burlew CC, Moore EE, Stahel PF, et al. Preperitoneal pelvic packing reduces mortality in patients with life-threatening hemorrhage due to unstable pelvic fractures. J Trauma Acute Care Surg 2017;82(2):233–42.

26. Hughes C. Use of an intra-aortic balloon catheter tamponade for controlling intra-abdominal hemorrhage in man. Surgery 1954;36(1):65–8.

27. Moore LJ, Brenner M, Kozar RA, et al. Implementation of resuscitative endovascular balloon occlusion of the aorta as an alternative to resuscitative thoracotomy

for noncompressible truncal hemorrhage. J Trauma Acute Care Surg 2015;79(4): 523–32.

28. Abe T, Uchida M, Nagata I, et al. Resuscitative endovascular balloon occlusion of the aorta versus aortic cross clamping among patients with critical trauma: a nationwide cohort study in Japan. Crit Care 2016;20(1):400.

29. Inoue J, Shiraishi A, Yoshiyuki A, et al. Resuscitative endovascular balloon occlusion of the aorta might be dangerous in patients with severe torso trauma: a propensity score analysis. J Trauma Acute Care Surg 2016;80(4):559–67.

30. Norii T, Crandall C, Terasaka Y. Survival of severe blunt trauma patients treated with resuscitative endovascular balloon occlusion of the aorta compared with propensity score/adjusted untreated patients. J Trauma Acute Care Surg 2015; 78(4):721–8.

31. Dubose JJ, Scalea TM, Brenner M, et al. The AAST prospective Aortic Occlusion for Resuscitation in Trauma and Acute Care Surgery (AORTA) registry: Data on contemporary utilization and outcomes of aortic occlusion and resuscitative balloon occlusion of the aorta (REBOA). J Trauma Acute Care Surg 2016;81(3): 409–19.

32. Dong J, Zhou D. Management and outcome of open pelvic fractures: a retrospective study of 41 cases. Injury 2019;42(2011):1003–7.

33. Cannada LK, Taylor RM, Reddix R, et al. The Jones-Powell classification of open pelvic fractures: a multicenter study evaluating mortality rates. J Trauma Acute Care Surg 2013;74(3):901–6.

34. Govaert G, Siriwardane M, Hatzifotis M, et al. Prevention of pelvic sepsis in major open pelviperineal injury. Injury 2019;43(2012):533–6.

35. Henry S, Brasel K, Stewart R. ATLS® advanced trauma life support; student course manual. 10th edition. American College of Surgeons; 2018.

36. Morey AF, Brandes S, David D, et al. Urotrauma: AUA guideline. J Urol 2014; 192(2):327–35.

37. Jeong S, Park S, Kim Y. Efficacy of urethral catheterisation with a hydrophilic guidewire in patients with urethral trauma for treating acute urinary bladder retention after failed attempt at blind catheterisation. Eur Radiol 2012;22(4):758–64.

38. Medina D, Lavery R, Ross SE, et al. Ureteral trauma: preoperative studies neither predict injury nor prevent missed injuries. J Am Coll Surg 1995;7515(98):641–4.

39. Nayagam S. Injuries of the hip and femur. In: Warwick D, Nayagam S, editors. Apley's system of orthopaedics and fractures. 9th edition. London: Hodder; 2010. p. 843–7.

40. Chiron P, Lafontan V, Reina N. Fracture-dislocations of the femoral head. Orthop Traumatol Surg Res 2013;99(1):S53–66.

41. Sahin V, Karakas E, Aksu S, et al. Traumatic dislocation and fracture-dislocation of the hip: a long-term follow-up study. J Trauma 2003;54(3):520–9.

42. Waddell BS, Mohamed S, Glomset JT, et al. A detailed review of hip reduction maneuvers: a focus on physician safety and introduction of the Waddell technique. Orthop Rev (Pavia) 2016;8(1):6253.

43. Hendey GW, Avila A. The captain morgan technique for the reduction of the dislocated hip. Ann Emerg Med 2011;58(6):536–40.

44. Walden PD, Hamr J. Whistler technique used to reduce traumatic dislocation of the hip in the emergency department setting. J Emerg Med 1999;17(3):441–4.

45. Kani K, Porrino J, Mulachy H, et al. Fragility fractures of the proximal femur: review and update for radiologists. Skeletal Radiol 2019;48(1):29–45.

46. Parker M, Johansen A. Clinical review Hip fracture. BMJ 2006;333(July):27–30.

47. Innocenti M, Civinini R, Carulli C, et al. Proximal femoral fractures: epidemiology. Clin Cases Miner Bone Metab 2009;6(2):117–9.
48. Kellam J, Meinberg E, Agel J, et al. Fracture and dislocation classification compendium — 2018. J Orthop Trauma 2018;32(1):1–10.
49. Trueta J, Harrison M. The normal vascular anatomy of the femoral head in adult man. J Bone Joint Surg Br 1953;35(3):442–61.
50. Leenen L, van der Werken C. Traumatic posterior luxation of the hip. Neth J Surg 1990;42(5):136–9.
51. Hougaard K, Thornsen P. Traumatic posterior fracture-dislocation of the hip with fracture of the femoral head or neck, or both. J Bone Joint Surg Am 1988;70(2): 223–39.
52. Abraham M, Bond M. Femur and hip. In: Walls RM, Hockberger R, Gausch-Hill M, editors. Rosen's emergency medicine concepts and clinical practice. 9th edition. Philadelphia: Elsevier, Inc; 2018. p. 593–613.
53. Sankey R, Turner J, Lee J, et al. The use of MRI to detect occult fractures of the proximal femur: a study of 102 consecutive cases over a ten-year period. J Bone Joint Surg Br 2009;91(8):1064–8.
54. Buord J, Flecher X, Parratte S, et al. Garden I femoral neck fractures in patients 65 years old and older: Is conservative functional treatment a viable option? Orthop Traumatol Surg Res 2010;96(3):228–34.
55. Van Embden D, Rhemrev SJ, Genelin F, et al. The reliability of a simplified Garden classification for intracapsular hip fractures. Orthop Traumatol Surg Res 2012; 98(4):405.
56. Eisler J, Cornwall R, Strauss E, et al. Outcomes of elderly patients with nondisplaced femoral neck fractures. Clin Orthop Relat Res 2002;399(399):52–8.
57. Hansen B, Solgaard S. Impacted fractures of the femoral neck treated by early mobilization and weight-bearing. Acta Orthop Scand 1978;49(2):180–5.
58. Godoy Monzon D, Iserson KV, Vazquez JA. Single fscia iliaca compartment block for post-hip fracture pain relief. J Emerg Med 2007 Apr;32(3):257–62.
59. Willeumier JJ, Schoones JW. Pathologic fractures of the distal femur: current concepts and treatment options. J Surg Oncol 2018;118(6):883–90.
60. Gehrchen PM, Nielsen J, Olesen B, et al. Seinsheimer's classification of subtrochanteric fractures: poor reproducibility of 4 observers' evaluation of 50 cases Seinsheimer's classification of subtrochanteric fractures. Acta Orthop Scand 1997;68(6):524–6.
61. Monzon D, Iserson K, Vazquez J. Single Fascia Iliaca compartment block for post-hip fracture pain relief. J Emerg Med 2007;32(3):257–62.
62. Monzon D, Vazquez J, Jaurequi J, et al. Pain treatment in post-traumatic hip fracture in the elderly: regional block vs. systemic nonsteroidal analgesics. Int J Emerg Med 2010;3(4):321–5.
63. Mavrogenis A, Panagopoulos G, Megaloikonomos P. Complications after hip nailing for fractures. Orthopedics 2016;39(1):e108–16.
64. Barnes R, Brown J, Garden R, et al. Subcapital fractures of the femur. J Bone Joint Surg Br 1976;58(1):2–24.

Knee and Leg Injuries

Moira Davenport, MD[a],*, Matthew P. Oczypok, MD[b]

KEYWORDS

- Knee injury • Leg injury • Posterolateral corner • Musculoskeletal ultrasonography
- Knee immobilizer

KEY POINTS

- Ligamentous knee injuries are commonly seen in the emergency department (ED). Appropriate management of the initial presentation can improve patient outcome.
- The posterolateral corner of the knee should be carefully evaluated during the secondary survey of the injured knee.
- Musculoskeletal ultrasonography can augment the ED evaluation of the acutely injured knee and leg.

INTRODUCTION

The knee is intricately involved in the various activities of daily living, from the seemingly benign act of self-care to higher-demand motion encountered in sports and employment. Based on the knee's role in weight bearing and multiplanar movement during these activities, the knee is subjected to a variety of different forces and thus a variety of injuries. Incidence varies greatly based on activity, but recent data report 229 knee injuries per 100,000 people presenting to emergency departments (EDs) of which 42.1% were strains/sprains, 3.9% dislocations, and 3.9% fractures.[1] Given the frequency of knee injuries, emergency physicians (EPs) should be familiar with the mechanisms of these injuries as well as the diagnosis and treatment of these conditions.

Knee Anatomy

Basic bony knee anatomy is straightforward, and it is not reviewed in this article. However, several anatomic considerations can help EPs in their knee evaluation. Recent research has focused on the anatomy of the posterolateral corner (PLC) of the knee and the role of this complex structure in overall knee stability. The PLC consists of 3 tissue layers: the deep, middle, and superficial layers. The deep layer (popliteus

Disclosure: The authors have no financial disclosures or conflicts of interest.
[a] Department of Emergency Medicine, Allegheny General Hospital, Temple University School of Medicine, 320 East North Avenue, Pittsburgh, PA 15212, USA; [b] Department of Emergency Medicine, Allegheny General Hospital, 320 East North Avenue, Pittsburgh, PA 15212, USA
* Corresponding author.
E-mail address: moira.davenport@ahn.org

Emerg Med Clin N Am 38 (2020) 143–165
https://doi.org/10.1016/j.emc.2019.09.012
0733-8627/20/Published by Elsevier Inc.

emed.theclinics.com

muscle, popliteofibular ligament, lateral collateral ligament [LCL], arcuate ligament, and the fabellofibular ligament)[2–4] plays a critical role in knee stability in varus and rotatory planes of motion.[5,6] PLC injuries rarely occur in isolation; they are commonly associated with anterior cruciate ligament (ACL) or posterior cruciate ligament (PCL) tears.[7] In addition, the anatomic relationship of the peroneal nerve to the proximal fibula and the PLC requires a thorough neurovascular examination because a missed injury to this nerve can result in significant morbidity (ie, foot drop).

Bony anatomy of the knee should be described using the 3-compartment model: the medial, lateral, and patellofemoral compartments. The medial femoral condyle–medial tibial plateau articulation forms the medial compartment, whereas the lateral compartment is the articulation of the lateral femoral condyle and the lateral tibial plateau. The final compartment is formed by the patella and its interface with the anterior femoral condyles. It is important to consider that the patella is the product of unification of several secondary centers of ossification. Failure of these centers to fully unify can result in a bipartite patella. This anatomic variant may be mistaken for a fracture, highlighting the importance of understanding the mechanism of injury when evaluating an acutely injured knee. This possible variant should prompt EPs to image the contralateral knee because the bipartite patella is typically seen in both knees.

Emergency department evaluation
A systematic approach to the knee examination ensures that EPs do not miss critical diagnoses.

History Patients may present with an apparently normal-appearing knee despite having sustained a significant knee injury, highlighting the need for an injury-specific history. Key historical considerations include the position of the extremity and the knee at the time of injury, the mechanism of injury, and the direction from which any force was applied. A patient's ability to ambulate after the injury as well as the subjective sensation of knee instability should be noted. It is also helpful for the EP to ascertain whether there is a prior history of knee injury/surgery, and any baseline functional deficits that resulted from those previous injuries.

Physical examination Close visual inspection can detect obvious deformities, including knee dislocation, patellar dislocation, skin disruption, and quadriceps/patellar tendon disruptions. The presence of any effusion, erythema, ecchymosis, abrasions, and lacerations should increase clinical suspicion for a significant injury. Effusions are typically associated with intraarticular fractures and ACL tears[8–10] (**Table 1**). Perform a thorough neurovascular examination. The presence of any neurovascular deficit is an indication for immediate reduction in order to reestablish normal blood flow to the injured extremity. If normal neurovascular parameters are restored, perform a complete evaluation to assess the full extent of the knee injury. Palpate all major bony joint structures, including the medial and lateral joint lines, quadriceps and patellar tendons, patella, tibial tubercle, the medial collateral ligament (MCL), and LCL.

Table 1 Conditions resulting in knee effusions	
Early Effusion	**Delayed Effusion**
ACL tear	Meniscal tear
Tibial plateau fracture	Cartilaginous loose bodies
PCL tear	
Femoral condyle fracture	
Patellar fracture	

Access active range of motion (ROM). If the patient is not able to actively range the knee joint, evaluate passive ROM. This assessment should include an evaluation of patellar movement within the trochlear groove. The uninjured patella should move in a relatively straight vertical line as the knee moves from full extension to full flexion. Patients with inherently weak quadriceps muscles or a disturbance of the patellofemoral complex may have patellae that move laterally and then vertically in a hockey stick–shaped track. The apprehension test can also be used to evaluate patellar instability. To perform this maneuver, extend the patient's knee and then apply a varus force to the patella. The test is positive if the patient tightens the quadriceps in an attempt to prevent dislocation. However, the sensitivity and specificity of this technique are still being evaluated.[11]

EPs should next focus on the examination of the ligamentous structures of the knee. However, EPs are not proficient at diagnosing ACL tears via physical examination,[12] possibly because of a lack of familiarity with the variety of tests available to examine the ACL. The Lachman test is performed with the injured knee in 20° to 30° of flexion. A gentle force is applied to the tibia to move the tibia anterior relative to the femur.[13] The anterior drawer test also assesses ACL stability with the anterior force applied to the tibia while the knee is in 90° flexion. However, with the knee positioned for the anterior drawer, both the MCL and the medial meniscus contribute to knee stability, significantly reducing the sensitivity of this maneuver.[14,15] The likelihood ratio of an ACL tear with a positive Lachman is 25, whereas for a positive anterior drawer it is only 3.8.[16]

The posterior drawer test is used to assess PCL integrity. Knee positioning is the same as for the anterior drawer, but apply the tibial force in a posterior direction. Varus and valgus forces should be applied to the knee to assess the LCL and MCL respectively. Apply a gentle force with the knee fully extended and with the knee at 30° flexion. The slight flexion effectively isolates the collateral ligaments because the ACL and PCL both contribute to the stability of the fully extended knee. Two variations of positive laxity may be detected: complete lack of an end point or delayed end point (relative laxity compared with the uninjured knee). This distinction highlights the need to examine both joints in order to establish the patient's baseline laxity.[17,18]

Use the external recurvatum maneuver to evaluate the PLC of the knee.[19] Place the patient supine on the stretcher with both legs extended. Hold the patient's toes and lift the extended leg while noting whether normal knee alignment is maintained. Suspect a PLC disruption if a varus deformity (bow leg) is found. Alternatively, the posterolateral drawer can be performed. Position the patient as if performing the posterior drawer test, but externally rotate the feet 15°, then apply a posterolaterally directed force to the tibia. Any laxity detected with this testing suggests a PLC injury along with a concurrent ligamentous injury, likely an ACL disruption. Repeat the maneuver with the knee flexed 30°; if laxity is noted in this position, an isolated PLC disruption is likely. Any examination that detects 2 or more lax ligaments should raise the possibility of a knee dislocation and prompt a repeat neurovascular examination.

Multiple examination techniques are available to evaluate meniscal integrity; however, the McMurray test is the most reliable. To perform this diagnostic test, place the patient supine on the stretcher. The examiner puts a thumb on either the medial or lateral joint line and the remaining fingers on the other joint line while holding the patient's leg with the other hand. The examiner should flex the patient's hip to 90° and then extend and rotate the knee while applying a varus force, effectively closing the medial joint line. While the leg is extending, the examiner is trying to appreciate a clunk as the suspected meniscal fragment is caught between and then extruded from the joint space. Repeat the maneuver while applying a valgus force to evaluate the lateral meniscus. A true positive McMurray test is the presence of a clunk, not just recreation of the patient's pain. When a clunk is appreciated, the sensitivity is 35.7% and the specificity 85.7% for isolated medial meniscal disorder and 22.2% and 100% for isolated lateral meniscal defects.[14] Both sensitivities decrease in the presence of a concurrent ACL tear[14] but increase with the presence of joint line tenderness.[16,20]

Imaging The thorough physical examination should be followed by imaging studies as needed. Analgesics may be required to allow a thorough examination and imaging to be performed. When possible, perform imaging without immobilization devices in place.

The standard knee radiograph series should include lateral, anterior-posterior (AP), and sunrise views. Verify the technique used for the radiograph, particularly for the lateral view. The knee should be flexed 20°-30° in a true lateral, whereas a cross-table lateral radiograph is taken with the knee fully extended. When possible, weight-bearing AP views should be obtained to allow a more realistic assessment of the joint spaces, particularly as affected by gravity. A commercially available device can be used to perform stress views at 30° and 80° of flexion in cases of suspected PCL injury.[21,22] If there is a concern for a tibial plateau fracture, obtain oblique views. Computed tomography (CT) provides better bony detail and is more reliable at detecting fractures with minimal to moderate depression, making it the preferred imaging modality for operative planning.

Two radiographic findings are pathognomonic for ligamentous injuries. The Segond fracture (capsular avulsion of the lateral tibial plateau) (**Figs. 1** and **2**) was classically associated with ACL disruption.[23–26] However, Segond fractures are now also associated with PLC disruptions[27] and MCL injuries.[24]

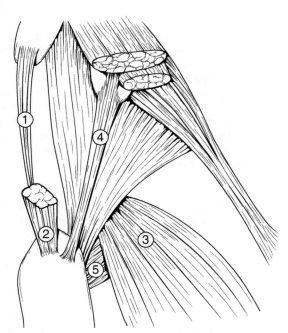

Fig. 1. Posterolateral corner of the knee anatomy. 1, LCL; 2, biceps femoris ligament; 3, popliteus muscle; 4, fabellofibular ligament; 5, popliteofibular ligament. (*Courtesy of* B. Lawner, DO. Pittsburgh, PA)

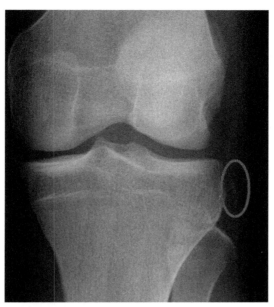

Fig. 2. A Segond fracture, a marker for ACL tears, is noted by the red ring. (*From* Wikimedia Commons. Available at: https://commons.wikimedia.org/wiki/File:SegondFracture.JPG.)

Calcification of the MCL on plain radiographs (**Fig. 3**) is known as the Pellegrini-Stieda (see **Fig. 3**) lesion and is historically thought to result from previous MCL injury.[28] Magnetic Resonance Imagery (MRI)-based research suggests that the forces required to injure the MCL may result in partial avulsion of the femoral periosteum, most importantly the PCL insertion. Thus, the Pellegrini-Stieda lesion may be found with PCL disruption.[29–31]

Point-of-care ultrasonography (US) and the dynamic studies produced have long made US the preferred musculoskeletal imaging modality in Europe; this practice has recently increased significantly in North America. Musculoskeletal US (MSK-US) is particularly relevant to EPs. The noninjured knee can easily be examined as a point of comparison, and the patient can be examined in a position of discomfort/laxity, further increasing the diagnostic yield. In addition, MSK-US can be performed at various phases of the ROM, thus correcting geometric averaging seen on MRI, which provides a more accurate evaluation.[32–35]

A variety of probes can be used in the course of an MSK-US examination, but the high-frequency linear transducer is preferred for the knee. Several critical physical examination findings can be evaluated with MSK-US, including the amount of tibial translation in ACL tears,[36] PCL thickness (particularly in the lateral plane),[37,38] and the PLC integrity.[39] Protocols are also being developed to incorporate MSK-US in the diagnosis of meniscal injuries.[40,41] Integration of MSK-US is particularly helpful for the evaluation of meniscal injuries, because MRI has been shown to have varying efficacy in making this diagnosis.[42–44]

Emergency Department Management

Anterior cruciate ligament injuries
Sports participation accounts for almost all ACL tears.[45,46] Both contact and noncontact tears are common, and the rate of tears is reaching epidemic numbers in some

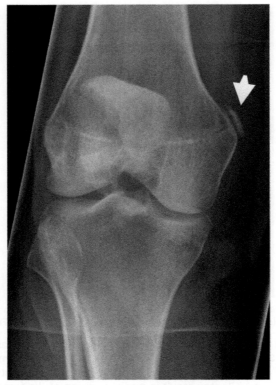

Fig. 3. Pellegrini-Stieda lesion (*white arrow*) is noted on this AP radiograph, which is associated with MCL injuries. (Photo by Paul Hellerhoff, MD. From Wikimedia Commons. Available at: https://commons.wikimedia.org/wiki/File:Zervikales_Web_Breischluck_001-00.jpg.)

sports.[47–50] According to recent data from the Multicenter ACL Revision Study (MARS), 76% of people in the study incurred ACL tears playing sports. Of the people enrolled, 71% of these tears occurred in a noncontact setting, with 31% jumping at the time of the injury, and 40% were cutting or changing direction.[51] Several mechanisms of injury can result in the athletic ACL tear. The most common mechanism of injury is when a valgus force is applied to an extended knee; a rotational component is often involved as well. Snowboarders are more likely to tear an ACL by landing flat on the board while the knee is flexed, leading to moderate to severe compression.[52] As high as 83% of people who tear their ACLs hear or feel a pop at the time of injury.[51] Interestingly, the patients with ACL injuries can often ambulate fairly normally immediately after the disruption. Moderate effusions are commonly seen within 2 to 3 hours of injury, significantly limiting unassisted ambulation. MRI is the preferred diagnostic test when an ACL injury is suspected; however, routine knee radiographs should be performed in an effort to evaluate for associated fractures, particularly the Segond fracture.[53] If MRI is obtained in the ED, it is essential to note whether the patient has had a prior ACL reconstruction, because MRI findings vary between native and reconstructed ACLs.[54] MSK-US is another imaging modality that can be used by EPs to diagnose ACL tears. In a recent meta-analysis, sensitivity and specificity of MSK-US evaluating for ACL tears were 90% and 97%, respectively. This finding shows the high diagnostic value and further shows that MSK-US should be part of the standard evaluation for ACL injury by EPs.[55] If an ACL tear is highly suspected, EPs should also evaluate for concurrent ligamentous or meniscal injuries. However, joint line tenderness, typically associated with meniscal tears, is not reliable in patients with concomitant ACL tears,[56] which is particularly relevant for tears of the posterolateral horn of the lateral meniscus.[43] Patients with isolated ACL tears and ACL/meniscal injury should be placed in a hinged knee brace and can be discharged from the ED. These patients can be weight bearing as tolerated with the brace, crutches, and 1-day to 3-day orthopedic referral.

Although not every patient with an ACL injury undergoes surgical reconstruction, orthopedic follow-up is recommended to better delineate a treatment plan. Patients with ACL injuries should have physical therapy initiated as soon as possible in order to optimize preoperative strength and ROM (particularly extension). Although age more than 50 years had been considered a relative contraindication to ACL reconstruction, age is no longer an absolute contraindication to surgery.[57] On the opposite end of the aging spectrum, the timing of ACL reconstruction in children has been controversial. Previous guidelines advised delayed reconstruction until skeletal maturity had been achieved. However, current recommendations encourage immediate reconstruction, because this approach has shown a significantly lower rate of postinjury meniscal tears.[58,59]

Orthopedic surgeons use a variety of ACL reconstruction techniques. Although the specifics are not relevant for EPs, some familiarity with these procedures is helpful, particularly when evaluating postoperative patients. The Achilles tendon is most commonly used in a cadaveric graft reconstruction, whereas the native hamstring or patellar tendon is commonly used for an autograft reconstruction. Consensus varies as to the optimum graft; however, the most commonly performed technique is a single-bundle patellar tendon reconstruction.[60–63] In addition to the integrity of the ACL reconstruction, EPs should consider complications at the site of autograft harvest. Patients that have undergone patellar tendon reconstruction may experience patellar tendon rupture, patellar fracture, and pain/inability to kneel,[64] whereas those who have had hamstring tendon reconstructions typically note hamstring weakness and a slower return to regular activity. Several infectious complications may arise after surgery, including operative site infection, wound dehiscence, septic arthritis,[65,66] and tuberculosis.[67]

If reconstruction is not performed, the patient is still at risk for complications. Alterations in knee anatomy can result in changes in the general mechanics of the knee, leading to both structural changes and injury to the MCL and LCL.[68] The increased instability that results from an ACL tear can lead to meniscal tears, leading to knee instability and advanced osteoarthrotic changes.[69,70] However, accelerated knee osteoarthrosis is also seen in the reconstructed ACL patient, although not typically at the rate seen in nonreconstructed knees.[71,72] The integrity of the meniscus likely plays a key role in the development of postoperative osteoarthropathy. One retrospective study showed that up to 61% of medial and 74% of lateral meniscal tears healed spontaneously during recovery from ACL reconstruction,[47] whereas a different group of investigators showed that meniscectomy performed at the time of ACL reconstruction resulted in greater arthritic changes than reconstruction alone.[73] Another retrospective review of knee injuries evaluated the effect of meniscectomy and ACL reconstruction on players' careers (defined as games played, games started, and years in the league). The investigators found that meniscectomy shortened players' careers significantly more than ACL reconstruction. Furthermore, athletes that had both meniscectomy and ACL reconstruction had all 3 parameters shortened more than either procedure in isolation.[74] These separate studies were further strengthened by a meta-analysis with similar conclusions.[75]

Posterior cruciate ligament injuries

The PCL is injured significantly less than the ACL. Most injuries to the PCL are seen in association with other ligamentous knee injuries. Injuries to the PCL alone are rarely seen.[76] The PCL is at highest risk for injury when a flexed knee is subjected to a posteriorly directed force, as seen when a knee strikes the dashboard during a motor vehicle crash or the flexed knee hits the ground during a fall. The extra-articular location of the PCL makes effusions rare.[77] The presence of an effusion should significantly increase clinician suspicion for concomitant ligamentous injury or knee dislocation; this also likely contributes to EPs missing the initial PCL injury. If a truly isolated PCL tear is suspected, patients can also be safely discharged from the ED in a hinged knee brace with weight bearing as tolerated while awaiting orthopedic follow-up. If the PCL injury is seen in conjunction with other ligamentous injuries, the patient may require emergent orthopedic consultation, particularly in cases of suspected dislocation or PLC injury.

PCL injuries were historically treated nonoperatively, but the current recommendations favor operative therapy.[78–81] As with ACL reconstruction, grafts can be autografts (eg, patellar tendon, quadriceps tendon) or allografts (eg, Achilles tendon, tibial tendon). Postoperative complications are also similar to those seen after ACL reconstruction. The evolution of PCL management has been driven by studies that further elucidated the role of the PCL in knee stability. Research showed the role of chronic PCL deficiency in the accelerated development of knee osteoarthropathy, particularly in the medial compartment.[82] Chronic PCL laxity also increases forces, and thus stretch, across the PLC, placing this complex at further injury risk.[83]

Posterolateral corner injuries

Injuries to the PLC can occur when a varus force is applied to the knee, regardless of the knee's position at the time of impact and the energy associated with the impact.[84] Any patient with a suspected PLC injury should be seen by orthopedics while in the ED. It is imperative that EPs consider PLC disruption in the differential diagnosis of acutely injured knees, because the timing of operative intervention is critical for the long-term stability of the knee. Chronic PLC instability has been identified as the most common cause of postoperative ACL failure.[85,86] Multiple studies have shown significantly reduced morbidity and higher functioning when repair/reconstruction of the PLC is performed within 10 to 14 days of injury.[87,88] The success of surgical attempts performed after this time is negatively affected by scarring and tissue degeneration, the combination of which makes proper identification of structures virtually impossible. Even if surgery is performed within the recommended time frame, several controversies exist. Recent studies seem to favor reconstruction rather than repair[89]; however, the preferred technique is still debated.[79,90–93]

Attention should be given to the neurovascular examination of the patients with PLC injury. Based on the anatomy of this area, there is an associated risk for peroneal nerve injury.[94] The presence of a concurrent fibular head avulsion or biceps femoris avulsion was found to increase the risk for peroneal nerve involvement.[94]

Lateral collateral ligament injuries

The position of the LCL within the PLC makes isolated LCL injuries uncommon.[95] Osteoarthrosis is also a risk factor for LCL compromise.[96] The knee examination should be performed, with a focus on the LCL, PLC, and neurovascular status. In addition to the standard knee radiographs, varus stress radiographs can be used to evaluate LCL integrity. More than 4 mm of widening relative to the standard views indicates a PLC injury, whereas 2.7 to 3.9 mm of laxity is typically associated with an isolated LCL injury.[97] If an isolated LCL injury is detected, the patient should be placed in a hinged knee brace, given crutches, and allowed to weight bear as tolerated. Arrange orthopedic follow-up within 2 to 3 days of injury to facilitate definitive imaging and the initiation of physical therapy. Although some investigators favor operative reconstruction with the semitendinous tendon as a graft,[98] the standard of care remains conservative management. A small study by Bushnell and colleagues[95] determined that the conservative approach resulted in a faster return to preinjury activity, including return to an elite level of competition.

Medial collateral ligament injuries

Of the 4 major knee ligaments, the MCL is the most commonly injured.[99] The classic mechanism of injury is a valgus force applied to the knee. MCL injuries have been reported with the knee in both extension and flexion. The MCL injury is unique among the ligamentous knee injuries, because multiple degrees of injury can occur. The extent of injury ranges from the disruption of a few fibers/simple stretch (grade I), to partial tear (grade II), and ultimately to complete tear (grade III). Although this distinction should be made definitively only from imaging studies, including MSK-US or MRI, clinical examination findings can be used to determine a preliminary diagnosis. A clearly appreciated end point with mild laxity on valgus stress testing relative to the uninjured knee is typically seen with grade I and II injuries, whereas significant laxity and no clear end point are classic findings in a grade III tear. Medial joint line tenderness and medial joint line laxity are typically found in MCL-injured knees. The intraarticular location of the MCL makes effusion rare in isolated MCL injuries.

Grade I and II MCL injuries are typically treated nonoperatively. Patients with isolated MCL injuries should be discharged with orthopedic follow-up while in a hinged knee brace with crutches and allowed to weight bear as tolerated.[99] As is the case with all ligamentous knee injuries, it is imperative that the patient not be sent home with a straight-leg knee immobilizer because this can hinder recovery by accelerating quadriceps wasting and subsequent weakness.[100] Patient education at ED discharge should focus on the need for physical therapy. Therapeutic US, early mobility, and early strengthening (particularly quadriceps) have been shown to shorten the recovery period.[101]

Management of grade III MCL injuries is slightly more complicated than the grade I and II conditions. Although complete MCL tears were previously treated operatively, nonoperative management is now preferred unless a large avulsion fracture is also found.[99,102–104] If surgery is necessary, primary repair is preferred, and the semitendinosus and gracilis tendons are used for both allografts and autografts.[99]

In cases of concomitant grade III MCL and ACL injuries, it is still advised to reconstruct the ACL but allow the MCL to heal nonoperatively. This approach is made easier by the typical 6-week to 8-week delay from the time of injury to ACL reconstruction enabling adequate MCL healing.[86] Multiple studies have failed to show a difference in postoperative ACL stability when this split approach is taken.[102–104] However, for this approach to be successful, the patient should be in physical therapy to maintain quadriceps strength and knee ROM (particularly full extension). This split approach is also recommended when the MCL, ACL, and PCL are injured; however, the literature regarding this is not as robust given the lower overall rate of this injury complex.[104]

In cases of MCL injury with the Pellegrini-Stieda lesion, surgical excision of the lesion is advised. However, by definition, with this lesion the surgery is delayed from the time of the initial injury.[105]

Meniscal injuries

Meniscal injuries are different than ligamentous disruptions. Because of their anatomic location and their role in shock absorption, the menisci are subjected to significantly more breakdown through normal activities than the other structures of the knee. Degenerative tears are almost as common as traumatic injuries; an MRI study of asymptomatic patients more than 50 years of age showed rates of meniscal tears ranging from 19% among those aged 50 to 59 years and 56% among those more than 70 years old.[106] Patients with meniscal abnormalities typically present with generalized knee pain localizing to either the medial or lateral joint lines. However, joint line tenderness (or lack thereof) is not a reliable finding in patients with chronic ACL deficiency.[56] Effusions may be seen, but usually do not develop until at least 4 to 6 hours from the time of the tear. Patients may notice a clicking sensation when walking, as the meniscal fragments slide between the tibia and the femur. Similarly, locking of the knee joint is possible if the fragment does not disengage from between the 2 bones. However, neither of these findings is definite because the location and the size of the tear affect the likelihood of developing these abnormalities. The presence of an acute meniscal injury should increase the concern for the possibility of a concurrent tibial plateau fracture. This relationship has been highlighted with the increased use of MRI.[107]

Patients with isolated meniscal injuries may be safely discharged from the ED with crutches or a cane as needed. If bracing is needed, a hinged knee brace may also be used; however, straight-leg knee immobilization is not indicated.[108] Outpatient orthopedic surgery referral is warranted. Treatment can be conservative (physical therapy) or operative (arthroscopic excision of the fragment). A small percentage of meniscal tears can be repaired; however, this depends on the anatomic location of the tear. It was initially thought that arthroscopy accelerated the development of knee osteoarthrosis more than conservative therapy. A recent study showed that nonoperatively managed meniscal tears also increase the rate of osteoarthrosis relative to the intact meniscus.[109]

Meniscal abnormalities are seen in children, with tears and discoid menisci being the most common.[110] In cases of discoid meniscus, the meniscus is typically larger than normal with a more oval morphology compared with the normal C-shaped morphology. Children with discoid menisci can note pain and snapping with ambulation. They may also present with tears because the morphologic changes result in more instability than is seen in the typical meniscus and predispose these patients to injury. Pediatric menisci have increased vascularity relative to the adult structure and are more amenable to surgical repair rather than excision.[110]

Knee dislocation

Disruption of at least 3 of the 4 major ligaments of the knee typically results in a knee dislocation. Because of the close proximity of the neurovascular bundle (ie, popliteal artery, popliteal vein, and peroneal nerve), this injury is considered a true orthopedic emergency. The popliteal artery is essentially tethered to the femur and tibia, making it particularly vulnerable to injury during a knee dislocation. Two disparate mechanisms of injury are responsible for knee dislocation: high-velocity trauma and apparently minor trauma in obese patients,[111] and the low-velocity mechanism may be more common.[112] Knee dislocations can be described either by the resting position of the tibia relative to the femur (eg, anterior, posterior, medial, lateral, or rotary) or by specifying the ligaments injured in the dislocation. The latter scheme is becoming increasingly common in clinical practice.[113]

Patient presentation varies along with the mechanism of injury. If a high-velocity injury occurs, the knee capsule is typically disrupted, making an effusion less likely. This capsular disruption usually allows the spontaneous reduction of the joint, making a visible deformity less likely.[113] However, if the joint capsule remains intact, the patient typically presents with a significant deformity. Both scenarios may have associated ecchymoses. Given that no significant effusion and no deformity may be seen, EPs should consider this diagnosis in the evaluation of patients with polytrauma. Knee laxity noted on the secondary survey should prompt further testing to better evaluate the popliteal artery and tibial nerve.[114]

If the patient presents with a significant deformity, reduction should be performed as quickly as possible to improve the status of the popliteal artery. While preparing for knee reduction, it is important to note the presence of a buttonhole deformity. With this condition, the medial femoral condyle is protruding through the joint capsule, essentially making closed reduction impossible. Inability to move the knee through a passive ROM assessment should heighten suspicion for this condition. Although this condition has been seen on MRI, it should be diagnosed clinically when possible.[115] To reduce the dislocated knee, apply longitudinal traction to the tibia to dislodge the tibia from the femur. Normal alignment can then be restored by applying a force opposite to the direction of the dislocation. If a rotary component of the dislocation is present, this should be corrected as well. As the reduction is performed, it is essential to avoid placing excess pressure on the popliteal fossa in order to protect the neurovascular structures. When the reduction is complete, the knee should be placed in a hinged knee brace with 15° to 20° of flexion; the brace should be locked in this position. If the reduced knee is unstable, external fixators may be used as a bridge to surgery.[116,117]

If possible, reduction should be performed within 6 hours of the injury to limit damage to the neurovascular structures and to decrease the likelihood of compartment syndrome.[114,118] As with all extremity injuries, perform a thorough neurovascular examination on the patient's arrival. The presence of hard signs of vascular injury (ie, absent pedal pulses, cool/mottled foot, expanding hematoma) is an indication for immediate operative intervention. If necessary, an angiogram may be performed if the patient's overall condition limits immediate surgery. Duplex US or angiogram can be used to evaluate patients with dorsolateral foot or leg paresthesia or asymmetric distal pulses. In patients with a normal neurovascular examination, an ankle-brachial index (ABI) should be performed.[119] Automatic angiography is no longer recommended following a knee dislocation and should only be performed on patients with neurovascular abnormalities or an abnormal ABI. An ABI less than 0.9 has a 100% positive predictive value for identifying vascular injuries requiring surgical exploration and repair.[120] If a patient has a normal initial neurovascular examination and a normal ABI, admission is recommended to allow for neurovascular checks every 2 to 3 hours for the first 24 hours after injury.[121] If the neurovascular examination changes during this time, immediate angiography is needed.[116] The ready availability of CT angiography (vs traditional angiography) has resulted in increasing use of this modality. In addition, Doppler studies are being used more frequently as an adjunct to the more traditional neurovascular examination.[122–126] The use of Doppler to identify a significant vascular injury has been found to have a specificity of 95% to 97% and an accuracy of 95% to 97%, resulting in increasing use of this modality as well. Note that the US examination can be made technically difficult, and thus less reliable, if large skin wounds, casts, hematomas, or subcutaneous air is present.[127]

Approximately 20% of patients sustaining a knee dislocation have a concomitant peroneal nerve injury leading to motor or sensory deficits.[128] Sensation should be carefully assessed in the first web space, the dorsum of the foot, and the lateral aspect of the leg. Weakness of the peroneal muscles, the tibialis anterior, and the extensor hallucis longus may be seen, manifesting as foot drop, weak ankle eversion, and decreased/weak great toe extension, respectively. If an acute peroneal nerve injury is suspected, the foot should be splinted in neutral position in order to minimize tension on the nerve and thus limit the progression of symptoms.

Operative intervention is typically done in a staggered fashion as opposed to 1 surgery.[129–132] Timing for surgery is the same time frame as an intervention on an isolated ligamentous injury. Similarly, reconstruction versus repair is the same as for an isolated ligamentous injury.[116,130]

Patellar dislocation

Patellar dislocations typically result from a varus force applied to a flexed knee. Dislocations can also occur from the forced contraction of a flexed quadriceps. Patellar dislocation has been reported following aggressive use of the Wii, resulting in the term Wii knee.[133] The lateral patellar retinaculum is significantly stronger than its medial counterpart, making lateral dislocations the more common injury. On arrival to the ED, the knee is typically flexed, with a visible lateral deformity; effusion and ecchymosis may also be present. Prereduction radiographs (AP, lateral, and sunrise views) are recommended to evaluate for concomitant fractures before the reduction attempt; osteochondral fractures are most commonly seen.[134,135] Sedation may be needed to achieve reduction, which is performed by extending the knee and simultaneously applying a valgus force to the dislocated patella. Once normal alignment is reestablished, the extensor mechanism should be assessed to ensure the integrity of the quadriceps and patellar tendons. The extremity should be placed in a straight-leg knee immobilizer and postreduction films performed. Patients with successful reductions may be discharged with the straight-leg knee immobilizer, crutches, and orthopedic follow-up.

The increased use of MRI has highlighted the higher-than-expected rate of injuries associated with patellar dislocation. Meniscal tears, MCL disruptions, and osteochondral fractures have all been associated with dislocations.[136] Classic complications following patellar dislocation include persistent instability, subluxation, repeat dislocation, and accelerated osteoarthrosis. Recent prospective studies comparing operative and nonoperative therapies showed a significant reduction in the redislocation rate in the surgically treated groups. However, the rates of return to baseline activity were similar between groups.[137,138] Surgical intervention is commonly recommended; however, the timing of the procedure varies. Immediate repair is generally recommended in physically active patients, whereas some surgeons advocate delaying surgical intervention until after a second dislocation.[139] If operative intervention is planned a variety of techniques may be used to reestablish the medial retinaculum and the medial patellofemoral ligament. The hamstring tendon is commonly used as the donor graft.[140,141] As with other knee injuries, surgical repair is still controversial in children, with recent literature advocating intervention before closure of the physes.[142]

Patellar fracture

Patellar fractures result from the same mechanisms as PCL injuries; fall onto a flexed knee and dashboard injury.[143] Several fracture patterns are possible (eg, transverse, horizontal, avulsion, and stellate) resulting in a variety of presentations. Effusion and ecchymosis are common with all fracture types; however, a palpable defect may or may not be detected. Although the neurovascular examination is typically benign, the critical physical examination finding is the status of the extensor mechanism.

Routine knee radiographs should be performed to further delineate the extent of the injury. Patients with intact extensor mechanisms can be discharged from the ED in a straight-leg knee immobilizer with crutches and orthopedic follow-up. Patients who cannot extend the leg should be seen by orthopedics immediately because internal fixation is often performed within 24 hours of the injury.[144,145]

A unique patellar fracture can be seen in pediatric patients: the sleeve fracture. The mechanism of injury is the same as in the traditional patellar fracture. However, in preteens the patellar tendon is typically stronger than the bone, resulting in an avulsion of the intact patellar tendon off the inferior aspect of the patella.[146,147] Extensor mechanism disruption is seen on clinical examination but effusion is rare. Orthopedic consultation is recommended before discharge from the ED to facilitate operative planning in order to limit the amount of retraction of the patellar tendon.

Quadriceps and patellar tendon rupture

The quadriceps and patellar tendons most commonly rupture because of trauma, particularly forced quadriceps contraction with a flexed knee. Tears can occur at any level from the quadriceps to the tibial tuberosity. Degenerative tears and disruptions secondary to chronic medical conditions (eg, diabetes, Lyme disease) are also seen but are significantly less common than traumatic mechanisms.[148] There is an age predilection for each injury, because patients more than 40 years of age tend to tear the quadriceps tendon, whereas younger patients are more likely to sustain patellar tendon disruptions.[46] Patients typically present with a large knee effusion and moderate pain. Although obvious tendon defects may be appreciable, it is imperative to assess the integrity of the extensor mechanism. The position of the patella on standard lateral knee radiographs may indicate a tendon rupture, with quadriceps tendon rupture resulting in low-riding patellae and patellar tendon rupture creating a high-riding patella (see **Fig. 1**). A minimally invasive technique to assess quadriceps tendon integrity has been proposed but has not gained clinical support.[149] MSK-US has also been shown to be reliable in diagnosing quadriceps rupture.[150,151] Patellar tendon disruptions were initially thought to be an isolated injury; however, a recent study indicates this may not be the case, highlighting the need for a complete knee examination.[152] Patients with tendon rupture should be placed in a straight-leg knee immobilizer and undergo orthopedic evaluation. Operative fixation within a month of injury has better clinical outcomes.[153]

Tibial plateau fractures

Tibial plateau fractures result when the knee is flexed and is subjected to varus or valgus forces. These fractures can be seen with or without an axial load being applied to the knee. As with knee dislocation, both low-velocity and high-velocity mechanisms may cause tibial plateau fractures.[154] The most common mechanism for tibial plateau fractures is an axial load combined with a valgus force applied to the knee, resulting in a lateral plateau fracture. Medial tibial plateau and bicondylar injuries are also possible but are less common. Patients with tibial plateau fractures typically have an effusion and joint line tenderness. Ecchymoses may be seen within a few hours of the injury. Larger fractures may have crepitance on examination. In addition to the standard knee radiographs, cross-table lateral and oblique views should be performed. Particular attention should be paid to the cross-table lateral view in an effort to identify a lipohemarthrosis. This layering of fat, blood, and synovial fluid is associated with an increased likelihood of tibial plateau fracture (see **Fig. 2**). This finding can be confirmed by direct visualization of fat cells and red blood cells on arthrocentesis or US. The preferred approach for MSK-US is to place the high-frequency probe on the midline suprapatellar bursa with the knee flexed to 30°. The probe should then be swept both medially and laterally to best evaluate the effusion. Fat cells in the effusion are echogenic relative to the hypoechoic blood and rest above the blood.[155] Identification of a lipohemarthrosis by any of these means should prompt further evaluation of the joint, preferably by CT using 2-mm slices.[156] CT is also recommended if a tibial plateau fracture is seen on plain radiographs, because it is imperative to determine the amount of fracture displacement (particularly fracture depression) (see **Fig. 3**; **Figs. 4** and **5**). Given the significant role of the tibial plateau in weight bearing, as little as 2 to 3 mm of displacement is an indication for operative repair. A variety of surgical options may be used to repair this injury, including external fixators, open reduction, and arthroscopic techniques.[157,158] Although the physical examination is often limited by pain, it is important to fully evaluate the injured extremity because compartment syndrome is common with tibial plateau fractures.[159,160] Concurrent ligamentous injuries are also seen with tibial plateau fractures; typically the collateral ligament opposite the fracture is injured. Meniscal injuries and knee dislocations have also been associated with tibial plateau fractures.[107,161] MRI is the preferred imaging modality if multiple associated injuries are suspected, but CT only misses 2% of ligamentous injuries associated with tibial plateau fractures.[162] Any patient with a tibial plateau fracture should be seen by orthopedics in the ED.

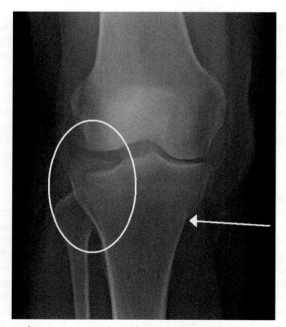

Fig. 4. Tibial plateau fracture is noted on this AP radiograph. The white circle shows the intraarticular fracture with depression of the medial plateau, whereas the white arrow denotes extension of the fracture along the medial cortex. (Photo by James Heilman. From Wikimedia Commons. Available at: https://commons.wikimedia.org/wiki/File:TibPlateauBadMark.png.)

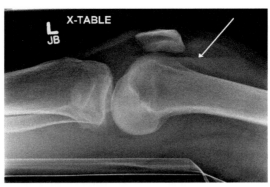

Fig. 5. Lipohemarthrosis (*white arrow*) is noted on this lateral radiograph. (Photo by James Heilman, MD. From Wikimedia Commons: https://commons.wikimedia.org/wiki/File: TibPlateauBadMark.png.)

SUMMARY

Knee injuries are seen on a daily basis by EPs. Use of a systematic approach to the knee examination and imaging studies allow EPs to properly manage these injuries and maximize patient outcomes.

REFERENCES

1. Gage BE, McIlvain NM, Collins CL, et al. Epidemiology of 6.6 million knee injuries presenting to United States emergency departments from 1999 through 2008. Acad Emerg Med 2012;19(4):378–85.
2. Maynard MJ, Deng X, Wickiewicz TL, et al. The popliteofibular ligament. Rediscovery of a key element in posterolateral stability. Am J Sports Med 1996;24(3): 311–6.
3. Seebacher JR, Inglis AE, Marshall JL, et al. The structure of the posterolateral aspect of the knee. J Bone Joint Surg Am 1982;64(4):536–41.
4. Watanabe Y, Moriya H, Takahashi K, et al. Functional anatomy of the posterolateral structures of the knee. Arthroscopy 1993;9(1):57–62.
5. Gollehon DL, Torzilli PA, Warren RF. The role of the posterolateral and cruciate ligaments in the stability of the human knee. A biomechanical study. J Bone Joint Surg Am 1987;69(2):233–42.
6. Hughston JC, Jacobson KE. Chronic posterolateral rotatory instability of the knee. J Bone Joint Surg Am 1985;67(3):351–9.
7. Vinson EN, Major NM, Helms CA. The posterolateral corner of the knee. AJR Am J Roentgenol 2008;190:449–58.
8. Maffulli N, Binfield PM, King JB, et al. Acute haemarthrosis of the knee in athletes A prospective study of 106 cases. J Bone Joint Surg Br 1993;75(6):945–9.
9. Noyes FR, Paulos L, Mooar LA, et al. Knee sprains and acute knee hemarthrosis: misdiagnosis of anterior cruciate ligament tears. Phys Ther 1980;60(12): 1596–601.
10. Hardaker WT Jr, Garrett WE Jr, Bassett FH 3rd. Evaluation of acute traumatic hemarthrosis of the knee joint. South Med J 1990;83(6):640–4.
11. Smith TO, Daview L, O'Driscoll ML, et al. An evaluation of the clinical tests and outcome measures used to assess patellar instability. Knee 2008;15(4):255–62.

12. Guillodo Y, Rannou N, Dubrana F, et al. Diagnosis of anterior cruciate ligament rupture in an emergency department. J Trauma 2009;65(5):1078–82.
13. Torg JS, Conrad W, Kalen V. Clinical diagnosis of anterior cruciate ligament instability in the athlete. Am J Sports Med 1976;4(2):84–93.
14. Jain DK, Amaravati R, Sharma G. Evaluation of the clinical signs of anterior cruciate ligament and meniscal injuries. Indian J Orthop 2009;43(4):375–8.
15. Benjaminse A, Gokeler A, van der Schans CP. Clinical diagnosis of an anterior cruciate ligament rupture: a meta-analysis. J Orthop Sports Phys Ther 2006; 36(5):267–88.
16. Solomon DH, Simel DL, Bates DW, et al. The rational clinical examination Does this patient have a torn meniscus or ligament of the knee? Value of the physical examination. JAMA 2001;286(13):1610–20.
17. Griffith CJ, LaPrade RF, Johansen S, et al. Medial knee injury: Part 1, static function of the individual components of the main medial knee structures. Am J Sports Med 2009;37(9):1762–70.
18. Wijdicks CA, Griffith CJ, LaPrade RF, et al. Medial knee injury: Part 2, load sharing between the posterior oblique ligament and superficial medial collateral ligament. Am J Sports Med 2009;37(9):1771–6.
19. Hughston JC, Norwood LA Jr. The posterolateral drawer test and external rotational recurvatum test for posterolateral rotatory instability of the knee. Clin Orthop Relat Res 1980;(147):82–7.
20. Konan S, Rayan F, Haddad FS. Do physical diagnostic tests accurately detect meniscal tears? Knee Surg Sports Traumatol Arthrosc 2009;17(7):806–11.
21. Garavaglia G, Lubbeke A, Dubois-Ferriere V, et al. Accuracy of stress radiography techniques in grading isolated and combined posterior knee injuries: A cadaveric study. Am J Sports Med 2007;35(12):2051–6.
22. Garofalo R, Fanelli GC, Cikes A, et al. Stress radiography and posterior pathological laxity of knee: Comparison between two different techniques. Knee 2009; 16(4):251–5.
23. Covey DC. Injuries of the posterolateral corner of the knee. J Bone Joint Surg Am 2001;83-A(1):106–18.
24. Albtoush OM, Horger M, Springer F, et al. Avulsion fracture of the medial collateral ligament association with Segond fracture. Clin Imaging 2019;53:32–4.
25. Kaplan PA, Walker CW, Kilcoyne RF, et al. Occult fracture patterns of the knee associated with anterior cruciate ligament tears: assessment with MR imaging. Radiology 1992;183(3):835–8.
26. Nawata K, Teshima R, Suzuki T. Osseous lesions associated with anterior cruciate ligament injuries Assessment by magnetic resonance imaging at various periods after injuries. Arch Orthop Trauma Surg 1993;113(1):1–4.
27. Harish S, O'Donnell P, Connell D, et al. Imaging of the posterolateral corner of the knee. Clin Radiol 2006;61:457–66.
28. Wang JC, Shapiro MS. Pellegrini-Stieda syndrome. Am J Orthop (Belle Mead NJ) 1995;24(6):493–7.
29. McAnally JL, Southam SL, Mlady GW. New thoughts on the origin of the pellegrini-stieda: The association of PCL injury and medial femoral epicondylar periosteal stripping. Skeletal Radiol 2009;38(2):193–8.
30. Tajima G, Nozaki M, Iriuchishima T, et al. Morphology of the tibial insertion of the posterior cruciate ligament. J Bone Joint Surg Am 2009;91(4):859–66.
31. Lorenz S, Elser F, Brucker PU, et al. Radiological evaluation of the anterolateral and posteromedial bundle insertion sites of the posterior cruciate ligament. Knee Surg Sports Traumatol Arthrosc 2009;17(6):683–90.

32. Blankenbaker DG, De Smet AA. The role of ultrasound in the evaluation of sports injuries of the lower extremities. Clin Sports Med 2006;25(4):867–97.
33. Finlay K, Friedman L. Ultrasonography of the lower extremity. Orthop Clin North Am 2006;37(3):245–75, v.
34. Jacobson JA. Musculoskeletal ultrasound and MRI: which do I choose? Semin Musculoskelet Radiol 2005;9(2):135–49.
35. Kaplan PA, Matamoros A Jr, Anderson JC. Sonography of the musculoskeletal system. AJR Am J Roentgenol 1990;155(2):237–45.
36. Palm HG, Bergenthal G, Ehry P, et al. Functional ultrasonography in the diagnosis of acute anterior cruciate ligament injuries: A field study. Knee 2009; 16(6):441–6.
37. Sorrentino F, Iovane A, Nicosia A, et al. Role of high-resolution ultrasonography without and with real-time spatial compound imaging in evaluating the injured posterior cruciate ligament: Preliminary study. Radiol Med 2009;114(2):312–20.
38. Karabay N, Sugun TS, Toros T. Ultrasonographic diagnosis of the posterior cruciate ligament injury in a 4-year old child: A case report. Emerg Radiol 2009; 16(5):415–7.
39. Barker RP, Lee JC, Healy JC. Normal sonographic anatomy of the posterolateral corner of the knee. AJR Am J Roentgenol 2009;192:73–9.
40. Shanbhogue AK, Sandhu MS, Singh P, et al. Real time spatial compound ultrasound in the evaluation of meniscal injuries: a comparison study with conventional ultrasound and MRI. Knee 2009;16(3):191–5.
41. Shetty AA, Tindall AJ, James KD, et al. Accuracy of hand-held ultrasound scanning in detecting meniscal tears. J Bone Joint Surg Br 2008;90(8):1045–8.
42. Venkatanarasimha N, Kamath A, Mukherjee K, et al. Potential pitfalls of a double PCL sign. Skeletal Radiol 2009;38(8):735–9.
43. Laundre BJ, Collins MS, Bond JR, et al. MRI accuracy for tears of the posterior horn of the lateral meniscus in patients with acute anterior cruciate ligament injury and the clinical relevance of missed tears. AJR Am J Roentgenol 2009; 193(2):515–23.
44. Krampla W, Roesel M, Svoboda K, et al. MRI of the knee: How do field strength and radiologist's experience influence diagnostic accuracy and interobserver correlation in assessing chondral and meniscal lesions and the integrity of the anterior cruciate ligament? Eur Radiol 2009;19(6):1519–28.
45. Gianotti SM, Marshall SW, Hume PA, et al. Incidence of anterior cruciate ligament injury and other knee ligament injuries: a national population-based study. J Sci Med Sport 2009;12(6):622–7.
46. Clayton RA, Court-Brown CM. The epidemiology of musculoskeletal tendinous and ligamentous injuries. Injury 2008;39(12):1338–44.
47. Agel J, Arendt EA, Bershadsky B. Anterior cruciate ligament injury in national collegiate athletic association basketball and soccer: a 13-year review. Am J Sports Med 2005;33(4):524–30.
48. Ireland ML. Anterior cruciate ligament injury in female athletes: epidemiology. J Athl Train 1999;34(2):150–4.
49. Mihata LC, Beutler AI, Boden BP. Comparing the incidence of anterior cruciate ligament injury in collegiate lacrosse, soccer, and basketball players: implications for anterior cruciate ligament mechanism and prevention. Am J Sports Med 2006;34(6):899–904.
50. Arendt EA, Agel J, Dick R. Anterior cruciate ligament injury patterns among collegiate men and women. J Athl Train 1999;34(2):86–92.

51. MARS Group, Wright RW, Huston LJ, Spindler KP, et al. Descriptive epidemiology of the Multicenter ACL Revision Study (MARS) cohort. Am J Sports Med 2010;38(10):1979–86.

52. Davies H, Tietjens B, Van Sterkenburg M, et al. Anterior cruciate ligament injuries in snowboarders: A quadriceps-induced injury. Knee Surg Sports Traumatol Arthrosc 2009;17(9):1048–51.

53. Behairy NH, Dorgham MA, Khaled SA. Accuracy of routine magnetic resonance imaging in meniscal and ligamentous injuries of the knee: Comparison with arthroscopy. Int Orthop 2009;33(4):961–7.

54. Kheder EM, Abd El-Bagi ME, El-Hosan MH. Anterior cruciate ligament graft tear. primary and secondary magnetic resonance signs. Saudi Med J 2009;30(4): 465–71.

55. Wang J, Wu H, Dong F, et al. The role of ultrasonography in the diagnosis of anterior cruciate ligament injury: A systematic review and meta-analysis. Eur J Sport Sci 2018;18(4):579–86.

56. Shelbourne KD, Benner RW. Correlation of joint line tenderness and meniscus pathology in patients with subacute and chronic anterior cruciate ligament injuries. J Knee Surg 2009;22(3):187–90.

57. Trojani C, Sane JC, Coste JS, et al. Four-strand hamstring tendon autograft for ACL reconstruction in patients aged 50 years or older. Orthop Traumatol Surg Res 2009;95(1):22–7.

58. Cohen M, Ferretti M, Quarteiro M, et al. Transphyseal anterior cruciate ligament reconstruction in patients with open physes. Arthroscopy 2009;25(8):831–8.

59. Henry J, Chotel F, Chouteau J, et al. Rupture of the anterior cruciate ligament in children: Early reconstruction with open physes or delayed reconstruction to skeletal maturity? Knee Surg Sports Traumatol Arthrosc 2009;17(7):748–55.

60. Duquin TR, Wind WM, Fineberg MS, et al. Current trends in anterior cruciate ligament reconstruction. J Knee Surg 2009;22(1):7–12.

61. Andersson D, Samuelsson K, Karlsson J. Treatment of anterior cruciate ligament injuries with special reference to surgical technique and rehabilitation: An assessment of randomized controlled trials. Arthroscopy 2009;25(6):653–85.

62. Cohen SB, Yucha DT, Ciccotti MC, et al. Factors affecting patient selection of graft type in anterior cruciate ligament reconstruction. Arthroscopy 2009; 25(9):1006–10.

63. Sun K, Tian SQ, Zhang JH, et al. Anterior cruciate ligament reconstruction with bone-patellar tendon-bone autograft versus allograft. Arthroscopy 2009;25(7): 750–9.

64. Piva SR, Clinds JD, Klucinec BM, et al. Patella fracture during rehabilitation after bone-patellar tendon-bone anterior cruciate ligament reconstruction: 2 case reports. J Orthop Sports Phys Ther 2009;39(4):278–86.

65. Mouzopoulos G, Fotopoulos VC, Tzurbakis M. Septic knee arthritis following ACL reconstruction: A systematic review. Knee Surg Sports Traumatol Arthrosc 2009;17(9):1033–42.

66. Wang C, Ao Y, Wang J, et al. Septic arthritis after arthroscopic anterior cruciate ligament reconstruction: A retrospective analysis of incidence, presentation, treatment, and cause. Arthroscopy 2009;25(3):243–9.

67. Nag HL, Negoi DS, Nataraj AR, et al. Tubercular infection after arthroscopic anterior cruciate ligament reconstruction. Arthroscopy 2009;25(2):131–6.

68. Van de Velde SK, DeFrate LE, Gill TJ, et al. The effect of anterior cruciate ligament deficiency on the in vivo elongation of the medial and lateral collateral ligaments. Am J Sports Med 2007;35(2):294–300.

69. Tayton E, Verma R, Higgins B, et al. A correlation of time with meniscal tears in anterior cruciate ligament deficiency; stratifying the risk of surgical delay. Knee Surg Sports Traumatol Arthrosc 2009;17(1):30–4.

70. Yoo JC, Ahn JH, Lee SH, et al. Increasing incidence of medial meniscal tears in nonoperatively treated anterior cruciate ligament insufficiency patients documented by serial magnetic resonance imaging studies. Am J Sports Med 2009;37(8):1478–83.

71. Louboutin H, Debarge R, Richou J, et al. Osteoarthritis in patients with anterior cruciate ligament rupture: A review of risk factors. Knee 2009;16(4):239–44.

72. Oiestad BE, Engebretsen L, Storheim K, et al. Knee osteoarthritis after anterior cruciate ligament injury: A systematic review. Am J Sports Med 2009;37(7):1434–43.

73. Palmieri-Smith RM, Thomas AC. A neuromuscular mechanism of posttraumatic osteoarthritis associated with ACL injury. Exerc Sport Sci Rev 2009;37(3):147–53.

74. Brophy RH, Gill CS, Lyman S, et al. Effect of anterior cruciate ligament reconstruction and meniscectomy and length of career in national football league athletes: A case control study. Am J Sports Med 2009;37(11):2102–7.

75. Beaufils P, Hulet C, Dhenain M, et al. Clinical practice guidelines for the management of meniscal lesions and isolated lesions of the anterior cruciate ligament of the knee in adults. Orthop Traumatol Surg Res 2009;95(6):437–42.

76. Hugston JC, Andrews JR, Cross MJ, et al. Classification of knee ligament instabilities. part II. the lateral compartment. J Bone Joint Surg Am 1976;58(2):173–9.

77. Ramos LA, de Carvalho RT, Cohen M, et al. Anatomic relation between the posterior cruciate ligament and the joint capsule. Arthroscopy 2008;24(12):1367–72.

78. Hermans S, Corten K, Bellemans J. Long-term results of isolated anterolateral bundle reconstructions of the posterior cruciate ligament: A 6- to 12- year follow-up study. Am J Sports Med 2009;37(8):1499–507.

79. Kim SJ, Kim TE, Jo SB, et al. Comparison of the clinical results of three posterior cruciate ligament reconstruction techniques. J Bone Joint Surg Am 2009;91(9):2543–9.

80. Matava MJ, Ellis E, Gruber B. Surgical treatment of posterior cruciate ligament tears: An evolving technique. J Am Acad Orthop Surg 2009;17(7):435–46.

81. McAllister DR, Miller MD, Sekiya JK, et al. Posterior cruciate ligament biomechanics and options for surgical treatment. Instr Course Lect 2009;58:377–88.

82. Van de Velde SK, Bingham JT, Gill TJ, et al. Analysis of tibiofemoral cartilage deformation in the posterior cruciate ligament-deficient knee. J Bone Joint Surg Am 2009;91(9):167–75.

83. Kozanek M, Fu EC, Van de Velde SK, et al. Posterolateral structures of the knee in posterior cruciate ligament deficiency. Am J Sports Med 2009;37(3):534–41.

84. Patel SC, Parker DA. Isolated rupture of the lateral collateral ligament during youga practice: A case report. J Orthop Surg 2008;16(3):378–80.

85. Chen FS, Rokito AS, Pitman ML. Acute and chronic posterolateral rotatory instability of the knee. J Am Acad Orthop Surg 2000;8:97–110.

86. O'Brien SJ, Warren RF, Pavlov H, et al. Reconstruction of the chronically insufficient anterior cruciate ligament with the central third of the patellar ligament. J Bone Joint Surg Am 1991;73:278–86.

87. Cooper JM, McAndrews PT, LaPrade RF. Posterolateral corner injuries of the knee: Anatomy, diagnosis, and treatment. Sports Med Arthrosc Rev 2006;14(4):213–20.

88. Malone AA, Dowd GSE, Saifuddin A. Injuries of the posterior cruciate ligament and posterolateral corner of the knee. Injury 2006;37:485–501.

89. Stannard JP, Brown SL, Farris RC, et al. The posterolateral corner of the knee: Repair versus reconstruction. Am J Sports Med 2005;33(6):881–8.

90. Apsingi S, Nguyen T, Bull AM, et al. A comparison of modified larson and 'anatomic' posterolateral corner reconstructions in knees with combined PCL and posterolateral corner deficiency. Knee Surg Sports Traumatol Arthrosc 2009;17(3):305–12.

91. Markolf KL, Graves BR, Sigward SM, et al. How well do anatomical reconstructions of the posterolateral corner restore varus stability to the posterior cruciate ligament-reconstructed knee? Am J Sports Med 2007;35(7):1117–22.

92. Shi SY, Ying XZ, Zheng Q, et al. Isometric reconstruction of the posterolateral corner of the knee. Acta Orthop Belg 2009;75(4):504–11.

93. Stannard JP, Brown SL, Robinson JT, et al. Reconstruction of the posterolateral corner of the knee. Arthroscopy 2005;21(9):1051–9.

94. Botomley N, Williams A, Birch R, et al. Displacement of the common peroneal nerve in posterolateral corner injuries of the knee. J Bone Joint Surg Br 2005; 87(9):1225–6.

95. Bushnell BD, Bitting SS, Crain JM, et al. Treatment of magnetic resonance imaging-documented isolated grade III lateral collateral ligament injuries in national football league athletes. Am J Sports Med 2010;38(1):86–91.

96. Chen YH, Carrino JA, Raman SP, et al. Atraumatic lateral collateral ligament complex signal abnormalities by magnetic resonance imaging in patients with osteoarthrosis of the knee. J Comput Assist Tomogr 2008;32(6):982–6.

97. LaPrade RF, Heikes C, Bakker AJ, et al. The reproducibility and repeatability of varus stress radiographs in the assessment of isolated fibular collateral ligament and grade-III posterolateral knee injuries. an in vitro biomechanical study. J Bone Joint Surg Am 2008;90(10):2069–76.

98. Coobs BR, LaPrade RF, Griffith CJ, et al. Biomechanical analysis of an isolated fibular (lateral) collateral ligament reconstruction using an autogenous semitendinous graft. Am J Sports Med 2007;35(9):521–7.

99. Miyamoto RG, Bosco JA, Sherman OH. Treatment of medial collateral ligament injuries. J Am Acad Orthop Surg 2009;17(3):152–61.

100. Thornton GM, Johnson JC, Maser RV, et al. Strength of medial structures of the knee joint are decreased by isolated injury to the medial collateral ligament and subsequent joint immobilization. J Orthop Res 2005;23:1191–8.

101. Sparrow KJ, Finucand SD, Owen JR, et al. The effects of low-intensity ultrasound on medial collateral ligament healing in the rabbit model. Am J Sports Med 2005;33:1048–56.

102. Petersen W, Laprell H. Combined injuries of the medial collateral ligament and the anterior cruciate ligament Early ACL reconstruction versus late ACL reconstruction. Arch Orthop Trauma Surg 1999;119(5–6):258–62.

103. Noyes FR, Barber-Westin SD. The treatment of acute combined ruptures of the anterior cruciate and medial ligaments of the knee. Am J Sports Med 1995; 23(4):380–9.

104. Kovachevich R, Shah JP, Arens AM, et al. Operative management of the medial collateral ligament in the multi-ligament injured knee: an evidence-based systematic review. Knee Surg Sports Traumatol Arthrosc 2009;17(7):823–9.

105. Theivendran K, Lever CJ, Hart WJ. Good result after surgical treatment of pellegrini-stieda syndrome. Knee Surg Sports Traumatol Arthrosc 2009;17(10): 1231–3.

106. Englund M, Guermazi A, Gale D, et al. Incidental meniscal findings on knee MRI in middle-aged and elderly persons. N Engl J Med 2008;359(11):1108–15.

107. Mustonen AOT, Koivikko MP, Lindhal J, et al. MRI of acute meniscal injury associated with tibial plateau fractures: Prevalence, type, and location. AJR Am J Roentgenol 2008;191:1002–9.

108. Gerbino P, Nielson JH. Knee injuries. In: Frontera WR, editor. Clinical sports medicine, medical management and rehabilitation. Philadelphia: Saunders/Elsevier; 2007. p. 421–39.

109. Englund M, Guermazi A, Roemer FW, et al. Meniscal tear in knees without surgery and the development of radiographic osteoarthritis among middle-aged and elderly persons: The multicenter osteoarthritis study. Arthritis Rheum 2009;60(3):831–9.

110. Kramer DE, Micheli LJ. Meniscal tears and discoid meniscus in children: diagnosis and treatment. J Am Acad Orthop Surg 2009;17(11):698–707.

111. Peltola EK, Lindahl J, Hietaranta H, et al. Knee dislocation in overweight patients. AJR Am J Roentgenol 2009;192:101–6.

112. Bui KL, Ilaslan H, Parker RD, et al. Knee dislocations: A magnetic resonance imaging study correlated with clinical and operative findings. Skeletal Radiol 2008; 37(7):653–61.

113. Robertson A, Nutton RW, Keating JF. Dislocation of the knee. J Bone Joint Surg Br 2006;88:706–11.

114. Seroyer ST, Musahl V, Harner CD. Management of the acute knee dislocation: The pittsburgh experience. Injury 2008;39:710–8.

115. Harb A, Lincold D, Michaelson J. The MR dimple sign in irreducible posterolateral knee dislocations. Skeletal Radiol 2009;38(11):1111–4.

116. Levy BA, Fanelli GC, Whelan DB, et al. Controversies in the treatment of knee dislocations and multiligament reconstruction. J Am Acad Orthop Surg 2009; 17(4):197–206.

117. Zaffagnini S, Iacono F, LoPresti M, et al. A new hinged dynamic distractor for immediate mobilization after knee dislocations: Technical note. Arch Orthop Trauma Surg 2008;128(11):1233–7.

118. Medvecky MJ, Zazulak BT, Hewett TE. A multidisciplinary approach to the evaluation, reconstruction and rehabilitation of the multi-ligament injured athlete. Sports Med 2007;37(2):169–87.

119. Nicandri GT, Dunbar RP, Wahl CJ. Are evidence-based protocols which identify vascular injury associated with knee dislocation underutilized? Knee Surg Sports Traumatol Arthrosc 2010;18(8):1005–12.

120. Mills WJ, Barei DP, McNair P. The value of the ankle-brachial index for diagnosing arterial injury after knee dislocation: A prospective study. J Trauma 2004;56:1261–5.

121. Johnson ME, Foster L, DeLee JC. Neurologic and vascular injuries associated with knee ligament injuries. Am J Sports Med 2008;36(12):2448–62.

122. Chapman J, Pallin D. Popliteal air following penetrating trauma. Am J Emerg Med 2006;24(5):638–9.

123. Miller-Thomas MM, West OC, Cohen AM. Diagnosing traumatic arterial injury in the extremities with CT angiography: pearls and pitfalls. Radiographics 2005; 25(Suppl 1):S133–42.

124. Peng PD, Spain DA, Tataria M, et al. CT angiography effectively evaluates extremity vascular trauma. Am Surg 2008;74(2):103–7.

125. Abou-Sayed H, Berger DL. Blunt lower-extremity trauma and popliteal artery injuries: revisiting the case for selective arteriography. Arch Surg 2002;137(5): 585–9.
126. Nicandri GT, Chamberlain AM, Wahl CJ. Practical management of knee dislocations: a selective angiography protocol to detect limb-threatening vascular injuries. Clin J Sport Med 2009;19(2):125–9.
127. Gaitini D, Razi NB, Ghersin E, et al. Sonographic evaluation of vascular injuries. J Ultrasound Med 2008;27:95–107.
128. Niall DM, Nutton RW, Keating JF. Palsy of the common peroneal nerve after traumatic dislocation of the knee. J Bone Joint Surg Br 2005;87:664–7.
129. Bin SI, Nam TS. Surgical outcome of 2-stage management of multiple knee ligament injuries after knee dislocation. Arthroscopy 2007;23(10):1066–72.
130. Fanelli GC, Edson CJ, Reinheimer KN. Evaluation and treatment of the multiligament-injured knee. Instr Course Lect 2009;58:389–95.
131. Ibrahim SA, Ahmad FH, Salah M, et al. Surgical management of traumatic knee dislocation. Arthroscopy 2008;24(2):178–87.
132. Levy BA, Dajani KA, Whelan DB, et al. Decision making in the multiligament-injured knee: An evidence-based systematic review. Arthroscopy 2009;25(4): 430–8.
133. Robinson RJ, Barron DA, Grainger AJ, et al. Wii knee. Emerg Radiol 2008;15(4): 255–7.
134. Felus J, Kowalczyk B, Lejman T. Sonographic evaluation of the injuries after traumatic patellar dislocation in adolescents. J Pediatr Orthop 2008;28(4):397–402.
135. Stefancin JJ, Parker RD. First-time traumatic patellar dislocation: a systematic review. Clin Orthop Relat Res 2007;455:93–101.
136. Guerrero P, Li X, Patel K, et al. Medial patellofemoral ligament injury patterns and associated pathology in lateral patella dislocation: An MRI study. Sports Med Arthrosc Rehabil Ther Technol 2009;1(1):17.
137. Camanho GL, Viegas Ade C, Bitar AC, et al. Conservative versus surgical treatment for repair of the medial patellofemoral ligament in acute dislocations of the patella. Arthroscopy 2009;25(6):620–5.
138. Sillanpaa PJ, Mattila VM, Maenpaa H, et al. Treatment with and without initial stabilizing surgery for primary traumatic patellar dislocation. A prospective randomized study. J Bone Joint Surg Am 2009;91:263–73.
139. Colvin AC, West RV. Patellar instability. J Bone Joint Surg Am 2008;90:2751–62.
140. Panagopoulos A, van Niekerk L, Triantafillopoulos IK. MPFL reconstruction for recurrent patella dislocation: A new surgical technique and review of the literature. Int J Sports Med 2008;29(5):359–65.
141. Ronga M, Oliva F, Longo UG, et al. Isolated medial patellofemoral ligament reconstruction for recurrent patellar dislocation. Am J Sports Med 2009;37(9): 1735–42.
142. Nietosvaara Y, Paukku R, Palmu S, et al. Acute patellar dislocation in children and adolescents. surgical technique. J Bone Joint Surg Am 2009;91(Supp 2): 139–45.
143. Atkinson PJ2001, Haut RC. Impact responses of the flexed human knee using a deformable impact interface. J Biomech Eng 2001;123(3):205–11.
144. Brostrom A. Fracture of the patella. A study of 422 patellar fractures. Acta Orthop Scand Suppl 1972;143:1–80.
145. Pritchett JW. Nonoperative treatment of widely displaced patella fractures. Am J Knee Surg 1997;10(3):145–7 [discussion: 147–8].

146. Lindor RA, Homme J. Patellar fracture with sleeve avulsion. N Engl J Med 2016; 375(24):e49.
147. Sullivan S, Maskell K, Knutson T. Patellar sleeve fracture. West J Emerg Med 2014;15(7):883–4.
148. Pandya NK, Zgonis M, Ahn J, et al. Patellar tendon rupture as a manifestation of lyme disease. Am J Orthop 2008;37(9):E167–70.
149. Jolles BM, Garofalo R, Gillain L, et al. New clinical test in diagnosing quadriceps tendon rupture. Ann R Coll Surg Engl 2007;89:259–61.
150. Heyde CE, Mahlfeld K, Stahel PF, et al. Ultrasonography as a reliable diagnostic tool in old quadriceps tendon ruptures: A prospective multicentre study. Knee Surg Sports Traumatol Arthrosc 2005;13(7):564–8.
151. LaRocco BG, Zlupko G, Sierzenski P. Ultrasound diagnosis of quadriceps tendon rupture. J Emerg Med 2008;35(3):293–5.
152. McKinney B, Cherney S, Penna J. Intra-articular knee injuries in patients with knee extensor mechanism ruptures. Knee Surg Sports Traumatol Arthrosc 2008;16(7):633–8.
153. Ramseier LE, Werner CML, Heinzelmann M. Quadriceps and patellar tendon rupture. Injury 2006;37:516–9.
154. Berkson EM, Virkus WW. High-energy tibial plateau fractures. J Am Acad Orthop Surg 2006;14(1):20–31.
155. Rippey J. Ultrasound for knee effusion: lipohaemarthrosis and tibial plateau fracture. Australas J Ultrasound Med 2015;17(4):159–66.
156. McEnery KW, Wilson AJ, Pilgram TK, et al. Fractures of the tibial plateau: value of spiral CT coronal plane reconstructions for detecting displacement in vitro. AJR Am J Roentgenol 1994;163(5):1177–81.
157. Duan XJ, Yang L, Guo L, et al. Arthroscopically assisted treatment for schatzker type I-V tibial plateau fractures. Chin J Traumatol 2008;11(5):288–92.
158. Papagelopoulos PJ, Partsinevelos AA, Themistocelous GS, et al. Complications after tibia plateau fracture surgery. Injury 2006;17:475–84.
159. Badhe S, Baiju D, Elliot R, et al. The 'silent' compartment syndrome. Injury 2009; 40(2):1879.
160. Stark E, stucken C, Trainer G, et al. Compartment syndrome in schatzker type VI plateau fractures and medial condylar fracture-dislocations treated with temporary external fixation. J Orthop Trauma 2009;23(7):502–6.
161. Abdel-Hamid MZ, Chang CH, Chan YS, et al. Arthroscopic evaluation of soft tissue injuries in tibial plateau fractures: Retrospective analysis of 98 cases. Arthroscopy 2006;22(6):669–75.
162. Mui LW, Engelsohn E, Umans H. Comparison of CT and MRI in patients with tibial plateau fracture: Can CT findings predict ligament tear or meniscal injury? Skeletal Radiol 2007;36(2):145–51.

The Emergent Evaluation and Treatment of Neck and Back Pain

Brian N. Corwell, MD[a,b],*, Natalie L. Davis, MD, MMSc[c]

KEYWORDS

- Epidural abscess • Cauda equina syndrome • Spinal stenosis
- Acute transverse myelitis • Vertebral osteomyelitis

KEY POINTS

- Most causes of neck and back pain are nonspecific or mechanical, but the goal of the emergency department (ED) assessment is to maintain a high index of suspicion for those rare emergent disorders that require prompt diagnosis and treatment to optimize outcomes.
- The presence of red flags on the history and examination should supplement, not replace, clinical judgment regarding further work-up in the ED; avoid focusing on a single feature in isolation, and instead combine red flags with additional clinical and examination findings to more accurately determine the likelihood of serious underlying disease.
- Blind diagnostic testing (so-called shotgunning) can lead to unnecessary therapies and interventions, so in the absence of serious disorders, should not be part of the diagnostic evaluation in the ED. Adhere to validated clinical decision rules when considering ordering imaging tests.
- If concern for spinal emergency exists (epidural compression syndrome, neoplasm, or spinal infection), obtain immediate advanced imaging, ideally MRI, and consult a spine surgeon.
- Given the overall good prognosis for recovery, conservative therapies are preferred for most patients with nonemergent pain.

Disclosure: The authors have no relationship with a commercial company that has a direct financial interest in subject matter or materials discussed in this article or with a company making a competing product. The authors have no relevant financial disclosures or conflicts of interest.

[a] Department of Emergency Medicine, University of Maryland School of Medicine, 110 S. Paca Street, 6th Floor, Suite 200, Baltimore, MD 21201, USA; [b] Department of Orthopaedics, University of Maryland School of Medicine, Baltimore, MD, USA; [c] Department of Pediatrics, University of Maryland School of Medicine, 110 S. Paca Street, 8th Floor, Baltimore, MD 21201, USA
* Corresponding author. Department of Emergency Medicine, 110 S. Paca Street, 6th Floor, Suite 200, Baltimore, MD 21201.
E-mail address: bcorwell@som.umaryland.edu

Emerg Med Clin N Am 38 (2020) 167–191
https://doi.org/10.1016/j.emc.2019.09.007
0733-8627/20/© 2019 Elsevier Inc. All rights reserved.

INTRODUCTION

Neck and back pain are two of the leading causes of disability worldwide. At some point in their lives, up to 60% of the population experience neck pain,[1] whereas up to 90% experience back pain. Back pain is the most common musculoskeletal complaint in the emergency department (ED). Neck and back pain lasting less than 6 weeks is termed acute pain. Most neck/back pain presenting to the ED is mechanical, lacking a specific concerning disorder (eg, cord compression, infection) and resolves without intervention in that time frame. In the ED, approximately 1 in 50 patients with back pain require hospitalization.[2] Origins of pain in the neck and back share similar mechanisms. Multiple conditions can occur together, making identification of a single cause challenging. Pain lasting greater than 3 months is defined as chronic pain and often results in persistence or recurrence within the next year.[3,4] Note that neck and back pain are symptoms rather than diseases that have numerous causes both benign and emergent. Pain may have mechanical, infectious, inflammatory, vascular, and visceral causes (**Table 1**). Thorough history and examination, with attention to concerning red flags (**Table 2**), are necessary for each patient in order to identify those at risk of more serious conditions that require further work-up and treatment. It is often impossible to determine the exact cause of the patient's neck or back pain. In the ED, the focus of the history and examination is to exclude those serious cases that do require identification and emergent treatment. Once excluded, the ED management of those nonemergent conditions consists of reassurance, pain control, and directing appropriate outpatient follow-up.

HISTORY

Most causes are nonspecific or mechanical, but the goal of the ED assessment is to identify rare emergent disorders that require prompt diagnosis and treatment to optimize outcomes. Considering an emergent cause is the key to diagnosis, and identifying key risk factors may move this higher on the differential, but be aware that few in isolation have useful diagnostic accuracy.[5]

Table 1
Causes of neck and back pain

Mechanical	Infectious	Malignancy	Visceral
• Muscle strain	• Epidural abscess	• Metastatic carcinoma	• Pelvic
• Intervertebral disc herniation	• Vertebral osteomyelitis	• Multiple myeloma	○ Endometriosis
• Osteoporosis	• Paraspinal abscess	• Leukemia	○ Pelvic inflammatory disease
• Ligamentous injury	• Spondylodiscitis	• Lymphoma	○ Prostatitis
• Spine curvature	Vascular	• Spinal cord tumor	• Myocardial ischemia
○ Lordosis	• Aortic dissection	Inflammatory	• Renal
○ Kyphosis	• AAA	• Osteoarthritis	○ Nephrolithiasis
• Spinal stenosis	Bone	• Psoriatic spondylitis	○ Pyelonephritis
• Spondylolisthesis	• Osteoid osteoma	• Ankylosing spondylitis	• GI
• Spondylolysis	• Fracture	• Reactive arthritis	○ Pancreatitis
• Facet joint arthritis		• Transverse myelitis	○ Cholecystitis
• Spondylosis			○ Perforated ulcer
			• Sickle cell crisis

Abbreviations: AAA, abdominal aortic aneurysm; GI, gastrointestinal.

Table 2
Red flags associated with neck and back pain

Red Flag	Pathologic Processes
Fevers/chills/night sweats	Infection Malignancy/tumor
Weight loss	Infection Malignancy/tumor
Recent bacterial infection (ie UTI, pneumonia, skin/ soft tissue infection)	Infection
Recent GU/GI procedures	Infection
Recent spinal surgery/ instrumentation	Infection
Pain >6 wk	Malignancy/tumor Infection Inflammatory Rheumatologic
History of malignancy	Malignancy/tumor
Morning stiffness	Ankylosing spondylitis (inflammatory back pain) Spondyloarthropathy
Pain that is severe or constant, occurs at night, is progressive, or interferes with activity	Malignancy/tumor Infection
Pain not relieved by rest, recumbency, or appropriate analgesic treatment	Malignancy/tumor Infection
Ripping/tearing sensation	Arterial dissection • Neck pain: carotid/vertebral dissection • Back pain: aortic dissection
IV drug use	Infection
Immunosuppression	Infection
Chronic corticosteroid	Infection Compression fracture
Pain worse with Valsalva, cough, sitting	Herniated disc (radiculopathy)
Down syndrome Rheumatoid arthritis	Atlantoaxial disruption/subluxation
Bowel or bladder dysfunction	Upper motor neuron disorder • Cord compression • Demyelinating process (ie, multiple sclerosis)
Sexual dysfunction	Cord compression
Severe, rapidly progressive neurologic deficit	Cord compression
Saddle anesthesia	Cord compression
Recent trauma	Fracture Spinal cord injury Ligamentous injury/disruption
Anterior neck pain	Myocardial ischemia/MI

(continued on next page)

Table 2 (continued)	
Red Flag	**Pathologic Processes**
<18 years old	Malignancy Infection Congenital defect (spina bifida) Spondylolysis Spondylolisthesis Osteoid osteoma Discitis
>50 years old	Malignancy Fracture Infection Extraspinal process (AAA, pancreatitis, MI) Spinal stenosis
Osteoporosis	Fracture
Associated chest or abdominal pain	Extraspinal process (AAA, aortic dissection, pancreatitis, MI)

Abbreviations: AAA, abdominal aortic aneurysm; GU, genitourinary; IV, intravenous; MI, myocardial infarction; UTI, urinary tract infection.

- Basing diagnostic work-up solely on the presence of a red flag leads to unnecessary diagnostic evaluations because most red flags are false-positives. For example, 80% of patients with low back pain (LBP) have at least 1 red flag present, but less than 1% have an emergent underlying disease.[6]
- The presence of red flags may raise the potential for, but does not predict the risk of, emergent causes.
  - Positive red flags should supplement, not replace, clinical judgment regarding further work-up in the ED.
  - The optimal approach in consideration of an emergent diagnosis is to avoid focusing on a single feature in isolation, and instead combine red flags with additional clinical and physical findings to more accurately determine the likelihood of a serious underlying disease.

When treating a patient with back pain, be sure to obtain a detailed history that addresses the red flags as noted in **Table 2**. Specific focus should be on onset, duration, severity, and associated neurologic symptoms (eg, weakness, sensory changes, bowel or bladder dysfunction, gait disturbance). **Table 3** highlights the typical signs and symptoms seen based on the nerve root involved.

A detailed physical examination needs to be completed, with particular attention to the neurologic examination (eg, gait, strength, sensory examination [particularly perineum sensation], reflexes). The physical examination should also look for signs of infection (eg, fever, rashes, septic emboli) and evidence of disorder outside the spinal canal (eg, abdominal aortic aneurysm, renal stones). Provocative testing (**Table 4**) should be performed in select patients.

DIAGNOSTIC TESTING

In general, if the history and physical examination (H&P) do not reveal any concerning findings for emergent disorder, no further testing is required. Testing is only needed if it will help guide specific management strategies. However, studies have shown

Table 3
Nerve root physiology and associated findings

Root	Associated Reflexes	Muscle Groups Innervated	Motor Weakness	Location of Pain	Sensory Deficits
C4	None	—	None	Upper-mid neck	Shoulder, cape distribution
C5	Deltoid Biceps Brachioradialis	Deltoid Supraspinatus Infraspinatus	Shoulder abduction, external shoulder rotation, elbow flexion	Neck Shoulder Scapula/interscapular region Anterior arm	Lateral Shoulder (over deltoid)
C6	Biceps Brachioradialis	Biceps brachii Brachialis Extensor carpi radialis longus and brevus	Elbow flexion Shoulder • External rotation • Abduction • Protraction Forearm • Supination • Pronation Wrist extension	Neck Shoulder Scapula/interscapular region Radial/lateral forearm Thumb and index finger	Radial/lateral forearm and hand Thumb and index finger
C7	Triceps Latissimus dorsi	Extensor carpi radialis longus and brevus Triceps brachii Flexor digitorum superficialis and profundus	Elbow extension Wrist (radial) extension Forearm pronation Wrist flexion	Lower neck Shoulder Scapula/interscapular Chest Forearm extensor surface Hand/middle finger	Palm, middle finger Can include parts of index, middle, and ring finger
C8	None	Triceps brachii	Wrist flexion Finger and thumb • Abduction • Adduction • Extension • Flexion	Lower neck Medial/ulnar forearm and hand Ring finger Little finger	Distal medial forearm to medial hand Ring finger Little finger

(continued on next page)

Table 3
(continued)

Root	Associated Reflexes	Muscle Groups Innervated	Motor Weakness	Location of Pain	Sensory Deficits
T1	None	Intrinsic muscles of hand Flexor digitorum superficialis and profundus Flexor policis longus Lumbricals, and interossei	Thumb abduction Distal thumb flexion Finger abduction and adduction	Neck Medial arm and forearm	Anterior arm and medial/ulnar forearm
L1–L3	None	Iliopsoas Adductor longus	Hip flexion (L2-3) Hip adductor (L3)	Back pain radiates to: • Groin (L1) • Anteromedial thigh (L2) • Anterior thigh to anterior leg (L3)	Anterior thigh
L4	Patellar	Vastus lateralis and medialis	Knee extension (quadriceps) Ankle inversion and dorsiflexion	Back pain radiates to anterior thigh to anterior leg	Medial lower leg/foot to medial surface great toe (not first web space)
L5	Semitendinosus/semimembranosus tendon	Extensor hallucis longus	Hip abduction Knee flexion Foot/ankle • Inversion • Eversion • Dorsiflexion Toe extension and flexion	Back radiating to buttock, lateral thigh and calf, dorsum foot, great toe	Lateral calf, dorsum foot, first web space (between great and second toe)
S1	Achilles tendon[a]	—	Hip extension Knee flexion Foot plantar flexion	Back radiating to buttock, lateral or posterior thigh, posterior calf, lateral or plantar foot	Posterior lower leg (calf) Lateral/plantar foot and ankle
S2-5	Bulbocavernosus (S2–S4) Anal wink (S2–S4)	—	Minimal weakness • Penile erection (S2–S4) • Rectal tone/retention (S2–S5) • Bladder dysfunction/retention (S2–S4)	Sacral/buttock pain radiates down posterior leg or into perineum	Medial buttock, perineal, perianal regions

[a] Ankle reflexes become increasingly absent with age, lost in nearly 50% of those more than 80 years old. This loss is usually symmetric, thus unilateral absence may signify disorder

Table 4
Provocative maneuvers

Provocative Maneuver	Description	Sensitivity/Specificity	Diagnosis
Lhermitte phenomenon	Forward neck flexion causes electric shock–like sensation in the neck, radiating down the spine and/or to the arms	Highly specific for compressive myelopathy (97%) Poor sensitivity (5%–15%) Positive test is helpful, but a negative test does not rule out myelopathy	Suggests lesion or compression of the cervical spinal cord (myelopathy) • Transverse myelitis • Cord compression caused by disc herniation, spondylosis, tumor, abscess • Multiple sclerosis

Spurling maneuver (neck compression test)
 	
Do not perform in patients who have potential cervical spine instability
	Performed by keeping the head in a neutral position and pressing down on the top of the head If this fails to reproduce the patient's pain, the procedure is repeated with the head extended and rotated and tilted to the affected side, followed by application of downward pressure on the head
	• Positive test
	  ○ Reproduction of symptoms (pain, paresthesias) beyond the shoulder toward the arm
	• Negative (nonspecific) test
	  ○ Reproduction of neck pain alone
		Highly specific for the presence of cervical root compression (89%–100%) Widely variable sensitivity (38%–97%). Positive test is helpful, but a negative test does not rule out radicular pain	Cervical radiculopathy

Shoulder abduction sign (abduction relief sign)	Patient raises symptomatic arm above head and rests hand on top of head
	• Positive test
	  ○ Pain is relieved (because of reducing tension on cervical root)
	  ○ Patient may also tilt head away from the painful side to relieve pain from radiculopathy
		Moderate to high specificity (85%) Low to moderate sensitivity (47%)	Cervical radiculopathy

(continued on next page)

Table 4 (continued)			
Provocative Maneuver	**Description**	**Sensitivity/Specificity**	**Diagnosis**
	• Negative test ○ Pain remains/worsens, more likely to be caused by shoulder disorder as opposed to cervical root disorder Can be taught as a therapeutic maneuver for pain relief in daily life		
Straight Leg Raise (SLR)	With patient supine and legs extended, clinician places 1 hand under ankle, other hand on top of knee to maintain leg extension (straight leg). Clinician lifts patient's leg by flexing at hip until pain elicited or end range reached • Positive test ○ Causes/reproduces radicular pain below the knee of the affected leg when the leg is increased between 30° and 70° • Negative test ○ Pain below 30°, above 70°, or with reproduction of pain only in the back, hamstring, or buttock region does not constitute a positive test Care should be taken that the patient is not actively helping in lifting the leg and that the knee remains straight throughout examination	Variable low-moderate specificity (11%–66%) Moderate to high sensitivity (72%–97%) Predictive value depends on pretest probability of radiculopathy High probability of radiculopathy: • PPV of 67%–89% • NPV of 33%–57% Low probability of radiculopathy (based on the absence of neurologic symptoms or sciatica) • PPV = 4%	Lumbar radiculopathy
Braggard sign	Following a positive SLR (see above), a further positive finding occurs if radicular symptoms (shooting pain, paresthesias) are elicited when the leg is then lowered until pain is eased and then the ipsilateral ankle is dorsiflexed	Moderate specificity (67%) Moderate sensitivity (70%) Moderate PPV (73%) and NPV (63%)	Lumbar radiculopathy

(continued on next page)

Table 4 *(continued)*			
Provocative Maneuver	**Description**	**Sensitivity/Specificity**	**Diagnosis**
Crossed SLR	During SLR, if pain is referred to the affected leg when the opposite asymptomatic leg is tested, this is positive test	High specificity (85%–100%) Low sensitivity (29%) PPV 79%–92%, NPV 22%–44%	Lumbar radiculopathy
Seated SLR (slump test)	Perform instead of SLR if patient is reluctant or unwilling to lie supine Patient sits at the edge of the examination table and slumps forward while flexing the neck and trunk, followed by knee extension and ankle dorsiflexion • Positive test reproduces radicular pain • Negative test, pain not reproduced, pain has nonradicular cause	Moderate to high specificity (70%–83%) High sensitivity (84%–91%)	Lumbar radiculopathy

Babinski test (plantar reflex)	The sole of the foot is stroked with a blunt instrument along the lateral side from the heel then curves medially along metatarsal pad below toes
	• Positive test
	  ○ Extension of the great toe with flexion and splaying of the other toes
	• Negative test
	  ○ Flexion of toes, inversion of foot
		High specificity (98%–100%) Low to moderate sensitivity (42%–60%) Presence of positive test helps rule in UMN disease, absence does not rule out	Suggests a lesion affecting the UMNs or corticospinal tract Present in normal newborns until ~12 mo of age; abnormal to persist beyond age ~2 y

Abbreviations: NPV, negative predictive value; PPV, Positive predictive value; SLR, straight leg raise; UMN, upper motor neuron.

that more than half of ED patients with LBP receive unnecessary imaging.[7] Blind diagnostic testing (so-called shotgunning) can lead to false-positive results and unnecessary therapies and interventions. In the absence of a serious or progressive neurologic deficit, concern for epidural compression syndrome, neoplasm, or spinal infection, advanced imaging should not be part of the diagnostic evaluation in the ED (**Fig. 1** shows a work-up algorithm).

- Laboratory studies
  - Rarely needed for the initial evaluation of acute LBP.
  - White blood cell count, erythrocyte sedimentation rate (ESR), and C-reactive protein (CRP) can be considered in cases of suspected infection, malignancy or nonspinal causes.

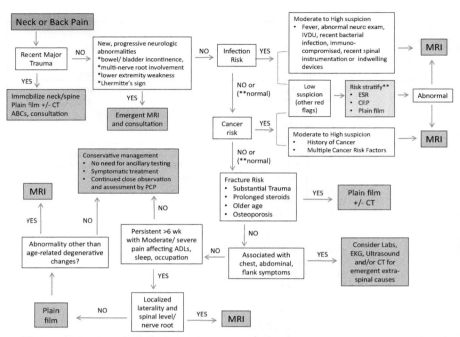

Fig. 1. Algorithm for the work-up of neck and back pain. * If the "Risk Stratify" ESR, CRP, plain films are normal, then can return to "NO" choice to "infection risk" and "cancer risk". ADLs, activities of daily living; CRP, C-reactive protein; CT, computed tomography; ECG, electrocardiogram; ESR, erythrocyte sedimentation rate; IVDU, intravenous drug use; PCP, primary care provider.

- Incorporating ESR and CRP values into an ED decision guideline may improve diagnostic delays and help distinguish patients in whom MRI may be performed on a nonemergent basis.[8]
  - Imaging
    - Plain radiographs
      - Plain films (anteroposterior and lateral) are helpful for suspected structural abnormalities such as spondylolisthesis and fractures
    - Computed tomography (CT)
      - Superior to plain radiographs for the detection of vertebral fractures, other bony disorders, bone fragments within the spinal canal, or spinal malalignment.
      - For atraumatic neck/back pain, CT should be performed only when MRI is not available or contraindicated (eg, metallic implants).
    - Magnetic Resonance Imagery (MRI)
      - The modality of choice for evaluation of myelopathy and progressive radiculopathy caused by spinal infections, malignancy, disc herniation, and epidural compression syndrome.
        - Obtain an MRI scan with contrast when there is suspicion for metastatic disease, osteomyelitis, abscess, inflammatory conditions.
      - There is no role for MRI in the setting of uncomplicated back pain in the ED population.
        - MRI is highly sensitive so may find asymptomatic degenerative changes in the cervical and lumbar spine.

- Patients in the ED who had an MRI scan were as likely to return to the ED within 1 week as those who did not receive an MRI scan.[9]

SPECIFIC CONDITIONS
Spinal Stenosis

Spinal stenosis, narrowing of the vertebral canal and foramina, can be caused by a variety of congenital and acquired conditions. It worsens with age. It is most commonly caused by spondylosis, loss of intervertebral disc height and space, deterioration of facet joints, and thickening and calcification of the ligamentum flavum, all of which can lead to nerve root compression.

- Stenosis can be asymptomatic, and there is poor correlation between the degree of narrowing on MRI and symptom severity.
- Symptoms can be caused by intermittent direct compression on the nerve root as well as nerve/cord ischemia resulting from decreased blood flow.
  - When symptomatic, the classic symptoms are neurogenic claudication, also called pseudoclaudication.
  - Unlike vascular claudication, symptoms are relieved when the patient flexes forward, such as when walking flexed with a cart (ie, shopping cart sign).
  - Symptoms are exacerbated by techniques that reduce canal size, such as erect posture or neck extension with prolonged standing without walking.
- Symptoms include stiffness, neck or back pain, paresthesias, and upper/lower extremity radicular pain depending on the affected nerve root, typically to the buttocks and posterolateral legs.
  - Unlike symptoms caused by disc herniation, pain is often bilateral and has an indolent onset.
  - Occasionally a more fixed nerve root injury occurs, causing radiculopathy or cauda equina syndrome (CES).
- Associated bilateral sensory changes may occur, such as numbness, tingling, or mild weakness affecting the arms or legs, which is often asymmetric.
- Focal weakness, sensory loss, or reflex changes may occur when spinal stenosis is associated with radiculopathy.
  - Physical examination may reveal single or multiple levels of radiculopathy with sensory loss, areflexia, or focal weakness in the distribution of the involved nerve roots.

Diagnosis

Presumptive diagnosis can be made based on clinical findings that suggest spinal stenosis, but definitive diagnosis requires correlation with neuroimaging that shows structural narrowing.

- A positive neuroimaging study without clinical correlation (ie, incidental finding of canal narrowing) is insufficient for a diagnosis. Radiographic spinal stenosis is an age-related population norm. More than 20% of asymptomatic persons above age 60 years may have findings of spinal stenosis on imaging studies.[10]
- ED management is conservative and focuses on pain control. In the absence of alarming findings (ie, progressive neurologic deficit or evidence of CES), these patients do not require any ancillary studies in the ED.
- Refer the patients back to their primary care providers (PCPs) to maximize medical management.

○ Consider outpatient surgical referral for those patients with severe, disabling symptoms or who have failed maximal medical therapy.

Disc Herniation

Disc herniation occurs when the nucleus pulposus prolapses through the tough outer annulus fibrosis. The posterior longitudinal ligament does not extend far enough laterally to fully reinforce the annulus, so the nucleus is more likely to herniate laterally rather than midline.

- Generally asymptomatic, often an incidental finding on MRI, but can lead to compression and inflammation of a nerve root and radicular symptoms.
  ○ Symptoms generally present more acutely than with spinal stenosis.
  ○ Herniation of a large disc in the midline can cause spinal cord compression and symptoms of myelopathy.
- Rare in children less than 18 years old and the elderly because of progressive fibrosis of the disc. Mean age at diagnosis ~48 years, incidence declines after age 60 years.

Radiculopathy

Radiculopathy is a clinical diagnosis of nerve root compression or irritation leading to symptoms such as pain, paresthesias, or weakness in the distribution of the affected nerve root (see **Table 3**). Most presentations have no identifiable trigger, although physical exertion or trauma have been reported.

- Most cases result from degenerative changes of the spine (spondylosis) such as from foraminal stenosis (with an indolent presentation) and disc herniation (with an acute presentation).
  ○ Symptoms of spinal stenosis worsen with walking, prolonged standing, and back extension, but are relieved with rest and forward flexion (sitting).
  ○ Symptoms of disc herniation worsen by Valsalva maneuvers, coughing, sneezing, and positions that produce increased pressure on annular fibers such as prolonged sitting, standing, and bending postures, but are relieved by lying supine.
- Nondegenerative radiculopathy can occur from disorders within the vertebral column, such as trauma, infection (ie, herpes zoster, Lyme disease), malignancy, or demyelination. Some patients have normal imaging.
- C7 is the most frequently affected cervical nerve root (60%–70%), followed by C6 (20%–25%), then C5, C8, and T1.[11]
- More than 90% of herniated lumbosacral discs occur at the L4 to L5 or L5 to S1 disc space, impinging L5 and S1 respectively.

Clinical features

The presentation is patient specific and may include isolated symptoms or a combination of typical symptoms:

- Neck/back pain with or without associated distal extremity involvement/radiation.
  ○ Symptoms of radiation to 1 or both upper/lower extremities usually along a single dermatome, but multidermatomal in more than half of cases, which can occur with spinal stenosis or a large or multilevel herniation.
  ○ Nerve root pain generally described as electrical, stabbing, sharp, and shooting, whereas peripheral nerve pain may be described as pins and needles.

- ○ Sciatica is radicular pain that travels down the legs in a lumbar or sacral nerve root distribution.
- ○ Pain exacerbated by turning the head ipsilateral to the pain source may indicate cervical radicular pain.
- Motor findings such as focal weakness occur less frequently than focal sensory or reflex changes. Weakness is seen in only ~15% of patients at presentation.[12]
- Sensory abnormalities such as numbness, paresthesias (described by about 90% of patients at presentation),[12] or dysesthesias.
  - ○ Sensory loss is typically mild or absent.
- Diminished deep tendon reflexes or areflexia may be seen.
  - ○ Asymmetric loss of a reflex is more suggestive of a specific root lesion than is the pattern of radicular pain.

Diagnosis
The diagnosis of radiculopathy is clinical. Imaging is not needed for the diagnosis and should not be obtained in the ED unless there is progressive neurologic impairment. Symptoms may persist for up to 6 to 8 weeks and may reoccur.

Management: 3 main groups of common presentations.

1. Patients with painful radicular symptoms and sensory dysfunction without other neurologic deficits or red flags.
   - ○ Typically self-limited and rarely progresses to a neurologic emergency
   - ○ No imaging or subspecialty referral needed
   - ○ Conservative management: treat similar to nonspecific neck/back pain
     - Appropriate effective analgesics (discussed later)
     - Avoid prolonged bed rest
     - Reassure patient that most people experience symptomatic resolution within 4 to 6 weeks with conservative, nonsurgical management.
   - ○ Follow up with PCP within 1 week
   - ○ Return for worsened neurologic symptoms
   - ○ Consider outpatient imaging if not resolved in 4 to 6 weeks
2. Patients with the symptoms discussed earlier plus a mild nonprogressive identifiable motor deficit with or without an associated reflex change.
   - Manage similarly to those without neurologic deficits (discussed earlier) unless progression occurs, then obtain imaging and consultation as appropriate.
3. Patients with the symptoms discussed earlier with severe or worsening motor deficits, urinary retention, saddle anesthesia, bilateral deficits, rapid progression, high risk of spinal infection or malignancy.
   - Urgent consultation and neuroimaging.

Myelopathy

Myelopathy refers to a spinal cord injury caused by direct compression or ischemia from compression of the arterial or venous supply to the cord. This injury can be secondary to degenerative disease/spondylosis (most commonly), stenosis, trauma, disc herniation, tumor, or abscess. There is no classic presentation, but upper motor neuron signs occur.

- Symptoms may be subtle and difficult for patients to describe.
  - ○ Onset is generally insidious and gradual with periods of quiescence followed by sudden or episodic worsening.
  - ○ Can occur in patients with previously known mild or unknown underlying cervical spondylosis. Rarely, this may be the first presentation.

○ Minor trauma involving sudden neck hyperextension can also cause sudden acute deterioration.
- Acute myelopathy is a neurologic emergency, requiring immediate consultation, neuroimaging, and administration of steroids.

Cervical myelopathy pearls

- C5 to C7 myotomes are most often affected.
- Cervical spondylotic myopathy: most common cause of myelopathy in adults greater than 55 years old and leads to progressive disability.
- Hand clumsiness (eg, loss of fine motor skills) and numbness/paresthesias of the hands/arms can be confused with distal median/ulnar mononeuropathies (eg, carpal tunnel syndrome).
- Sensory loss can be seen in a dermatomal or nonspecific distribution.
- May have:
  ○ Pain/stiffness in the neck, subscapular region, or shoulder that can radiate to the arms.
  ○ Lhermitte sign: forward neck flexion causes an electric shock–like sensation in the neck, radiating down the spine or to the arms.
  ○ Lower motor neuron findings in a myotomal distribution in the arms/hands (ie, weakness, atrophy, decreased reflexes).

Management

- Treatment options are controversial and best left to the consulting spine surgeon.
  ○ If, after consultation, the decision is made to discharge, return precautions should include worsening bowel or bladder dysfunction, weakness, sensory loss, or gait instability.
  ○ Patients who return should have repeat imaging and consultation with strong consideration of admission.
- In general, surgical decompression is offered to patients with moderate to severe myelopathy, progressive deterioration, or disabling neurologic deficits.
  ○ There is no consensus regarding the indications and timing of surgical decompression.

Acute Transverse Myelitis

Acute transverse myelitis (ATM) refers to inflammation of gray and white matter in 1 or more adjacent spinal cord segments leading to acute/subacute dysfunction of all cord functions (ie, motor, sensory, and autonomic). There is a bimodal peak between ages 10 and 19 years and ages 30 and 39 years.[13] It is a rare disorder, and most cases are idiopathic.[14] Young adults may develop ATM as the initial presentation of multiple sclerosis (MS). A significant association exists between ATM and recent preceding viral infection (eg, herpes, cytomegalovirus, Epstein-Barr virus, varicella), either related to infection or postinfectious inflammation. Causes are also associated with bacterial infections (eg, mycoplasma, syphilis, tuberculosis, Lyme disease), autoimmune disorders (eg, lupus, antiphospholipid syndrome), vasculitis, and certain drugs. The thoracic cord is most frequently involved, followed by the lumbosacral area, and rarely the cervical cord. The presentation is variable depending on the spinal segment involved. Other emergent causes of back pain may mimic the presentation, such as infection, malignancy, and compressive lesions. In an ED population eventually confirmed to have ATM, it was the initial diagnostic impression in fewer than 10% of cases, with more common initial impressions being disc herniation, stroke, Guillain-Barré syndrome, and CES.[15] Despite its low incidence, when a patient presents with a classic constellation of symptoms, ED providers must include ATM in the differential diagnosis because rapid identification and early initiation of treatment predicts the best outcomes.

Clinical features
Onset is characterized by acute/subacute development of neurologic signs and symptoms consistent with motor weakness, sensory changes, or autonomic dysfunction. Additional details are as discussed earlier in relation to myelopathy.

- ATM localizes to 1 or more contiguous spinal cord levels and is not caused by an underlying compressive lesion.
- Motor and sensory changes occur below the level of the lesion and are most likely to be bilateral. Motor symptoms include a rapidly progressing paraparesis.
- Autonomic dysfunction may include urinary urgency or difficulty voiding, bowel or bladder incontinence, tenesmus, constipation, and sexual dysfunction. As with the other causes of myelopathy discussed earlier, urinary retention is a major red flag for underlying myelopathy.

Most patients with idiopathic ATM have at least partial recovery, although some degree of persistent disability is common. Recovery usually begins within 1 to 3 months and can proceed for years.

Diagnosis
Whole-spine MRI with and without gadolinium usually makes the diagnosis. In cases of diagnostic uncertainty, a lumbar puncture showing cerebrospinal fluid inflammation can be helpful. Nonemergent MRI of the brain with and without gadolinium to evaluate for MS may also be performed.

Management
Goals include reducing cord inflammation, alleviating symptoms, and treating underlying causes (eg, infections, autoimmune) as appropriate.

- Reducing inflammation
  - Start intravenous (IV) glucocorticoids as first-line therapy to decrease swelling and inflammation.
  - Consider plasma exchange in patients who do not respond to steroids.
  - Consider IV immunoglobulin
- Symptom management
  - Pain management
  - Bladder decompression
- Otherwise, treatment is with supportive measures and correction of underlying causes and consultation as appropriate

Epidural Spinal Cord Compression Syndromes

Epidural spinal cord compression (ESCC) is a collective term encompassing compression of the spinal cord, conus medullaris, and cauda equina. These pathologic entities are grouped because they share a similar ED presentation, evaluation, and management. They differ on the level of neurologic deficit noted at the time of presentation.

Cauda Equina Syndrome

CES is a constellation of variable signs and symptoms that occur from compression of the nerves in the cauda equina. The most common cause is a herniated L4/L5 or L5/S1 disc. Other causes include tumor, epidural abscess, spinal canal hematoma, or lumbar spine spondylosis.

Clinical features

Clinical presentations vary, and there is no sign/symptom combination that can reliably diagnose or exclude CES. Only 56% of patients with positive MRI for CES were accurately identified by senior neurosurgical residents based on H&P findings, which shows the challenge of an accurate diagnosis.[16] In the setting of presumed CES, a sensory-level deficit or a positive Babinski reflex suggests the involvement of the conus medullaris. Disorder in this region can produce both upper and lower motor neuron signs; a mixture of spinal cord and nerve root dysfunction.

The 5 classic characteristic features include[17]:

- Bilateral radiculopathy
  - Progressively worsening back pain is often the first symptom, although complaints of leg pain and neurologic symptoms may predominate.
    - Unlike other causes of back pain, pain is worse with recumbent positioning secondary to epidural venous plexus distention.
  - Bilateral lower extremity pain and associated unilateral or bilateral radiculopathy may develop.
    - Weakness is common at the time of diagnosis. It is generally bilateral and symmetric, and may progress to the point of gait disturbance or paralysis.
    - Lower extremity reflexes can be decreased.
  - Although less common than motor findings, abnormal sensory findings may include bilateral lower extremity paresthesias and anesthesia.
- Saddle anesthesia
  - Loss of sensation around the anus, genitals, perineum, buttocks, and posterosuperior thighs.
  - Saddle sensory deficits were the only clinical feature associated with a positive MRI in one series.[18]
- Altered bladder function (ie, incontinence and retention)
  - A common late finding is urinary retention with overflow incontinence (sensitivity 90%, specificity 95%).
  - Patients can deteriorate rapidly, developing urinary retention at a rate of 1% per hour in the first 24 hours following medical contact.[19]
- Loss of anal tone
  - May include fecal incontinence caused by sphincter laxity.
  - Found in 60% to 80% of patients with CES.
- Sexual dysfunction

The functional status of the patient on arrival predicts neurologic outcomes. Patients who are ambulatory on arrival are likely to remain ambulatory. Patients who are too weak to walk but not paraplegic have an approximately 50% chance of walking again. Patients who are paraplegic on arrival are unlikely to walk again. Hence, early detection and treatment is needed in order to maximize the patient's functional status.

Diagnosis

Obtain an MRI of the lumbar and sacral spine without contrast to make the diagnosis. Because clinical certainty only becomes apparent with the classic symptoms, which are generally late findings, waiting to initiate MRI delays decompressive surgery and can lead to worse functional outcomes, which leads to increased MRI demand with more negative MRI findings. Only ~20% of MRI scans for suspected CES are positive,[18] although this has the benefit of diagnosing this condition promptly. Cases of suspected CES with negative MRI are usually caused by functional neurologic disorders, psychiatric comorbidities, and chronic pain.[20]

Management
Management depends on the cause of CES/ESCC. With emergent conditions such as abscess, malignancy/tumor, and hematoma, appropriate referrals should be made (discussed elsewhere in relation to the individual topics). General treatment guidelines involve systemic steroids and providing analgesia.

- Glucocorticoid therapy
  - Generally considered to be part of the standard regimen for symptomatic ESCC as a bridge to definitive treatment and palliation of pain.
  - Minimizes ongoing neurologic damage from compression/edema.
  - Administer the first dose as soon as ESCC syndrome is suspected. Do not wait for confirmatory diagnostic testing, which can take hours to complete, while epidural compression progresses.
- Pain management (discussed later)
  - Pain control is the most pressing need from the patient's perspective.
  - Glucocorticoids usually improve the pain within several hours, but many patients require opioid analgesics to tolerate the physical examination and necessary diagnostic studies.

Neoplastic Epidural Spinal Cord Compression
Neoplastic ESCC is a common complication of cancer that can cause pain, mechanical instability of the spine, and potentially irreversible loss of neurologic function. Both benign and malignant tumors can cause myelopathy as a result of compression. The most common syndrome involves metastatic spread to the vertebrae causing variable spinal cord compression. The most common primary sources in adults are lung, breast, and prostate cancers, and multiple myeloma.[21] Metastatic cord compression is an oncologic emergency that affects 5 to 10 in every 200 patients with terminal cancer. Almost two-thirds of the cases affect the thoracic spine.[22] The tumors responsible for ESCC in children include sarcomas (especially Ewing sarcoma) and neuroblastomas. ESCC is the initial manifestation of malignancy in ~20% of patients.[23]

Clinical features
- Suspect in patients with a history of cancer with new-onset neck or back pain (thoracic most common).
- Severe local pain is the initial symptom of spinal metastasis in 85% to 90% of presentations.
  - Pain described as dull, constant, and aching.
  - Pain is not relieved by rest and may worsen with recumbency.
  - Severe nighttime pain is also characteristic.
  - Pain may precede other neurologic symptoms by several weeks.
- New gait ataxia in the setting of back pain in a patient with cancer should raise suspicion of ESCC.
- Pathologic compression fractures may present with abrupt worsening of back pain.

- Late findings.
  - Radicular symptoms and progressive weakness with accompanying sensory loss.
  - Rapid progression to paraplegia may occur secondary to vascular compression.
  - Bladdery dysfunction/urinary retention is a common finding but rarely seen in isolation. Opiates for pain management also contribute to urinary retention.

Diagnosis

Timely diagnosis and treatment are essential because the ultimate prognosis depends on the neurologic function at the time of intervention. The diagnosis of ESCC requires the demonstration of a neoplastic mass that extrinsically compresses the thecal sac. MRI with gadolinium is preferred and should include the entire spine if there is a concern of metastatic compression. Imaging should be obtained as soon as possible.

Similar to the pathologic appearance of a spinal epidural abscess on MRI, multiple locations of disorder often coexist. Bone metastases are rarely restricted to a single site, and multiple epidural tumor deposits can be present. Clinical localization is imprecise for spinal cord levels. The compressive lesion may be several levels higher than is suggested by a sensory level. When a spinal sensory level is present, it is typically 1 to 5 levels below the level of cord compression. Referred pain from ESCC is common and can be misleading in terms of localizing the lesion.

Management

As with other causes of ESCC, IV glucocorticoids, appropriate consultation (eg, oncology, spine surgeon), pain management, and inpatient admission are the mainstays of ED management.

Spinal Infections

Spinal infections, including vertebral osteomyelitis and spinal epidural abscess (SEA), are rare but potentially catastrophic causes of neck and back pain. They are challenging to diagnose because the presentation is often subtle, insidious, and nonspecific. Initial manifestations can include nonspecific symptoms such as malaise, nausea, fatigue, and mild back pain. In 1 series on vertebral osteomyelitis, the mean duration of symptoms was 48 ± 40 days.[24] Diagnosis may be obscured or delayed in patients with a history of degenerative spinal disease or recent trauma because the typical early presentation consists of neck or back pain with tenderness to palpation and associated muscle spasm. Symptoms may initially respond to conservative management such as bed rest, which may lead clinicians to diagnose a noninfectious source such as musculoskeletal back pain or minor trauma. More than half of patients with SEA presented to the ED 2 or more times before being diagnosed, with 10% presenting 3 or more times.[25] The mean duration of symptoms in SEA between onset and the first ED visit or admission was 5 and 9 days, respectively.[25] Incidence is increasing because of an aging population and more health care–associated intravascular devices, instrumentation, and procedures.

Spinal infections occur by 3 basic routes:

- Hematogenous spread from a distant site of infection (most common mechanism)
- Direct inoculation from trauma or spinal surgery/instrumentation

- 14% to 22% of SEAs occur as a result of percutaneous spine procedures/surgery[26]
- Contiguous spread from an adjacent soft tissue infection

The most important infecting organisms in spinal infections are:

- *Staphylococcus aureus* (>50% of cases) is the leading pathogen of both SEA and vertebral osteomyelitis
- Other pathogens include:
  - *Streptococcus* species
  - Coagulase-negative *staphylococci* associated with spinal surgery and foreign bodies
  - Enteric gram-negative bacilli (eg, *Escherichia coli* in the setting of urinary tract infection)
  - *Candida* species in immunocompromised patients and those with recent spinal surgery
  - *Pseudomonas aeruginosa* seen in IV drug use (IVDU)
  - *Mycobacterium tuberculosis* in the immunocompromised
  - Anaerobes (rare)
- ~One-third of patients with SEA have no identifiable source for the infection.
- Empiric treatment should therefore begin with agents that cover most common organisms based on H&P; tailor the patient's treatment once a pathogen is identified.

Clinical features

- Suspect infection with new or worsening neck or back pain, with or without neurologic symptoms, in the setting of known risk factors:
  - Intravenous drug use (IVDU)
    - One retrospective review of patients with IVDU presenting to the ED with acute back pain (new or worsening within 24 hours) showed evidence of spinal infection in almost 40% of the patients[27]
  - Recent bacterial infection or bacteremia
  - Immunosuppressed state
  - Multiple chronic medical conditions
  - Recent surgery/instrumentation
  - Presence of foreign bodies/intravascular devices
- The most common clinical finding of spinal infection is local tenderness to percussion over the involved spinous processes, but this is nonspecific
- Back/neck pain
  - Presentation is insidious and progressively worsens
  - Generally localized to the infected area/disc space
  - Worse with physical activity, may be relieved by rest
  - Worse at night, pain interferes with sleep
- Classic triad of SEA is fever, pain, and focal neurologic deficit, but this is seen in only 15% of patients[25]
  - One or more features of the classic triad of SEA were present in 98% of patients with SEA compared with only 21% of controls[25]

Diagnosis

- CBC (poorly sensitive or specific)[28]
  - Increased leukocyte count or bandemia may or may not be present[25]

- ESR and CRP
  - Increased ESR and CRP level observed in greater than 80% of patients with vertebral osteomyelitis
  - Sensitive for infection, but not specific[25,29]
  - ESR
    - Most sensitive and specific serum marker usually increased in both SEA and vertebral osteomyelitis
    - ESR was increased (>20 mm/h) in 94% to 100% of patients with SEA versus only 33% of patients without SEA
    - Mean ESR in patients with SEA was significantly increased (51–77 mm/h)[8,26]
  - CRP
    - Less useful for acute diagnosis because CRP levels increase faster and return to baseline faster than ESR (increased CRP seen in 87% of patients with SEA as well as in 50% of patients with spine pain not caused by SEA)[26]
    - Better used as a marker of response to treatment
  - Risk stratify need for emergent MRI using ESR/CRP and red flags (see algorithm in **Fig. 1**)
    - In the setting of low to moderate pretest probability, obtain ESR/CRP to evaluate need for emergent MRI[8,30]
    - In setting of moderate to high pretest probability (eg, new-onset neck/back pain with neurologic deficit, or with fever and IVDU), obtain emergent MRI[8,29,30]
- Collect 2 sets of blood cultures
  - Isolates the causative pathogen in ~50% to 60% of patients[31]
- Lumbar puncture is not recommended; the diagnostic yield is low and it has a high risk of spreading infection

Imaging: once the diagnosis of spinal infection is seriously considered, obtain spinal imaging urgently.

- MRI with gadolinium is the gold standard for the diagnosis of spinal infections (sensitivity and specificity >90%).[32]
  - Image the entire spinal column even with focal signs/symptoms because of the risk of multiple skip lesions that may be asymptomatic
- CT is the alternative imaging modality, although MRI is preferred. High false-negative rate for SEA.
- Plain films, poor sensitivity/specificity, not recommended for initial work-up. Negative films do not rule out SEA.
- CT myelogram: high sensitivity for detecting SEA but is invasive, with the risk of spreading infection into the subarachnoid space; now largely obsolete.

Vertebral Osteomyelitis and Spondylodiscitis

Infection of the vertebral bodies (osteomyelitis) can spread to the intervertebral spaces and discs, leading to spondylodiscitis (infection/inflammation of vertebrae and vertebral disc spaces). Diagnosis and management of vertebral osteomyelitis and spondylodiscitis are similar.

- The risk increases with age and is more common in men.
- The lumbar spine is the most common site, followed by the thoracic and cervical spine.
- If left untreated can lead to pathologic fractures.
- Infection can spread to the epidural space, leading to abscesses.

Management

- Hold on initiating antimicrobial treatment until pathogen identified, if possible.
  - Diagnosis/pathogen confirmed via CT-guided biopsy of involved vertebral bone or disc space.
  - Clinical exceptions include neurologic compromise and sepsis; in these circumstances, start empiric therapy.
- Once the pathogen is isolated, begin antimicrobial treatment.
  - If highly suspicious but negative culture results, begin empiric treatment of most likely causal organisms.
- Surgical intervention indicated for:
  - Threatened or actual cord compression caused by spinal instability or vertebral collapse.
  - Neurologic deficits.
  - Presence of epidural or paravertebral abscess.
  - Progression, persistence, or recurrence of disease (persistent positive blood cultures or worsening pain) despite appropriate antimicrobial therapy.
- If positive blood cultures for gram-positive organisms, evaluate for concurrent infective endocarditis in patients with underlying valve disease or new-onset heart failure.

Spinal Epidural Abscess

SEA is an abscess that forms in the epidural space (vertical sheath that extends down the length of the spinal canal, containing blood vessels and infection-prone fat tissue). The median age of onset of SEA is ~50 years.

- SEAs are most common in the thoracolumbar region, and least common in the cervical region.
- Extension to additional vertebral levels is common.
  - Average extent is 3 to 5 spinal cord segments, but the whole length of the spinal column may be involved.[33]
  - Noncontiguous abscesses (ie, skip lesions) may also occur.
- If left untreated, symptoms follow a typical progression from neck/back pain to radiculopathy to severe weakness and sensory changes, bowel/bladder dysfunction, and eventual paralysis.[31]

Management

- Immediately begin IV antibiotic therapy; do not wait for pathogen identification.
  - ~5% of patients with SEA die of uncontrolled sepsis or other complications.[28]
- Consult spine surgeon to evaluate for surgical decompression and drainage of abscess.
  - Emergent surgical intervention for patients with neurologic deficits, progressive weakness, paralysis, or cord compression (threatened or actual).
  - Degree of neurologic recovery after surgery is related to the duration of the neurologic deficit.

NECK AND BACK PAIN TREATMENT

An important goal of ED management is to provide an acceptable level of analgesia. Given the overall good prognosis for recovery, conservative therapies are preferred.

- Mild to moderate pain

- ○ Nonsteroidal anti-inflammatory drugs (NSAIDs)
  - First-line treatment, unless contraindicated
- ○ Acetaminophen is of little benefit to ED patients with acute nonradicular back pain[34] but may be prescribed if there is a contraindication to NSAIDs
- Moderate to severe pain
  - ○ Opioid analgesics or tramadol
    - Reasonable in the acute phase as second-line treatment of pain that is severe, debilitating, or refractory to first-line medications
      - Early opioid prescription for acute occupational LBP in the ED increases long-term opioid use, medical costs, and disability[35]
    - Prescribe the smallest quantity possible for the shortest duration possible
      - Wide variation in opioid prescribing practices for back pain exist among ED physicians[36]
      - Use of prescription drug monitoring programs and prescriber practice guidelines can assist with physician/patient concerns
- Other medications
  - ○ Lidocaine patch
    - Topical option to treat neck and back pain, especially in patients with primary or secondary paraspinal muscle involvement
  - ○ Muscle relaxants (eg, cyclobenzaprine)
    - Evidence for the effectiveness of muscle relaxants in the relief of neck pain is weak compared with NSAIDs
      - Limit to patients who cannot tolerate NSAIDs but can tolerate the side effect profile of muscle relaxants, which include dizziness, drowsiness, and sedation
    - Muscle relaxants provide pain relief in patients with acute LBP but there is insufficient evidence to support their use in chronic back pain[37]
  - ○ Combination therapy does not seem to be better than monotherapy
    - Compared with NSAIDs alone, adding muscle relaxants or opioids for acute nonradicular pain does not improve functional outcomes or pain within 3 months[38–41]
  - ○ Oral corticosteroids
    - There is no role for corticosteroids in the treatment of musculoskeletal pain in ED patients[42]
    - Radiculopathy: limited evidence to support use
      - There may be small, short-term, unsustained benefit in ED patients with cervical and lumbar radiculopathy[43]

SUMMARY

In the ED, the goal is not to establish the presence of a benign disease process, but rather to exclude those cases that require immediate identification and emergent treatment, as previously discussed. Once excluded, the ED management of those nonemergent conditions includes education, reassurance, pain control, and appropriate outpatient follow-up. During the visit, focus on patient education (eg, why they are not undergoing laboratory or radiographic testing) and reassurance of the likely benign cause of the pain. This approach helps avoid misperceptions of substandard care as well as unnecessary return visits when symptoms persist for an expected amount of time.

Carefully selected and presented advice and information about neck/back pain can have a positive effect on patients' beliefs and clinical outcomes. ED physicians should reassure their patients by acknowledging their pain and being supportive. Avoid language that may scare medically naive patients by implying a serious abnormality when none exists (eg, ruptured disc). Consider using the term "common" or "mechanical" neck/back pain because "nonspecific" may not engender patient confidence.[44] The final and perhaps most important aspect of ED management of acute neck/back pain involves discharge instructions. All patients should be given clear discharge instructions with specific indications to return to an ED with symptoms such as new or progressive weakness, bowel or bladder dysfunction, or saddle anesthesia, because the absence of findings is common in early presentations of emergent disorders.

ACKNOWLEDGMENTS

The authors thank Roy Hatch for his invaluable assistance in preparing this article.

REFERENCES

1. Binder A. Neck pain. Clin Evid 2006;15:1654–75.
2. Waterman BR, Belmont PJ Jr, Schoenfeld AJ. Low back pain in the United States: incidence and risk factors for presentation in the emergency setting. Spine J 2012;12:63–70.
3. Axen I, Leboeuf-Yde C. Trajectories of low back pain. Best Pract Res Clin Rheumatol 2013;27:601–12.
4. da C Menezes Costa L, Maher CG, Hancock MJ, et al. The prognosis of acute and persistent low-back pain: a meta-analysis. CMAJ 2012;184:E613–24.
5. Cook CE, George SZ, Reiman MP. Red flag screening for low back pain: nothing to see here, move along: a narrative review. Br J Sports Med 2018;52:493–6.
6. Henschke N, Maher CG, Refshauge KM, et al. Prevalence of and screening for serious spinal pathology in patients presenting to primary care settings with acute low back pain. Arthritis Rheum 2009;60:3072–80.
7. Schlemmer E, Mitchiner JC, Brown M, et al. Imaging during low back pain ED visits: a claims-based descriptive analysis. Am J Emerg Med 2015;33:414–8.
8. Davis DP, Salazar A, Chan TC, et al. Prospective evaluation of a clinical decision guideline to diagnose spinal epidural abscess in patients who present to the emergency department with spine pain. J Neurosurg Spine 2011;14:765–70.
9. Aaronson EL, Yun BJ, Mort E, et al. Association of magnetic resonance imaging for back pain on seven-day return visit to the Emergency Department. Emerg Med J 2017;34:677–9.
10. Katz JN, Harris MB. Clinical practice. Lumbar spinal stenosis. N Engl J Med 2008; 358:818–25.
11. Radhakrishnan K, Litchy WJ, O'Fallon WM, et al. Epidemiology of cervical radiculopathy. A population-based study from Rochester, Minnesota, 1976 through 1990. Brain 1994;117(Pt 2):325–35.
12. Evans G. Identifying and treating the causes of neck pain. Med Clin North Am 2014;98:645–61.
13. Jacob A, Weinshenker BG. An approach to the diagnosis of acute transverse myelitis. Semin Neurol 2008;28:105–20.
14. Krishnan C, Kaplin AI, Pardo CA, et al. Demyelinating disorders: update on transverse myelitis. Curr Neurol Neurosci Rep 2006;6:236–43.
15. Huh Y, Park EJ, Jung JW, et al. Clinical insights for early detection of acute transverse myelitis in the emergency department. Clin Exp Emerg Med 2015;2:44–50.

16. Bell DA, Collie D, Statham PF. Cauda equina syndrome: what is the correlation between clinical assessment and MRI scanning? Br J Neurosurg 2007;21:201–3.

17. Todd NV. Guidelines for cauda equina syndrome. Red flags and white flags. Systematic review and implications for triage. Br J Neurosurg 2017;31:336–9.

18. Balasubramanian K, Kalsi P, Greenough CG, et al. Reliability of clinical assessment in diagnosing cauda equina syndrome. Br J Neurosurg 2010;24:383–6.

19. Todd NV. Cauda equina syndrome: is the current management of patients presenting to district general hospitals fit for purpose? A personal view based on a review of the literature and a medicolegal experience. Bone Joint J 2015; 97-B:1390–4.

20. Hoeritzauer I, Pronin S, Carson A, et al. The clinical features and outcome of scan-negative and scan-positive cases in suspected cauda equina syndrome: a retrospective study of 276 patients. J Neurol 2018;265:2916–26.

21. Mak KS, Lee LK, Mak RH, et al. Incidence and treatment patterns in hospitalizations for malignant spinal cord compression in the United States, 1998-2006. Int J Radiat Oncol Biol Phys 2011;80:824–31.

22. Al-Qurainy R, Collis E. Metastatic spinal cord compression: diagnosis and management. BMJ 2016;353:i2539.

23. Savage P, Sharkey R, Kua T, et al. Malignant spinal cord compression: NICE guidance, improvements and challenges. QJM 2014;107:277–82.

24. Nolla JM, Ariza J, Gomez-Vaquero C, et al. Spontaneous pyogenic vertebral osteomyelitis in nondrug users. Semin Arthritis Rheum 2002;31:271–8.

25. Davis DP, Wold RM, Patel RJ, et al. The clinical presentation and impact of diagnostic delays on emergency department patients with spinal epidural abscess. J Emerg Med 2004;26:285–91.

26. Reihsaus E, Waldbaur H, Seeling W. Spinal epidural abscess: a meta-analysis of 915 patients. Neurosurg Rev 2000;23(175):204 [discussion: 205].

27. Colip CG, Lotfi M, Buch K, et al. Emergent spinal MRI in IVDU patients presenting with back pain: do we need an MRI in every case? Emerg Radiol 2018;25:247–56.

28. Darouiche RO. Spinal epidural abscess. N Engl J Med 2006;355:2012–20.

29. Edlow JA. Managing nontraumatic acute back pain. Ann Emerg Med 2015;66(2): 148–53.

30. Alerhand S, Wood S, Long B, et al. The time-sensitive challenge of diagnosing spinal epidural abscess in the emergency department. Intern Emerg Med 2017;12:1179–83.

31. Tompkins M, Panuncialman I, Lucas P, et al. Spinal epidural abscess. J Emerg Med 2010;39:384–90.

32. Tali ET, Oner AY, Koc AM. Pyogenic spinal infections. Neuroimaging Clin N Am 2015;25:193–208.

33. Darouiche RO, Hamill RJ, Greenberg SB, et al. Bacterial spinal epidural abscess. Review of 43 cases and literature survey. Medicine (Baltimore) 1992;71:369–85.

34. Saragiotto BT, Machado GC, Ferreira ML, et al. Paracetamol for low back pain. Cochrane Database Syst Rev 2016;(6):CD012230.

35. Lee SS, Choi Y, Pransky GS. Extent and impact of opioid prescribing for acute occupational low back pain in the emergency department. J Emerg Med 2016; 50:376–84.e1-2.

36. Hoppe JA, McStay C, Sun BC, et al. Emergency department attending physician variation in opioid prescribing in low acuity back pain. West J Emerg Med 2017; 18:1135–42.

37. Abdel Shaheed C, Maher CG, Williams KA, et al. Efficacy and tolerability of muscle relaxants for low back pain: systematic review and meta-analysis. Eur J Pain 2017;21:228–37.
38. Friedman BW, Dym AA, Davitt M, et al. Naproxen with cyclobenzaprine, oxycodone/acetaminophen, or placebo for treating acute low back pain: a randomized clinical trial. JAMA 2015;314:1572–80.
39. Friedman BW, Cisewski D, Irizarry E, et al. A randomized, double-blind, placebo-controlled trial of naproxen with or without orphenadrine or methocarbamol for acute low back pain. Ann Emerg Med 2018;71:348–56.e5.
40. Khwaja SM, Minnerop M, Singer AJ. Comparison of ibuprofen, cyclobenzaprine or both in patients with acute cervical strain: a randomized controlled trial. CJEM 2010;12:39–44.
41. Turturro MA, Frater CR, D'Amico FJ. Cyclobenzaprine with ibuprofen versus ibuprofen alone in acute myofascial strain: a randomized, double-blind clinical trial. Ann Emerg Med 2003;41:818–26.
42. Eskin B, Shih RD, Fiesseler FW, et al. Prednisone for emergency department low back pain: a randomized controlled trial. J Emerg Med 2014;47:65–70.
43. Balakrishnamoorthy R, Horgan I, Perez S, et al. Does a single dose of intravenous dexamethasone reduce Symptoms in Emergency department patients with low Back pain and RAdiculopathy (SEBRA)? A double-blind randomised controlled trial. Emerg Med J 2015;32(7):525–30.
44. Bardin LD, King P, Maher CG. Diagnostic triage for low back pain: a practical approach for primary care. Med J Aust 2017;206:268–73.

Risk Management and Avoiding Legal Pitfalls in the Emergency Treatment of High-Risk Orthopedic Injuries

Michael C. Bond, MD*, George C. Willis, MD

KEYWORDS

- Compartment syndrome • Medicolegal • Malpractice • Epidural abscess
- High-pressure • Tendon laceration • Foreign body

KEY POINTS

- High-pressure injuries often seem very benign but often lead to significant disability. Do not overlook these injuries and manage them appropriately with imaging, antibiotics, and consultation with hand surgery.
- Tendon lacerations are often missed in the evaluation of hand lacerations. Providers need to examine the extremity in a bloodless field, through the full range of motion, and possibly through an extension of the wound to not miss this diagnosis.
- Spinal epidural abscesses are commonly missed on their initial presentation. Patients do not need to have the triad of fever, back pain, and neurologic deficit. Consider in patients with red flags for back pain.
- Delays in the diagnosis and treatment of compartment syndrome can result in permanent disability. Single compartment pressure measurements can be unreliable. Refer patients suspected of having the diagnosis to an appropriate surgeon quickly.

INTRODUCTION

Medical liability often results from poor physician-patient communication, and errors in patient management.[1,2] Missed myocardial infarction (MI) is often thought of as one of the highest areas for litigation in emergency medicine (EM), and although missed MI results in higher payouts, orthopedic injuries are associated with more cases filed. Multiple reviews of closed malpractice claims have shown the leading causes of liability for EM practitioners are chest pain, abdominal pain, fractures,

Disclosure Statement: The authors have nothing to disclose.
Department of Emergency Medicine, University of Maryland School of Medicine, 110 South Paca Street, Sixth Floor, Suite 200, Baltimore, MD 21201, USA
* Corresponding author.
E-mail address: mbond@som.umaryland.edu
Twitter: @Docbond007 (M.C.B.); @DocWillisMD (G.C.W.)

Emerg Med Clin N Am 38 (2020) 193–206
https://doi.org/10.1016/j.emc.2019.09.008
0733-8627/20/© 2019 Elsevier Inc. All rights reserved.

emed.theclinics.com

wounds, pediatric fever/meningitis, subarachnoid hemorrhage, aortic aneurysm, and epiglottitis.[3,4] A study by Kachalia and colleagues[5] showed that missed or delayed diagnosis of fracture was almost twice that of MI. Therefore, EM practitioners are more likely to be named in a lawsuit for an orthopedic complaint than chest pain.

This article focuses on high-risk orthopedic complaints that the authors have noted an uptick in the number of lawsuits or the chance of a successful plaintiff's verdict. We will highlight difficulties and limitations in making the diagnosis and provide recommendations on how to improve the patient's care.

COMPARTMENT SYNDROME

One of the most challenging orthopedic emergencies to diagnose is acute compartment syndrome (ACS). ACS is often the result of trauma (eg, long bone fractures, crush injuries, rhabdomyolysis, burns, vascular injury) but also can be second to nontraumatic causes (eg, extravasation of intravenous fluids, contrast dye, or medications; thrombosis; intravenous drug abuse; hematomas from anticoagulation use). Fractures account for 70% to 75% of ACS cases with fractures of the tibia being the leading cause followed by the radius.[6,7] Patients with ACS not due to a fracture are at higher risk for delayed diagnosis. Patients who undergo open reduction and internal fixation of their fracture have a peak incidence of ACS at the time of their surgery, and it decreases over the next 24 to 36 hours.[8,9] However, they can still develop it days later, and the risk is not zero. The incidence of ACS is higher in male versus female patients, and younger patients versus older patients. This is thought to be related to muscle mass and soft tissue pliability.

The differential diagnosis often can be broad with symptoms often overlapping with other less emergent diagnoses. The treatment, an emergent fasciotomy, can result in complications (ie, infection, permanent scarring, muscle loss). As such, the decision to perform one is not to be taken lightly. The diagnostic challenges and permanent disability that can result from these cases make them favorites of plaintiff attorneys. One study even noted that although only approximately 20% of general malpractice cases result in a settlement or plaintiff's verdict, 57% of ACS cases ultimately result in a plaintiff verdict or settlement. These cases are very high risk for orthopedic surgeons, as it is one of a few true emergencies that they have to deal with, but current trends show that they are very high risk for EM practitioners, as delays in diagnosis or in arranging for definitive treatment are often placed on the shoulders of the EM practitioner.

To avoid the pitfalls of ACS, we must first start with an understanding of the pathophysiology and physical examination findings that are typically seen. ACS results when the pressure in a muscular compartment exceeds the perfusion pressure, resulting in muscle ischemia and death. The muscle compartments of the human body are surrounded by fascial membranes that are unyielding and prevent expansion. The perfusion pressure is the pressure at the local tissue level that is affected by arterial pressure and venous pressure. In patients who develop ACS, there is initially decreased capillary flow that results in local ischemia that leads to increased permeability of the blood vessels. As the compartment pressure increases, venous and lymphatic flow is hindered, and there is increased third spacing of fluid that further increases the compartment pressure, leading to more ischemia.[6] Unless corrective action is taken, a vicious cycle results, leading to higher pressures and additional ischemia. It is exceedingly rare for the pressure to get high enough to hinder arterial flow, but capillary, lymphatic, and venous flow are compromised early.

The symptoms of ACS have traditionally been taught to be the 6 Ps (ie, pain, paresthesia, pallor, pulselessness, paralysis, and poikilothermia); however, most of these symptoms are not seen clinically and are more specific for arterial insufficiency, which is often not present in ACS. None of the symptoms of ACS have good sensitivity or specificity, but the most widely accepted are pain out of proportion to the examination or injury and increased pain with passive stretch of the compartment.[10] A hardwood like feel to the compartment is also suggestive of ACS; however, one must remember that this is subjective, and not all compartments can be palpated easily to be able to appreciate this finding. One cadaveric study found that manual palpation of a compartment had a sensitivity of 24%, specificity of 55%, positive predictive value of 19%, and negative predictive value of 63% in detecting an elevated compartment pressure.[11] Therefore, manual palpation for compartment firmness is a poor predictor of the actual compartment pressure. To improve one's skills, emergency practitioners should routinely palpate compartments in musculoskeletal complaints to help keep ACS in the differential and develop a sense of the spectrum of normal. The most common symptoms that are reported are pain out of proportion to the injury, a deep ache in the affected limb, and paresthesias. Muscle weakness or paralysis is a late finding, and if seen immediately after an injury is more suggestive of a direct nerve injury than ischemia. If concerned about compartment syndrome, it is ideal to test sensation with pinprick and 2-point discrimination. This testing will allow comparison between examinations to see if there is progression of disease.

Some investigators state that the diagnosis of ACS must be made by measuring compartment pressures. This procedure is within the purvey of EM physicians; however, there are several reasons why it is not a gold standard for the diagnosis.[12] First, the procedure is not done often by EM physicians so the reproducibility and reliability of the results are often called into question. Large and colleagues[13] studied 38 participants (ie, orthopaedists, general surgeons, and EM physicians) on their ability to measure compartment pressures of the lower leg. They found that a catastrophic error was committed on 30% of the recorded measurements and that only 6 of the 38 subjects were able to measure all 4 compartments of the lower leg correctly. The diagnosis is further complicated by the fact that ACS exists along a continuum and there is no exact compartment pressure reading that can make the diagnosis. The currently accepted pressure definition of ACS is when the diastolic blood pressure is within 30 mm Hg of the compartment pressure. When the delta pressure (ΔP) is greater than 30 mm Hg, capillary flow is not compromised. For example, if the measured compartment pressure is 40 mm Hg and the diastolic blood pressure is 80 mm Hg (80 mm Hg – 40 mm Hg = 40), the patient would not meet the pressure criteria for ACS, but if the diastolic blood pressure decreased to 60 mm Hg (60 mm Hg – 40 mm Hg = 20), they would meet the pressure criteria for ACS. Finally, Whitney and colleagues[14] found that one-time measurements of compartment pressure resulted in a 35% false-positive rate when using a delta P of 30 mm Hg. Obtaining a pressure reading can be helpful in convincing a trauma surgeon or orthopedist to evaluate the patient, but it is our experience that an EM physician's readings are rarely used to mobilize the operating room. Often the readings are repeated by the surgeon or the patient is personally evaluated by the surgeon first.

If measuring compartment pressures, a few steps can help ensure you obtain the most accurate pressure reading:

1. The pressure monitor should be zeroed at the same angle as the needle will enter the skin.
2. Be sure to inject 0.1 mL of normal saline through the needle to clear out any tissue that might obscure the pressure reading.

3. Measure each compartment separately and re-zero the monitor between measurements. For instance, when measuring the superficial compartment of the lower leg, avoid advancing the needle into the deep compartment for a second reading. Although this might provide an accurate reading, there is a higher likelihood that the needle's angle may have changed, resulting in an inaccurate measurement.

There are no laboratory values that have sufficient specificity or sensitivity to diagnose ACS, although in later stages patients may have elevated creatine kinase, myoglobin, and lactate levels.[15]

The initial treatment of ACS is important and some simple steps can help reduce compartment pressures:

1. Remove all restrictive dressings, splints, and casts. It has been shown that bivalving a cast and spreading it can reduce compartment pressures by 65%, and an additional 10% to 20% pressure reduction can be achieved by cutting the cotton padding (Webril).[16]
2. Keep the legs neutral. Elevating the limb, although it can help reduce edema, actually impedes arterial flow, which can exacerbate the ischemia, whereas keeping the limb dependent can increase edema and compartmental pressures.[17,18]
3. Arrange for orthopedic or trauma surgeon consultation for consideration of an urgent fasciotomy.

A few final pitfalls in the diagnosis of ACS. Although it is generally considered in the differential diagnosis of patients who have had a recent fracture, it also should be considered in patients who have crush injuries, rhabdomyolysis, or have been "found down" after a prolonged period. In fact, patients with altered mental status are at increased risk for delayed diagnosis of ACS, as they often cannot report pain, nor cooperate with the examination to know if there is any weakness or pain with passive stretch. These patients should have serial examinations documented.

Bhattacharyya and Vrahas[19] looked at 23 years of closed malpractice claims data involving compartment syndrome and found 2 things that were associated with an indemnity payment. They included poor physician-patient communication and increased time from onset of symptoms to the fasciotomy. They also found a linear correlation of the number of cardinal signs (Ps) that the patient had at presentation with the amount of the indemnity that was awarded. A fasciotomy performed within 8 hours of presentation of symptoms was universally associated with a defense verdict.

Compartment Syndrome Medicolegal Pearls

- Ensure you document the date and time of all your examinations, conversations, and attempts to mobilize your resources to treat your patient.
- Document 2-point discrimination, and in patients with altered mental status be sure to document reflexes as evidence that motor and sensory function is present.
- Ensure you document the reasons for any delays in care and how you attempted to address them.
- Although many community orthopaedists may ask that the patient be transferred to a trauma or referral center, it is prudent to have this discussion with your on-call consultant and document his or her decision in the case.
- Ensure you document the removal of all restrictive clothing, dressings, and splints/casts, and if there is any change in the patient's condition (eg, improvement).

SPINAL EPIDURAL ABSCESS

Back pain is one of the most common diagnoses seen in emergency departments (EDs) and accounts for 2% to 3% of ED visits.[20,21] The vast majority of cases will be secondary to musculoskeletal causes; however, the EM practitioner must always be on the lookout for more serious causes of back pain. One of these, spinal epidural abscess (SEA), is a particularly challenging diagnosis to make. It has been estimated that the diagnosis is missed on 75% of initial presentations.[22,23] One retrospective review of 119 SEA outpatient cases showed that 66 (55.5%) of the cases had a diagnostic error, and the median time to diagnosis was 12 days as opposed to 4 days in those without a diagnostic error.[22] Davis and colleagues[23] conducted a case-control study of 74 ED patients with SEA. They found that diagnostic delays were present in 75% of patients with SEA; the classic triad of fever, back pain, and a neurologic deficit was present in only 13% of cases; and the median number of ED visits before a diagnosis was made was 2, with a maximum of 8 in one patient. Plaintiff attorneys also favor these cases, as approximately 60% of cases result in a plaintiff ruling or settlement with a mean award of approximately $5 million (range $4551 to $22,903,000).[24,25] Paralysis, delays in diagnosis, or delays in treatment were the 3 most common factors associated with a plaintiff verdict.[24,25]

The incidence of SEA, although historically reported as 0.2 to 1.2 cases per 10,000 hospital admissions, has had a marked increase in its prevalence (12.5 per 10,000) admissions. Many factors (ie, diabetes mellitus, intravenous drug abuse, immunosuppression, and invasive spinal procedures [eg, epidural injections, discectomies]) have attributed to the increased prevalence.[26]

EM practitioners should consider the diagnosis in patients who have any red flags, as shown in **Table 1**. The red flags have been used to identify secondary causes of back pain (eg, cancer, infection, or abdominal aortic aneurysm); however, the items denoted with "a" are more specific for infectious causes like SEA. **Table 2** denotes the prevalence of risk factors and red flags in patients with SEA.[22,23] Patients with no red flags and a normal neurologic examination are at extremely low risk of a serious cause of back pain, and no further testing needs to be done.[27] However, care should be taken to do a thorough neurologic examination that includes testing sensation of the perineum and a Babinski sign. If the patient has any urinary complaints, a post

Table 1	
Red flags of back pain	
Historical Red Flags	**Physical Examination Red Flags**

• Age <18 or >50
• Pain lasting more than 6 wk
• History of cancer
• Fever[a]
• Night sweats
• Unexplained weight loss
• Recent bacterial infection[a]
• Recent endoscopy, colonoscopy, or cystoscopy[a]
• Recent back surgery or injection[a]
• Intravenous drug abuse[a]
• Pain that is increased at night
• Pain not relieved by typical pain regimen
	• Fever[a]
	• Neurologic finding[a]
	  ○ Bowel or bladder incontinence
	  ○ Saddle anesthesia or abnormal rectal tone
	  ○ Neurologic defect (eg, weakness, diminished reflexes)
	• Diminished or absent peripheral pulses in the legs

[a] Indicates items more specific for spinal epidural abscess and osteomyelitis.

Table 2
Prevalence of a priori risk factors and red flags for patients with spinal epidural abscess

Emergency Department Study[23]		Outpatient Study[22]	
Risk Factor	Percent	Red Flags	Percent
Intravenous drug use	60	Unexplained Fever	86.4
Immunocompromised	21	Focal neurologic deficit	81.8
Alcohol abuse	19	Active infection	81.8
Recent spine procedure	16	Immunosuppression	54.5
Distant site of infection	14	Intravenous drug use	30.3
Diabetes	13	Prolonged use of corticosteroids	24.2
Indwelling catheter	11	Unexplained weight loss	19.7
Chronic renal failure	3	Back pain >6 wk	19.7
Cancer	3	Cancer	13.6
Recent spine fracture	3		
Presence of 1 or more of the above	98		

void residual should be checked. Any red flag should prompt an additional evaluation, but this does not necessarily mean an MRI examination. Because MRI is not readily available at all institutions, if SEA is considered low risk, the patient can be further risk stratified by obtaining a white blood cell count (WBC), erythrocyte sedimentation rate (ESR), and C-reactive protein (CRP). If all 3 of these studies are normal, it is highly unlikely that the patient has an SEA or osteomyelitis.[27,28] Obtaining an ESR and CRP is also associated with a decrease in diagnostic delays (84% to 10%).[28]

If suspicion is moderate to high or the patient's laboratory tests show an ESR >20 mm/h or elevated CRP, the patient will require MRI imaging. If not a candidate for MRI imaging, computed tomography (CT) should be considered along with documenting a discussion with the patient on the decreased sensitivity of this modality. CT myelography should be avoided because of the risk of seeding the subarachnoid space with bacteria if the patient does have an SEA. Because most cases of SEA are from hematogenous spread, it is not uncommon for a patient to have multiple lesions along the spinal canal. It is also difficult to isolate the level of the SEA based on the patient's symptoms. Because of the time it takes to obtain a full-spine MRI, it is not uncommon for MRI techs and radiologists to try to limit the amount of the spine imaged; however, a full-spine MRI with gadolinium is warranted to identify skip lesions and for proper operative planning. A missed skipped lesion can result in continued neurologic decline and sepsis. One single-center retrospective case-control study of 233 cases of SEA from 1993 to 2011 identified 3 factors that were associated with skip lesions. They are (1) concomitant area of infection outside the spine or paraspinal region, (2) an ESR greater than 95 mm/h, and (3) a delayed presentation with symptoms ≥7 days. The predicted probability for the presence of a skip lesion (seen in 22 of their 233 cases) was 73% for patients possessing all 3 predictors, 13% for 2, 2% for 1, and 0% for zero predictors.[29] This single-center study, however, should not change the recommendation of obtaining a full-spine MRI, as the risk of continued sepsis, paralysis, and death is too high if a lesion is missed without other studies validating these findings.

For patients in whom there is suspicion for an SEA, but the patient is felt to be low risk (ie, no neuro deficits) it is acceptable to withhold antibiotics until the MRI results are known. Osteomyelitis treatment is best tailored by the results of a bone biopsy, which can be affected by the administration of empiric antibiotics. If suspicion is very high or there is a neurologic deficit, the patient should be started on antibiotics to prevent worsening of symptoms.

If empiric treatment is started, the patient should be placed on broad-spectrum antibiotics that covers methicillin-resistant *Staphylococcus aureus*, anaerobes, skin flora, and gram-negative rods. A common combination is cefepime or piperacillin/tazobactam plus vancomycin. There has been no reported cross-reactivity between penicillin and third and fourth generation cephalosporins, so cefepime can be given to individuals with a reported penicillin allergy.[30]

Spinal Epidural Abscess Medicolegal Pearls

- Be sure to perform and document a thorough neurologic examination in patients with back pain that includes evaluation of perineal sensation and Babinski reflexes.
- If there are any red flags, strongly consider radiologic or laboratory testing to exclude more serious causes of back pain.
  - A normal WBC, ESR, and CRP essentially excludes the diagnosis of SEA.
- If obtaining an MRI, image the entire spine, as skip lesions are not uncommon.
- Document the time and the reason for any delays in treatment or diagnosis and your attempts to address the situation.

TENDON LACERATIONS

Tendon lacerations are a diagnostic challenge and are often missed on initial presentation to the ED. Mismanagement of these injuries often leads to impaired usage of the extremity and significant disability. The most common pitfall in the evaluation of these injuries is the failure to diagnose. In one study, EM practitioners, as well as hand surgeons, were prone to missing this diagnosis, 36% and 16% of the time, respectively.[31] As a result, hand injuries are the second-most common malpractice claims.[31,32] Although tendons on any extremity may be injured during a traumatic event, the hand is addressed primarily, as it has the most associated disability and the highest propensity to be missed.

Tendon injuries are common in traumatic injuries to the hand. The hands are very susceptible to trauma and hand injuries compromise about 20% of all patients presenting to EDs with a traumatic injury.[33–35] Subsequently, hand injuries are among the most common occupational injuries treated in EDs and among the most common cause of lost workdays.[36] Tendon injuries account for approximately 5% of hand injuries encountered in one large study of 50,272 hand injuries.[33,37] Male individuals are more likely to experience a tendon laceration, and the age group most affected is the 20-year-old to 29-year-old population.[33,34,38] The most common injuring instruments are knives, glass, and trade tools, such as saws and other machinery. Anatomically, the extensor tendons are more superficial to the skin compared with the flexor tendons and are, therefore, more at risk. Consequently, extensor tendons are more commonly injured than flexor tendons.[33,34,39]

In the evaluation of patients with an injury with a laceration, it is important for the EM practitioners to assume there is damage to deeper structures until proven otherwise. The history should include the weapon, the mechanism of injury (ie, stab, slice, puncture), and hand dominance, for the purposes of functionality. A thorough distal neurovascular examination is recommended to assess for any nerve or vascular damage at the site of the wound. Once that has been ascertained, a comprehensive functional examination of the tendons is required and should precede wound exploration, as it may direct the EM practitioners toward a previously unrecognized tendon laceration. This is performed by testing the active and passive motion of all joints distal to the laceration against resistance. For example, a laceration over the dorsum of the hand necessitates the examination of the metacarpal phalangeal (MCP), proximal interphalangeal (PIP), and distal interphalangeal (DIP) joints distal to the wound. The provider should be sure to evaluate the extensor tendons while the digits are in full extension, as the lumbricals assist in the extension of the fingers. In addition, the extensor tendons are attached in the hand to the juncturae tendinum, which can mask an extensor tendon injury. Flexor tendons should be tested while the digits are in flexion. Remember that a partial tendon laceration can still appear to have full function, which is why it must be tested against resistance to examine for weakness. Examine the contralateral hand for comparison. Any weakness or lack of movement on the functional tendon examination warrants evaluation for tendon injury.

Exploration of the wound is where the diagnosis of a tendon laceration is made. Wound exploration should occur in a bloodless field. Local anesthesia with lidocaine with epinephrine is recommended, as it helps vasoconstrict the small blood vessels surrounding the injury to minimize blood loss. The use of lidocaine with epinephrine in digits has been shown to decrease bleeding compared with lidocaine alone, as well as prolonging the time of anesthesia.[40] In addition, use of a tourniquet locally near the wound or a blood pressure cuff more proximally will compress the vessels further and minimize blood in the wound. If there is no visible fascial defect and no signs of weakness or injury on functional examination, it is safe to assume there is no tendon laceration and the wound can be closed as appropriate. Any defect in the fascia overlying the tendon warrants evaluation for tendon laceration. Search the entirety of the wound for any partial or full-thickness tendon injury. Remember that tendons tend to retract proximally when injured. As tendons move, one needs to put the hand through its full range of motion while visualizing the tendon, to ensure the injury has not moved out of the visible field.

All flexor tendon lacerations should be referred to a hand surgeon on an outpatient basis for definitive management. Flexor tendon repairs are at risk for complications, such as adhesion formation limiting the range of motion, stiffness, and contractures.[41] For the management of these injuries in the ED, thorough irrigation of the wound is recommended to remove debris and blood from the wound for ample exploration and to lessen the risk of infection. The wound should then be loosely approximated to minimize the risk of infection to the underlying exposed tissue. The finger or hand should be splinted to prevent further disruption of partial tendon injuries and to prevent further displacement of the proximal portion of the tendon. A dorsal blocking splint is an ideal splint for flexor tendon lacerations. The splint is placed dorsally from the wrist to the distal fingers with the MCP flexed at 60° and the PIP flexed at 40°. Prompt follow-up with hand surgery within a week is recommended, as later repairs are associated with worse outcomes.

Extensor tendon lacerations can be managed by the EM practitioners depending on where the injury lies. The hand is divided into Verdan zones (**Fig. 1**). ED repair can be performed in zones II, III, IV, and VI, which encompass from the DIP joint up to the MCP joint and anything involving the dorsum of the hand.[38] Other zones should be managed by a hand surgeon on an outpatient basis. In general, lacerations that are greater than 50% will require repair. Nonabsorbable sutures are recommended, as absorbable sutures will dissolve before the complete healing of the tendon. If the EM practitioner is not comfortable with tendon repair in the ED, loose approximation of the wound and follow-up with hand surgery is an acceptable alternative. The hand should be splinted whether a repair is done in the ED or not. Tendon lacerations distal

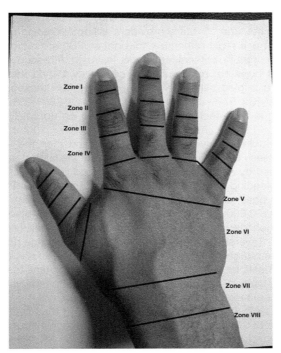

Fig. 1. Verdan zones. Extensor zones of the hand. (*Courtesy of* G.C. Willis, MD, Baltimore, MD.)

to and including the PIP should be splinted with finger splints in full extension. Tendon lacerations proximal to the PIP should be placed in a volar splint in full extension from the wrist to the distal fingertips. All patients should have a prompt referral within a week with a hand surgeon.

Tendon Laceration Medicolegal Pearls

- Make sure to examine all joints distal to a skin laceration against resistance to evaluate for a tendon injury. Any weakness or absence of movement is a tendon injury until proven otherwise.
- The wound should be examined in a bloodless field to evaluate if a tendon injury is present. This can be done by using lidocaine with epinephrine for anesthesia and a tourniquet or blood pressure cuff.
- Flexor tendon injuries need prompt referral to a hand surgeon. Extensor tendon injuries can be repaired in the ED depending on the location and comfort of the provider with the procedure. Splinting is recommended regardless of whether the injury is repaired in the ED.

RETAINED FOREIGN BODY

Retained foreign bodies (FBs) are another area ripe for litigation. Injuries that bring patients to the ED or urgent care center are often prone to be contaminated with an FB, whether it is the gravel from the road, glass from a broken window, or organic material due to a wayward chainsaw accident. It is estimated that retained FBs are found in 7% to 15% of wounds in the ED, and they can be missed on initial presentation up to 38% of the time.[3,42] Many providers will obtain radiographs of all wounds to look for FBs, but one must remember that not all FBs are radiopaque (ie, certain plastics, glass, and organic material [eg, wood, leaves]). Ultrasound also can be used to identify FBs but does not have sufficient sensitivity to find them all. One meta-analysis reported a pooled sensitivity and specificity for ultrasound of 72% (95% confidence interval [CI] 57%–83%) and 92% (95% CI 88%–95%), respectively.[43] Therefore, imaging is imperfect and cannot be relied on up solely for identification of an FB.

Wound care should begin with ample irrigation, and then the wound should be explored in a bloodless field to improve the chance of visualizing an FB. A bloodless field can be obtained by applying a tourniquet or blood pressure cuff to the affected limb to minimize bleeding during the visualization of the wound. The wound should be explored to its base with good directed light into the wound. Finally, lidocaine with epinephrine 1:100,000 can and should be used to minimize bleeding and improve visualization. Epinephrine can even be used in the hands, feet, fingers, and toes to minimize bleeding. Several studies have shown that epinephrine does not cause the necrosis that was suspected in the 1950s.[44,45] In fact, the effects of epinephrine on digital arteries only lasts for 90 minutes, which is not enough time to cause necrosis.[46] Caution should be used in patients who have severe peripheral vascular disease or Raynaud, as this could exacerbate a period of ischemia.

Despite the best efforts of an EM practitioner, an FB may be retained. Patients should be informed of this risk and provided clear discharge instructions on the signs of infection and to return if they feel there is a retained FB. Patients also can be informed of the limitations of ultrasound and plain radiographs. CT can help in the localization of an FB but it is not recommended on the initial evaluation of all patients with wounds, except in patients in whom an FB is highly suspected and not seen with conventional methods.

With the increased incidence of intravenous drug abuse (IVDA) in some areas, it is not uncommon to have patients present suspecting that they had a needle break off in their body. Similar to bullets from gunshot wounds, these should generally be left in place and if really troublesome referred to a surgeon for removal. One retrospective review of 50 patients with neck needles from IVDA showed that only 10% of patients with a retained needle in their neck developed a complication when the event occurred and that there were no delayed complications.[47] Therefore, observation is recommended over surgical removal. Removal in the ED can result in increased soft tissue damage, infection, and inability to remove the FB. These are best removed electively with the assistance of fluoroscopy in the operating room. Most never need to be removed.

HIGH-PRESSURE INJURIES

High-pressure injuries of the hand are another source of litigation. Initially, these injuries appear very benign; however, if not recognized and managed early, they have the potential for devastating functional disability for the patient, as it often results in amputation or requiring multiple surgical washouts and debridements. It is incumbent on EM practitioners to recognize these injuries and involve the hand surgical team promptly.

Most patients involved in high-pressure injuries are male patients who are laborers by trade. The patients use power injectors or paint guns and injure themselves by attempting to use their finger or hand to wipe off the nozzle while it is still running. These tools can contain and subsequently inject paint, paint thinner, fuel, grease, or even water or air and can propel the substance at between 3000 and 10,000 psi.[48,49] The index finger of the nondominant hand is the most commonly injured finger. However, these injuries are not limited to just the laboring population, as there is a case report of an e-cigarette explosion causing a high-pressure injury to a finger.[50] Therefore, any harm to the hand or finger from a high-velocity injection of noxious substances can lead to high-pressure injuries.

The natural progression of the disease varies based on the chemical. The initial presentation is often delayed because of the benign appearance of the wound, and some providers might not recognize the severity of the wound and predicted complications. The initial wound may be a tiny punctate wound on the hand or digit; however, the damage comes from the high pressure dissecting through the planes of tissue, along vascular structures, or within tendon sheaths deep to the puncture wound that is not visible to the naked eye. In some cases, the damage extended up the arm and into the mediastinum.[51–53] Subsequently, the area becomes edematous, and a resultant compartment syndrome develops leading to decreased perfusion and capillary leaking leading to further edema. The chemical causes an inflammatory reaction that further increases edema worsening the perfusion and causing resultant ischemia.[48] Secondary infections occur up to 42% of the time and are most commonly polymicrobial infections.[48,53–55]

Clinical presentations vary, but any small wound that is either painful out of proportion to the examination or with a history of a high-pressure tool or explosion should raise suspicion for high-pressure injury. The average time to initial presentation can be delayed up to 9 hours.[48,56] The EM practitioner should inquire about the substance in the tool, approximate pressure of the tool, and timing of the injury. Organic substances, such as paint thinner and fuel, have the worst outcomes, often leading to amputation, whereas air and water have the best outcomes.[48,55] Grease leads to fewer amputations, but there is still scarring from granuloma formation.[48,55] Tools that injected at greater than 1000 psi were more likely to require amputation. The timing of the injury is also important. One study showed that a delay of more than 6 hours from the initial injury to surgical debridement had higher rates of amputation.[54] The location is also crucial, as the more distal the injury, the higher the percentage of amputation, as there is less space for tissue expansion and a higher likelihood of compartment syndrome.

Management involves radiographs, broad-spectrum antibiotics, and prompt consultation with hand surgery. Preoperative laboratory samples can be drawn, but no laboratory value rules in or rules out a high-pressure injury. The extremity should be elevated to decrease inflammation and swelling, and tetanus prophylaxis should be updated. Radiographs can help with localizing the extent of the damage, especially in cases of radiopaque substances. Radiolucent substances are less likely to be visualized on radiographs; however, air in the soft tissue can sometimes be visualized. Avoid digital nerve blocks, as this may increase compartment pressures, and do not close any wounds. Provide analgesia as needed. Steroids are controversial and have not been shown to improve outcomes despite their known anti-inflammatory properties.[54,55] Patients who have had air or water injected without developing compartment syndrome can be managed conservatively and should be observed overnight to monitor for development of compartment syndrome. Hand consultation for surgical debridement and washout is paramount in the management of all other patients. Hand surgeons will inquire about the substance, the pressure, the timing of the injury, the location of the wound, and extent of the damage. If hand surgery is not available, a transfer to the nearest surgical hand center is necessary to facilitate care.

High-Pressure Injuries Medicolegal Pearls

- Do not downplay the benign nature of the wound of a high-pressure injury, as the damage often extends well past the initial point of entry.
- Obtain radiographs to look for the extent of the injury; however, the absence of findings does not indicate lack of injury, as some substances are radiolucent.
- It is essential to find the type of substance injected, as well as the time initially injured.
- Broad-spectrum antibiotics and prompt hand consultation are paramount for the management of these patients.

SUMMARY

In a busy ED, it is easy to become complacent and assume that patients do not have any serious pathology and that they only have musculoskeletal back pain, a simple laceration, or a simple fracture. EM practitioners must remain vigilant and on the lookout for more severe injuries. Not only will this result in better patient outcomes, but it will decrease medicolegal risk.

REFERENCES

1. Gould MT, Langworthy MJ, Santore R, et al. An analysis of orthopaedic liability in the acute care setting. Clin Orthop Relat Res 2003;407:59–66.
2. Oetgen WJ, Parikh PD, Cacchione JG, et al. Characteristics of medical professional liability claims in patients with cardiovascular diseases. Am J Cardiol 2010;105(5):745–52.
3. Karcz A, Korn R, Burke MC, et al. Malpractice claims against emergency physicians in Massachusetts: 1975-1993. Am J Emerg Med 1996;14(4):341–5.
4. Oetgen ME, Parikh PD. Characteristics of orthopaedic malpractice claims of pediatric and adult patients in private practice. J Pediatr Orthop 2016;36(2):213–7.
5. Kachalia A, Gandhi TK, Puopolo AL, et al. Missed and delayed diagnoses in the emergency department: a study of closed malpractice claims from 4 liability insurers. Ann Emerg Med 2007;49(2):196–205.
6. Elliott KG, Johnstone AJ. Diagnosing acute compartment syndrome. J Bone Joint Surg Br 2003;85(5):625–32.
7. McQueen MM, Gaston P, Court-Brown CM. Acute compartment syndrome. Who is at risk? J Bone Joint Surg Br 2000;82(2):200–3.
8. Fuller DA, Barrett M, Marburger RK, et al. Carpal canal pressures after volar plating of distal radius fractures. J Hand Surg Br 2006;31(2):236–9.
9. McQueen MM, Christie J, Court-Brown CM. Compartment pressures after intramedullary nailing of the tibia. J Bone Joint Surg Br 1990;72(3):395–7.
10. Ulmer T. The clinical diagnosis of compartment syndrome of the lower leg: are clinical findings predictive of the disorder? J Orthop Trauma 2002;16(8):572–7.
11. Shuler FD, Dietz MJ. Physicians' ability to manually detect isolated elevations in leg intracompartmental pressure. J Bone Joint Surg Am 2010;92(2):361–7.
12. Nelson JA. Compartment pressure measurements have poor specificity for compartment syndrome in the traumatized limb. J Emerg Med 2013;44(5):1039–44.
13. Large TM, Agel J, Holtzman DJ, et al. Interobserver variability in the measurement of lower leg compartment pressures. J Orthop Trauma 2015;29(7):316–21.

14. Whitney A, O'Toole RV, Hui E, et al. Do one-time intracompartmental pressure measurements have a high false-positive rate in diagnosing compartment syndrome? J Trauma Acute Care Surg 2014;76(2):479–83.
15. Valdez C, Schroeder E, Amdur R, et al. Serum creatine kinase levels are associated with extremity compartment syndrome. J Trauma Acute Care Surg 2013; 74(2):441–5 [discussion: 445–7].
16. Garfin SR, Mubarak SJ, Evans KL, et al. Quantification of intracompartmental pressure and volume under plaster casts. J Bone Joint Surg Am 1981;63(3): 449–53.
17. Styf J, Wiger P. Abnormally increased intramuscular pressure in human legs: comparison of two experimental models. J Trauma 1998;45(1):133–9.
18. Wiger P, Styf JR. Effects of limb elevation on abnormally increased intramuscular pressure, blood perfusion pressure, and foot sensation: an experimental study in humans. J Orthop Trauma 1998;12(5):343–7.
19. Bhattacharyya T, Vrahas MS. The medical-legal aspects of compartment syndrome. J Bone Joint Surg Am 2004;86-A(4):864–8.
20. Pitts SR, Niska RW, Xu J, et al. National Hospital Ambulatory Medical Care Survey: 2006 emergency department summary. Natl Health Stat Rep 2008;(7):1–38.
21. Friedman BW, Chilstrom M, Bijur PE, et al. Diagnostic testing and treatment of low back pain in United States emergency departments: a national perspective. Spine (Phila Pa 1976) 2010;35(24):E1406–11.
22. Bhise V, Meyer AND, Singh H, et al. Errors in diagnosis of spinal epidural abscesses in the era of electronic health records. Am J Med 2017;130(8):975–81.
23. Davis DP, Wold RM, Patel RJ, et al. The clinical presentation and impact of diagnostic delays on emergency department patients with spinal epidural abscess. J Emerg Med 2004;26(3):285–91.
24. Shantharam G, DePasse JM, Eltorai AEM, et al. Physician and patients factors associated with outcome of spinal epidural abscess related malpractice litigation. Orthop Rev (Pavia) 2018;10(3):7693.
25. DePasse JM, Ruttiman R, Eltorai AEM, et al. Assessment of malpractice claims due to spinal epidural abscess. J Neurosurg Spine 2017;27(4):476–80.
26. Singleton J, Edlow JA. Acute nontraumatic back pain: risk stratification, emergency department management, and review of serious pathologies. Emerg Med Clin North Am 2016;34(4):743–57.
27. Edlow JA. Managing nontraumatic acute back pain. Ann Emerg Med 2015;66(2): 148–53.
28. Davis DP, Salazar A, Chan TC, et al. Prospective evaluation of a clinical decision guideline to diagnose spinal epidural abscess in patients who present to the emergency department with spine pain. J Neurosurg Spine 2011;14(6):765–70.
29. Ju KL, Kim SD, Melikian R, et al. Predicting patients with concurrent noncontiguous spinal epidural abscess lesions. Spine J 2015;15(1):95–101.
30. Campagna JD, Bond MC, Schabelman E, et al. The use of cephalosporins in penicillin-allergic patients: a literature review. J Emerg Med 2012;42(5):612–20.
31. Patel J, Couli R, Harris PA, et al. Hand lacerations. An audit of clinical examination. J Hand Surg 1998;23(4):482–4.
32. Riggs L Jr. Medical-legal problems in the emergency department related to hand injuries. Emerg Med Clin North Am 1985;3(2):415–8.
33. Tuncali D, Yavuz N, Terzioglu A, et al. The rate of upper-extremity deep-structure injuries through small penetrating lacerations. Ann Plast Surg 2005;55(2):146–8.

34. de Jong JP, Nguyen JT, Sonnema AJ, et al. The incidence of acute traumatic tendon injuries in the hand and wrist: a 10-year population-based study. Clin Orthop Surg 2014;6(2):196–202.
35. Clark DP, Scott RN, Anderson IW. Hand problems in an accident and emergency department. J Hand Surg 1985;10(3):297–9.
36. Sorock GS, Lombardi DA, Courtney TK, et al. Epidemiology of occupational acute traumatic hand injuries: a literature review. Saf Sci 2001;38(3):241–56.
37. Angermann P, Lohmann M. Injuries to the hand and wrist. A study of 50,272 injuries. J Hand Surg 1993;18(5):642–4.
38. Bowen WT, Slaven EM. Evidence-based management of acute hand injuries in the emergency department. Emerg Med Pract 2014;16(12):1–25 [quiz: 26–7].
39. Patillo D, Rayan GM. Open extensor tendon injuries: an epidemiologic study. Hand Surg 2012;17(1):37–42.
40. Prabhakar H, Rath S, Kalaivani M, et al. Adrenaline with lidocaine for digital nerve blocks. Cochrane Database Syst Rev 2015;(3):CD010645.
41. Lilly SI, Messer TM. Complications after treatment of flexor tendon injuries. J Am Acad Orthop Surg 2006;14(7):387–96.
42. Tibbles CD, Porcaro W. Procedural applications of ultrasound. Emerg Med Clin North Am 2004;22(3):797–815.
43. Davis J, Czerniski B, Au A, et al. Diagnostic accuracy of ultrasonography in retained soft tissue foreign bodies: a systematic review and meta-analysis. Acad Emerg Med 2015;22(7):777–87.
44. Thomson CJ, Lalonde DH, Denkler KA, et al. A critical look at the evidence for and against elective epinephrine use in the finger. Plast Reconstr Surg 2007;119(1):260–6.
45. Muck AE, Bebarta VS, Borys DJ, et al. Six years of epinephrine digital injections: absence of significant local or systemic effects. Ann Emerg Med 2010;56(3):270–4.
46. Altinyazar HC, Ozdemir H, Koca R, et al. Epinephrine in digital block: color Doppler flow imaging. Dermatol Surg 2004;30(4 Pt 1):508–11.
47. Williams MF, Eisele DW, Wyatt SH. Neck needle foreign bodies in intravenous drug abusers. Laryngoscope 1993;103(1 Pt 1):59–63.
48. Rosenwasser MP, Wei DH. High-pressure injection injuries to the hand. J Am Acad Orthop Surg 2014;22(1):38–45.
49. Bean B, Cook S, Loeffler BJ, et al. High-pressure water injection injuries of the hand may not be trivial. Orthopedics 2018;41(2):e245–51.
50. Foran I, Oak NR, Meunier MJ. High-pressure injection injury caused by electronic cigarette explosion: a case report. JBJS Case Connect 2017;7(2):e36.
51. Kennedy J, Harrington P. Pneumomediastinum following high pressure air injection to the hand. Ir Med J 2010;103(4):118–9.
52. Temple CL, Richards RS, Dawson WB. Pneumomediastinum after injection injury to the hand. Ann Plast Surg 2000;45(1):64–6.
53. Amsdell SL, Hammert WC. High-pressure injection injuries in the hand: current treatment concepts. Plast Reconstr Surg 2013;132(4):586e–91e.
54. Hogan CJ, Ruland RT. High-pressure injection injuries to the upper extremity: a review of the literature. J Orthop Trauma 2006;20(7):503–11.
55. Cannon TA. High-pressure injection injuries of the hand. Orthop Clin North Am 2016;47(3):617–24.
56. Verhoeven N, Hierner R. High-pressure injection injury of the hand: an often underestimated trauma: case report with study of the literature. Strategies Trauma Limb Reconstr 2008;3(1):27–33.

Sports Medicine Update
Concussion

Michael Robert Misch, MD, CCFP-CAC(EM)[a],[*],
Neha P. Raukar, MD, MS, CAQ Primary Care Sports Medicine[b]

KEYWORDS

- Concussion • Mild traumatic brain injury • Return to play • Head injury
- Persistent postconcussion symptoms

KEY POINTS

- A concussion is a form of traumatic brain injury with both functional and structural disturbances, both of which occur at a level that precludes detection with standard imaging modalities available in the emergency department.
- A systematic approach is necessary when assessing a patient in whom a concussion is suspected. Although standardized tools help in the assessment of patients with concussion, the diagnosis of concussion remains a clinical one.
- Patients diagnosed with a concussion should be given both a verbal and written review of the common symptoms of concussion, expected course of recovery, and symptom-management strategies.
- Most patients with a concussion benefit from a brief (24–48 hours) period of rest followed by gradual reintroduction of activities as tolerated. A graduated return-to-sport protocol should be recommended.
- Patients with prolonged recovery from a concussion may benefit from exercise, vestibular, and cognitive rehabilitation programs delivered by multiprofessional teams.

INTRODUCTION

Traumatic brain injury (TBI) is commonly encountered in emergency departments (EDs), with an annual incidence of more than 2.5 million in the United States.[1] Of the patients presenting to an ED with a head injury, most are diagnosed with a minor head injury or concussion.[2] Although emergency physicians (EPs) are often proficient with the emergent evaluation and management of the more severely head-injured patients, most providers are less familiar with the appropriate diagnosis and

Disclosures: None.
[a] Division of Emergency Medicine, Department of Family and Community Medicine, University of Toronto, Toronto, Canada; [b] Department of Emergency Medicine, Mayo Clinic, 200 First Street, Southwest, Rochester, MN 55905, USA
* Corresponding author. North York General Hospital, 1NW-126, 4001 Leslie Street, North York, Ontario M2K 1E1, Canada.
E-mail address: Michael.r.misch@gmail.com

Emerg Med Clin N Am 38 (2020) 207–222
https://doi.org/10.1016/j.emc.2019.09.010
emed.theclinics.com

management of patients with suspected concussion. Increasing public awareness of concussion in recent years has led to community-based initiatives to enhance the prevention and recognition of concussion, but this has also been associated with increasing misconceptions and controversies in the management of this diverse patient population. Although most patients who sustain a concussion experience complete symptom resolution within weeks of injury, some patients have protracted symptoms causing prolonged disability and reduced quality of life. Given that a large proportion of patients with concussion are evaluated in an ED, it is incumbent on EPs to be aware of the intricacies in the evaluation and management of patients with suspected concussion, and to be able to educate them on how to manage their symptoms and prevent further injury in order to facilitate a complete recovery.

PATHOPHYSIOLOGY

The basic pathophysiology of concussion is still being investigated, and although much work has been done, there is no unifying theory. It is often simplistically stated that a concussion is the result of a functional abnormality and not a structural one, but it is more likely that it is both functional and structural. However, despite this, the structural changes are often not visible on standard imaging techniques such as computed tomography (CT) and magnetic resonance imagery (MRI).

A concussion can be caused by a direct head impact or by nonhead impact mechanisms that result in rapid acceleration and deceleration.[3] Another biomechanical perspective includes the contribution of rotational versus linear acceleration, and considerations must be made of the effect of each type of acceleration on neural tissue, and their clinical relevance.[4,5] It is known that the clinical correlation between linear and rotational acceleration depends on the vector of the force through the center of gravity of the head that results in the appearance of symptoms, but the threshold of injury to precipitate symptoms is not known.[6]

Local deformation of brain tissue (strain) initiates a variety of microscopic and macroscopic changes. The threshold to initiate these changes is not known, and efforts to convert global head acceleration and velocity to distortion in a particular location are underway. It has been suggested that this threshold differs between men and women, and that athletes of different sports also have different thresholds to experience a concussion.[7]

On a cellular level, there is a change in the neurochemical cascade following a TBI.[8] The sequence of events that occurs after a concussive event is thought to be similar to those observed after a more major traumatic event, just at a lower magnitude. The normal cell has a variety of processes in place to maintain cellular equilibrium with a membrane potential between -40 and -80 mV. After a percussive force, changes in the permeability of the membrane result in an influx of calcium and an efflux of potassium and glutamate. The extracellular glutamate causes depolarization of the brain cells. To restore the ionic balance, the sodium-potassium pumps require ATP, resulting in a transient increase in glucose uptake in the brain. This disruption in the ionic balance prevents the cells from being depolarized again and renders the cells useless during this prolonged refractory period. Simultaneously, while the cell tries to buffer the intracellular calcium there is an increase in free radical production by the mitochondria. These free radicals cause oxidative damage to lipids, DNA, and protein.

On a more macroscopic level, research has found a variety of pathways that have been affected by the percussive forces on the brain. There is neurofilament misalignment and breakage, disruption of axonal transport, and eventual disconnection.

The effects on a macroscopic level after a single concussion are not readily apparent, but the effects after a career of both concussive and subconcussive impacts (a head injury that does not lead to a concussion) are summarized here. However, the interdependence and the relationship between these changes continue to be elucidated.[9]

1. There is an abnormal deposition of abnormally phosphorylated tau protein in the depth of the cortical sulci. Abnormal phosphorylation of tau protein is part of the normal aging process but it is seen in the brains of young, healthy athletes who sustain head injuries.[10] In healthy brain tissue, the role of tau is to stabilize axonal microtubules used for neuronal communication, but, when abnormally deposited, this leads to cell death and destruction, and a loss in the neuronal network connectivity.
2. There is an alteration of myelin, the white matter of the brain, used to coordinate and accelerate neuronal communication.[11] After concussions, there is an increase in varicosities around the subcortical white matter microstructure leading to an overall decrease in brain volume, reduced diffusivity, and diffuse axonal injury.
3. There is atrophy of the gray matter in the brain leading to overall shrinkage of the hippocampus and the thalamus, structures important for memory and cognition.[12]
4. Experimental imaging techniques show a dramatic reduction in neural connectivity delaying communication between brain regions, a loss in cognition, and an increase in symptoms that rely on a coordinated neural communication.[13]
5. There is a change in cerebral perfusion seen after concussion, the clinical effects of which are not clear.[14]

CLINICAL FEATURES

The most commonly cited definition states that a concussion is a TBI induced by biomechanical forces.[15] Common features that help to define concussions clinically include:

- Concussions can be caused by a direct blow to the head, face, or neck, or elsewhere on the body with the impulsive force transmitted to the head.
- Concussions typically result in a rapid onset of short-lived neurologic impairment that resolves spontaneously but may evolve over several minutes to hours.
- The symptoms of concussion result primarily from a functional disturbance of the brain rather than an overt structural injury, which is not detectable with standard neuroimaging modalities.
- Concussions result in a range of clinical symptoms whose resolution typically follows a sequential course. However, in some cases, symptoms may be protracted.[15]

Importantly, based on this definition, the patient does not need to sustain a direct injury to the head to have a concussion. Force transmitted to the head, such as in a whiplash-type injury, is sufficient to cause a concussion.

The clinical presentation of concussion can be extremely variable both in terms of the constellation of symptoms (**Table 1**) and symptom severity. Concussive head injuries may be associated with a loss of consciousness. Shortly after a concussion, the patient may develop slurred speech, inattention, and incoordination. Retrograde and anterograde amnesia around the time of the head injury are also possible.

Table 1 Common concussion symptoms	
Somatic	Headache
	Nausea
	Tinnitus
	Photophobia
	Phonophobia
	Vertigo
Cognitive	Feeling in fog
	Difficulty concentrating
	Decreased reaction time
Emotional/Behavioral	Lability
	Depressed mood
	Anxiety
	Fatigue
Balance	Dizziness
	Gait instability
Sleep/Wake Disturbance	Somnolence
	Drowsiness
	Insomnia

ASSESSMENT

Head-injured patients should first be evaluated to rule out more severe injuries. The Canadian CT Head rules can help to reduce the number of unnecessary CTs performed while identifying disorder that requires intervention.[16] In addition, the use of the Canadian C-spine Rule or National Emergency X-Radiography Utilization Study (NEXUS) criteria can help to identify patients who require cervical spine imaging.[17] After a more serious disorder, such as an intracranial or spinal cord injury, is ruled out, the diagnosis of concussion should be entertained.

The diagnosis of concussion is not made by a single historical or physical examination finding. Although there are many physical examination findings and provocative tests that can suggest the diagnosis, only when these are considered in the framework of a complete history, and symptoms are consistent with a concussion, can the diagnosis be made. Although many athletes offer their health care providers the benefit of baseline computerized neurocognitive testing, these are often not available to EPs.

History

In patients with a suspected concussion, a thorough review of the possible concussion symptoms should be obtained (see **Table 1**). Given the breadth of symptoms, a standardized symptom checklist may be helpful. This checklist also allows tracking of symptoms during follow-up with the patient's primary care provider (PCP). It is particularly important to obtain information regarding historical features that put the patient at risk of delayed recovery of prolonged symptoms because this may prompt closer follow-up. (**Table 2**). Although there are multiple factors thought to influence recovery from a concussion, the strongest predictor of a slower recovery is the severity of the initial concussion symptom burden.[15]

Physical Examination and Standardized Assessment Tools

Given that a concussion affects different domains, these should be specifically investigated in a systematic fashion. The Sport Concussion Assessment Tool (SCAT) 5 is a validated aid that can be used to systematically guide EPs through their evaluation of

Table 2	
Risk factors for prolonged recovery	
Injury Factors	**Contextual Factors**
Anterograde or retrograde Amnesia	Previous concussions
Severe initial symptom burden	Mental illness
Prominent dizziness	History of migraines
Prominent cognitive symptoms	Learning disability
	Older age
	Social isolation
	Litigation surrounding injury

Data from Refs.[15,18,19]

acutely head-injured patients.[20] The SCAT5 can be found at http://bjsm.bmj.com/content/bjsports/early/2017/04/26/bjsports-2017-097506SCAT5.full.pdf and is used to assess athletes aged 13 years and older, whereas athletes aged 12 years and younger should be evaluated using the Child SCAT5.[21] The SCAT5 queries red flags, observable signs of concussion, immediate memory, Glasgow Coma Scale score, cervical spine assessment, athlete history, symptom evaluation, cognitive screening, neurologic screen, and delayed memory. The cervical spine assessment prompted by the SCAT5 should be augmented by following the Canadian C-spine rules or the NEXUS criteria to help identify patients who require imaging. The SCAT5 continues with a cognitive evaluation (part 3). Serial subtraction can assess concentration and working memory, and can be done by starting at 100 and having the patient subtract 7 until they reach 65, serial 3s from 100 can be used for patients 14 to 18 years old, and serial 1s from 10 for children aged 7 to 14 years. It is important to recognize that baseline cognitive status needs to be considered.

The neurologic examination on the SCAT5 also includes balance testing. The Romberg test is a simple test often used to assess balance. Developed initially to test posterior column disease, as can be seen with tabes dorsalis, the Romberg test assesses the interaction between the visual system, the vestibular system, and proprioception, and serves as an initial test of balance dysfunction in concussed patients. A more sensitive test, which is also inexpensive and quick (can be done in <2 minutes), making it an ideal for the ED, is the Balance Error Scoring System, which more accurately identifies concussed patients.[22] Traditionally, this is done by testing balance on both a hard surface, such as the floor, and while the patient stands on a foam mat. The patient stands in 3 different poses, each lasting 20 seconds. All 3 are completed with the eyes closed and scored based on the number of errors across trials. First, the patient does the double-leg stance, in which the patient stands with the feet narrowly together, hands on the hips, and eyes closed. The second pose is the single-leg stance, in which the patient stands on the nondominant foot and lifts the dominant foot. The third and final pose is the heel-toe tandem pose, in which the patient stands with the dominant foot in front of the nondominant foot. The patient holds each stance for 20 seconds while the number of errors is recorded. Errors include opening the eyes, taking hands off the hips, moving the hips more than 30°, taking a step, stumbling or falling, lifting the forefoot or heel, and remaining out of testing position for more than 5 seconds.

The SCAT5 does not include a detailed oculomotor examination; however, there is evidence to suggest that this is a very sensitive measure of head injury. The vestibulo-ocular system is assessed using the Vestibular Ocular Motor Screening (VOMS) tool, a test that can be completed in less than 5 minutes.[23] The VOMS test is composed of

Smooth Pursuits, Horizontal and Vertical Saccades, Convergence, and the Horizontal and Vertical Vestibulo-Ocular Reflex tests. More details can be found at https://www.physiotherapyalberta.ca/files/vomstool.pdf (**Box 1**).

MANAGEMENT

Recommendations regarding concussion management are often based on low-quality evidence and expert opinion. It is increasingly understood that patients' recovery from concussion is highly variable, requiring individualized recommendations, and there will likely never be a one-size-fits-all management strategy. Although most patients benefit from an initial period of rest, others benefit from an early, more active rehabilitation strategy. Although recommendations as to best practice can be given, these strategies have to be tailored to the individual patient based on the symptom severity, treatment goals, and previous experiences with concussion.

Initial Management and Rest

The recommendation of rest following a concussion has been a cornerstone of concussion management for many years, but the evidence to support the duration of rest has been conflicting.[24–31]

The rationale for recommending rest following a concussion is 3-fold. First, rest mitigates the possibility of additional injury from returning to sports while still symptomatic. Second, it is thought to lessen the severity of symptoms during the recovery period. Third, it is thought to decrease the metabolic demands on the healing brain, which may improve recovery. Although there is consensus that avoiding a repeat head injury while experiencing concussion symptoms is essential to prevent worsening brain injury, there are no strong data to support the idea that complete rest lessens symptom severity or improves brain recovery following a concussion.[15,32] There have been few randomized controlled trials of prescribing rest to patients with concussion in the ED.[33] A randomized controlled trial of adult patients with concussion found that patients prescribed strict bed rest for 6 days reported less severe dizziness in the first 2 weeks but showed no difference in symptom burden at 3 months compared with those who were instructed not to take bed rest.[34] In contrast, a study of pediatric and adolescent patients prescribed strict rest for 5 days had more postconcussive symptoms and a longer time to symptom resolution compared with those prescribed only 1 to 2 days of rest.[35] In addition, a study of adult patients with concussion presenting to an ED found that advising rest followed by a graduated

---

Box 1
Key components of the emergency department concussion assessment

- Obtain directed history
- Assess for traumatic intracranial injury risk factors and obtain head CT when appropriate
- Assess for risk factors of prolonged recovery
- Assess current concussive symptoms
- Perform concussion-focused physical examination by assessing
  - Awareness and alertness
  - Cervical spine and head
  - Cognitive function (attention, memory, and concentration)
  - Vestibular function (balance and eye movements)
  - Near vision (accommodation and convergence)

return to physical activity did not reduce concussion symptom severity at 2 or 4 weeks compared with usual head injury precautions.[36] Meta-analyses have shown that the role of rest is unclear but may be beneficial.[33,37]

What defines rest has also been an evolving concept. Previously, the prescription of strict rest, also called cocoon or sensory deprivation therapy necessitated bed rest with strict avoidance of exercise as well as electronics, books, reading, and other potentially cognitively stimulating activities. However, increasingly, this is now thought to cause symptoms of anxiety, self-perpetuation of symptoms, and social isolation, and is no longer recommended.[15,32] Current recommendations suggest that cognitive and physical rest may be beneficial following a concussion, but should be limited to 24 to 48 hours.[15,32,38] During this time period, patients should be counseled that cognitively demanding tasks such as reading, watching television, or using electronics may exacerbate their symptoms. However, if these activities do not worsen the patient's symptoms, then strict avoidance of them has not been shown to have a benefit and may be associated with harm.[32] After this 24 to 48 hours, a gradual reintroduction of these activities can be encouraged as tolerated, provided the patient's cognitive and physical activity remain below the symptom-exacerbation thresholds. That is, the activities can be done provided they do not worsen symptoms.

Patient Education and Symptom Management

Although associated with disability as well as absence from work, school, or athletics, almost all patients recover within 1 month.[15,19,38,39] One of the few interventions that may reduce the potential for persistent symptoms is early education interventions and patient counseling.[40–43] Although the benefits of such interventions have not been consistently shown,[36,44] patients who have negative expectations toward their recovery from concussion are more likely to have persistent symptoms.[45] As such, it is recommended that both a verbal and written review of the common symptoms of concussion, expected course of recovery, and symptom-management strategies be provided to patients diagnosed with concussion in the ED.[15,19,38,39] A sample handout is available at https://www.cdc.gov/traumaticbraininjury/pdf/tbi_patient_instructions-a.pdf.

Initially, most concussion symptoms are addressed with patient education and reassurance regarding their transient nature and expected resolution with time. Nonpharmacologic strategies for managing headaches, such as encouraging regular sleep, meals, and hydration, as well as avoiding triggers, should be recommended. Patients can use acetaminophen or nonsteroidal antiinflammatories for headaches as required but should be warned regarding the potential for rebound headaches with overuse of these medications. Avoid opioid analgesics when possible. Importantly, medications should never be used to expedite return to play in athletes by masking concussion symptoms because of the risks of reinjury following a concussion.[15]

Return to Play

There is clear consensus that athletes diagnosed with concussion are not to return to play the same day.[15,19,38,39] Second-impact syndrome (SIS), purported to occur when a patient with concussion symptoms sustains a second head injury, resulting in severe and often fatal cerebral swelling, is often cited as a reason for athletes to not return to sport following a concussion.[46] The incidence of SIS is unknown, and many investigators question the existence of such a phenomenon. Regardless, cognitive and balance deficits following concussion place the athletes at greater risk of additional concussive injuries if they engage in sport while still symptomatic.[47–49] Up to 90% of repeat concussions occur within 10 days of the initial concussion.[48] In addition, patients who have multiple concussions are more likely to have more severe symptoms and a more prolonged recovery. As such, a period of physical rest for 24 to 48 hours is recommended by most guidelines.[15,19,38,39]

Interestingly, both prolonged absence from physical activity and vigorous exertion following a concussion have been associated with prolonged recovery, and both of these extremes should be avoided in most patients.[28,50] After this initial period of physical rest, light physical activity can be reintroduced as tolerated, provided it does not exacerbate symptoms. This approach is referred to as a subthreshold exercise program.[15,51]

When athletes are asymptomatic at rest, they may initiate a graduated return-to-sport strategy.[15] A 6-stage return-to-sport strategy that is commonly used is shown in **Table 3**. In general, each stage has gradually increasing physical intensity, with progression through each stage occurring when the patient completes the current stage without symptoms. Each stage should be at least 24 hours. If concussion symptoms occur at a given stage, the athlete should return to the previous stage for a period of at least 24 hours. Following this strategy, athletes diagnosed with concussion often return to full-contact sports no sooner than 5 to 6 days following the initial injury. Patients with recurrent concussions or a history of prolonged recovery following concussion are likely to require a more prolonged return-to-play strategy and may benefit from a formal subthreshold physical rehabilitation program.[15,33]

SPECIAL CONSIDERATIONS
Persistent Postconcussion Symptoms

Persistent postconcussion symptoms (PPCSs) refers to symptoms that persist beyond what would be considered the normal recovery period. There is debate as to when recovery is considered prolonged, ranging from 2 weeks to 3 months.[15,19,38] Given the likely benefit of earlier identification and intervention for patients at risk of prolonged recovery, it is reasonable to consider a diagnosis of PPCS when symptoms persist for more than one month. The cause of prolonged symptoms is debated and likely represents a combination of brain injury with confounding psychological and social factors.[15,19,52] It is often difficult to ascertain whether PPCSs are attributable to the initial brain injury or caused by symptoms of mood or anxiety disorders that can result

Table 3		
Graduate return-to-sport strategy		
Stage	**Aim**	**Activity**
1	Symptom-limited activity	Daily activities that do not provoke symptoms
2	Light aerobic exercise	Walking or stationary cycling at a slow pace. No resistance training
3	Sport-specific exercise	Running or skating drills. No head impact activities
4	Noncontact training drills	Harder training drills. Start progressive resistance activities
5	Full-contact practice	Following medical clearance, participate in normal training activities
6	Return to play	Normal game play

From McCrory P, Meeuwisse W, Dvorak J, et al. Consensus statement on concussion in sport. Br J Sports Med. 2017;51(21):1557-1558; with permission.

from absence from academic, athletic, occupational, and social activities that result from a concussion.

The mainstay of treatment of most persistent symptoms is education and reassurance that most patients can expect a full recovery. Also, cognitive behavior therapy, as well as exercise, vestibular, and cognitive rehabilitation programs, show promise in managing symptoms and improving quality of life.[33,52] Patients experiencing persisting symptoms are likely to benefit from referral to a specialized concussion clinic. Referral should be made earlier in patients with risk factors for prolonged recovery, including high initial symptom burden, previous concussions, comorbid psychiatric illness, and poor social support.[53,54]

Patients who believe that their symptoms will have an ongoing negative impact on their lives are more likely to have persistent symptoms.[45] Although EPs are likely to have little role in the ongoing management of PPCSs, the messaging patients receive when diagnosed with a concussion may influence their recovery.[41–44] As such, patient education and expectation setting regarding the nature of their symptoms and their expected recovery is an important role of the EP.

Chronic Traumatic Encephalopathy

There is increasing public awareness of the potential harms of repetitive concussions. Chronic traumatic encephalopathy (CTE) is used to describe the constellation of attention, memory, and psychiatric symptoms along with characteristic neuropathologic findings, including the regional deposition of tau proteins.[55,56] Although the classic CTE syndrome was elucidated from studying boxers in the United Kingdom in the 1920s, more recent descriptions of CTE come from studying the implications of repetitive concussions in contact sports such as American football.[57] There is evidence that cumulative concussions can cause persistent neuropsychological deficits and are associated with Alzheimer disease, Parkinson disease, depression, and suicide. This relationship likely represents an interaction between repetitive brain injury and biological predispositions.[56–63] Although this remains an ongoing area of research, recommendations meant to reduce the harm from repetitive concussions in competitive sport are a priority.

Pediatrics

Pediatric patients presenting to the ED with head injury should be risk stratified for the need for imaging. CT is the imaging modality of choice for initial investigation of pediatric head trauma.[64] There are several low-risk criteria to guide the decision to perform CT imaging in pediatric patients, including Pediatric Emergency Care Applied Research Network (PECARN), Children's *Head Injury* Algorithm for the Prediction of Important Clinical Events (CHALICE), and Canadian Assessment of Tomography for Childhood Head injury (CATCH).[65–67] Although all 3 rules have excellent negative predictive values, PECARN is thought to have greater sensitivity and may be the preferred tool.[68,69]

As with adults, a systematic approach guided by the SCAT5 (patients aged 13 years and older) or the Child SCAT5 (patients aged 12 years and younger) to the history and physical examination helps to identify concussed patients.[21] A brief period of cognitive and physical rest (24–48 hours) may be helpful for pediatric patients with concussion.[15] Electronics, reading, and other cognitively demanding tasks do not need to be strictly avoided provided they do not worsen symptoms. After this period, cognitively demanding tasks and exercise can be gradually reintroduced as tolerated.

Return to school and return to play are important considerations in pediatric populations. Prolonged absence from school and athletics can cause symptoms of anxiety and depression, which can overlap with those of a concussion and make it difficult to assess recovery in these patients.[70,71] Following the initial period of rest, a graduated return-to-learn protocol should be followed.[15] This protocol includes performing school-based activities such as reading or homework at home before return to school at reduced hours as tolerated. Such a protocol requires academic accommodations to be provided by the patient's school and should be monitored by the patient's PCP.[39] Return-to-play strategies in pediatric patients follow the same graduated protocol as in adults. Although subsymptom threshold exercise is permitted during recovery, patients should not return to competitive sports until they have fully returned to school and completed the return-to-play protocol.[15,39]

Some adolescents are thought to be at particularly high risk for a prolonged recovery, which is likely multifactorial and may be related to a higher frequency of mental illness, more rigorous academic requirements, as well as more anxiety regarding school performance in this age group.[72] Other factors that have been associated with prolonged recovery are female gender, history of migraines, and history of previous prolonged recovery from a concussion.[39] Patients with multiple risk factors for a prolonged recovery may benefit from more intensive follow-up and early referral to specialized concussion clinics.

Gender Considerations

Although men have a higher incidence of concussion, when controlling for the type of sport, women sustain more concussions relative to men.[73] The reasons for this are multifactorial: physiologic, biomechanical, and social.

Physiologically, it has been suggested that a decrease in neck strength may increase concussion risk. As a result of smaller head mass, women generate greater acceleration when exposed to or trying to generate the same force, as when heading a ball in soccer.[74,75] The weaker neck muscles are less able to absorb the forces sustained by the body, translating to greater forces experienced by the head. For every 450-g (1 pound) increase in neck strength, there is a 5% reduction in the odds of a concussion.[76] There also seems to be a difference in the threshold of linear and rotational acceleration required to precipitate a concussion, with women having a lower threshold.[7]

When considering the constellation of symptoms that can be expressed when a patient is concussed, women tend to experience symptoms that affect their activities of daily living more than men do, especially neurocognitive symptoms.[77] Also, it has been suggested that women report their symptoms more than men, or hide their symptoms less, because they are more concerned about their future health.[78]

The potential protective effect of female hormones on neural injury has not been definitively shown. Some investigators have found that estrogen protects the brain, whereas others have found no protective effect.[79,80]

PREVENTION

Concussion prevention can be grouped into education initiatives, rule changes, and legislative changes, as well as the use of protective equipment.

Changing the rules in sports has been found to achieve the desired effect of reducing the incidence of head injuries. For example, eliminating body checking in youth hockey in Canada, or eliminating drills involving full-speed and head-on blocking or tackling as well as limiting full-contact practice time in high school and youth football, have reduced rates of concussion.[81–84] The Centers for Disease Control and Prevention (CDC) has led the way with the dissemination of educational materials relating to concussion to a variety of audiences and it has been suggested that these educational interventions have led to better recognition and management of concussion.[85–87]

The goal of protective equipment is to alter the biomechanical forces, linear or rotational, experienced by the brain. Helmets were originally designed to reduce the incidence of skull fractures, which are generally caused by linear acceleration, but they were found to also reduce rotational forces by up to 30%.[88] As helmet technology responds to the science of concussion, they are evolving to better absorb both linear and rotational acceleration. One unfortunate result of helmet use that has been observed is risk compensation, in which helmet wearers take additional risks because they are wearing protective equipment.[89] Other protective devices have also proclaimed protective effects against concussion, such as soccer headbands, mouthguards, and neck braces. Although mouthguards have been shown to reduce the incidence of dental and maxillofacial injuries, their ability to mitigate the forces transmitted to the skull base is controversial, as is the clinical relevance of this theoretic effect.[90]

Changes in the playing surface on playgrounds have been found to reduce the risk of head injuries. Changes such as not placing playground equipment over untested asphalt, concrete, dirt, grass, or carpet, and instead using rubber mulch, rubber tiles, or loose fill materials at an approved depth, have reduced the rate of playground injuries.[91] In contrast, the use of synthetic surfaces such as turf, which are harder than natural surfaces and result in faster speeds of impact, has resulted in a significantly higher incidence of head/neck injuries, including concussions, compared with grass. However, the effect of these surfaces on the rates of concussion has not been consistently shown, and the rate of concussion while playing on synthetic surfaces, such as turf, seems to be dependent on infill weight.[92,93]

As evidence is published regarding the effectiveness of each of these technologies, there is pressure to approve these devices for public use. However, although many of the studies lack the methodological rigor to draw appropriate conclusions, the media and the consumer market are strongly influenced by sensational marketing techniques capitalizing on increasing public concern regarding head injuries. This influence complicates efforts to find the best strategies to reduce head injuries and concussion in sport.

SUMMARY

Patients commonly present to the ED with head injuries. A systematic approach is required for patients with suspected concussion, and although standardized tools can aid in assessment, the diagnosis of concussion remains a clinical one. At the time of diagnosis, patients should be given both a verbal and written review of the common symptoms of concussion as well as symptom-management strategies. Most patients benefit from a brief (24–48 hours) period of rest, followed by a gradual reintroduction of activities as tolerated. Patients diagnosed with concussion should never return to sport the same day and should follow a graduated return-to sport protocol. Patients with prolonged recovery from concussion may benefit from exercise, vestibular, and cognitive rehabilitation programs. EPs play an important role in patient education and expectation setting at the time of diagnosis. By helping patients to manage their symptoms and prevent further injury, EPs can help to ensure a full recovery in patients with concussion.

REFERENCES

1. Taylor CA, Bell JM, Breiding MJ, et al. Traumatic brain injury-related emergency department visits, hospitalizations, and deaths - United States, 2007 and 2013. MMWR Surveill Summ 2017;66(9):1–16.

2. Jagoda AS, Bazarian JJ, Bruns JJ, et al. Clinical policy: neuroimaging and decisionmaking in adult mild traumatic brain injury in the acute setting. J Emerg Nurs 2009;35(2):e5–40.

3. Ommaya AK, Goldsmith W, Thibault L. Biomechanics and neuropathology of adult and pediatric head injury. Br J Neurosurg 2002;16(3):220–42.

4. King AI, Yang KH, Zhang L, et al. Is head injury caused by linear or angular acceleration? IRCOBI Conference. *Lisbon, Portugal,September* 25-26, *2003.* p. 1–12.

5. Rowson S, Brolinson G, Goforth M, et al. Linear and angular head acceleration measurements in collegiate football. J Biomech Eng 2009;131(6):061016.

6. Zhang L, Yang KH, King AI. A proposed injury threshold for mild traumatic brain injury. J Biomech Eng 2004;126(2):226–36.

7. Wilcox BJ, Beckwith JG, Greenwald RM, et al. Biomechanics of head impacts associated with diagnosed concussion in female collegiate ice hockey players. J Biomech 2015;48(10):2201–4.

8. Giza CC, Hovda DA. The new neurometabolic cascade of concussion. Neurosurgery 2014;75(Suppl 4):S24–33.

9. Satarasinghe P, Hamilton DK, Buchanan RJ, et al. Unifying pathophysiological explanations for sports-related concussion and concussion protocol management: literature review. J Exp Neurosci 2019;13. 1179069518824125.

10. Safinia C, Bershad EM, Clark HB, et al. Chronic traumatic encephalopathy in athletes involved with high-impact sports. J Vasc Interv Neurol 2016;9:34–48.

11. Wright AD, Jarrett M, Vavasour I, et al. Myelin water fraction is transiently reduced after a single mild traumatic brain injury–a prospective cohort study in collegiate hockey players. PLoS One 2016;11(2):e0150215.

12. Goswami R, Dufort P, Tartaglia MC, et al. Frontotemporal correlates of impulsivity and machine learning in retired professional athletes with a history of multiple concussions. Brain Struct Funct 2016;221(4):1911–25.

13. Mcallister TW, Ford JC, Ji S, et al. Maximum principal strain and strain rate associated with concussion diagnosis correlates with changes in corpus callosum white matter indices. Ann Biomed Eng 2012;40(1):127–40.

14. Slobounov SM, Walter A, Breiter HC, et al. The effect of repetitive subconcussive collisions on brain integrity in collegiate football players over a single football season: a multi-modal neuroimaging study. Neuroimage Clin 2017;14:708–18.

15. McCrory P, Meeuwisse W, Dvorak J, et al. Consensus statement on concussion in sport. Br J Sports Med 2017;51(21):1557–8.

16. Stiell IG, Wells GA, Vandemheen K, et al. The Canadian CT Head Rule for patients with minor head injury. Lancet 2001;357(9266):1391–6.

17. Stiell IG, Clement CM, Mcknight RD, et al. The Canadian C-spine rule versus the NEXUS low-risk criteria in patients with trauma. N Engl J Med 2003;349(26):2510–8.

18. Makdissi M, Darby D, Maruff P, et al. Natural history of concussion in sport: markers of severity and implications for management. Am J Sports Med 2010;38(3):464–71.

19. Guidelines for Concussion/mTBI and Persistent Symptoms, Second Edition. Available at: http://onf.org/documents/guidelines-for-concussion-mtbi-persistent-symptoms-second-edition. Accessed November 20, 2017.

20. Echemendia RJ, Meeuwisse W, Mccrory P, et al. The Sport Concussion Assessment Tool 5th Edition (SCAT5): background and rationale. Br J Sports Med 2017;51(11):848–50.

21. Davis GA, Purcell L, Schneider KJ, et al. The Child Sport Concussion Assessment Tool 5th Edition (Child SCAT5): background and rationale. Br J Sports Med 2017; 51(11):859–61.
22. Furman GR, Lin CC, Bellanca JL, et al. Comparison of the balance accelerometer measure and balance error scoring system in adolescent concussions in sports. Am J Sports Med 2013;41(6):1404–10.
23. Mucha A, Collins MW, Elbin RJ, et al. A Brief Vestibular/Ocular Motor Screening (VOMS) assessment to evaluate concussions: preliminary findings. Am J Sports Med 2014;42(10):2479–86.
24. Brown NJ, Mannix RC, O'brien MJ, et al. Effect of cognitive activity level on duration of post-concussion symptoms. Pediatrics 2014;133(2):e299–304.
25. Corwin DJ, Zonfrillo MR, Master CL, et al. Characteristics of prolonged concussion recovery in a pediatric subspecialty referral population. J Pediatr 2014; 165(6):1207–15.
26. Eisenberg MA, Andrea J, Meehan W, et al. Time interval between concussions and symptom duration. Pediatrics 2013;132(1):8–17.
27. Gibson S, Nigrovic LE, O'brien M, et al. The effect of recommending cognitive rest on recovery from sport-related concussion. Brain Inj 2013;27(7–8):839–42.
28. Grool AM, Aglipay M, Momoli F, et al. Association between early participation in physical activity following acute concussion and persistent postconcussive symptoms in children and adolescents. JAMA 2016;316(23):2504–14.
29. Howell DR, Mannix RC, Quinn B, et al. Physical activity level and symptom duration are not associated after concussion. Am J Sports Med 2016;44(4):1040–6.
30. Moor HM, Eisenhauer RC, Killian KD, et al. The relationship between adherence behaviors and recovery time in adolescents after a sports-related concussion: an observational study. Int J Sports Phys Ther 2015;10(2):225–33.
31. Moser RS, Schatz P, Glenn M, et al. Examining prescribed rest as treatment for adolescents who are slow to recover from concussion. Brain Inj 2015;29(1): 58–63.
32. Collins MW, Kontos AP, Okonkwo DO, et al. Statements of agreement from the targeted evaluation and active management (TEAM) approaches to treating concussion meeting held in Pittsburgh, October 15-16, 2015. Neurosurgery 2016;79(6):912–29.
33. Schneider KJ, Leddy JJ, Guskiewicz KM, et al. Rest and treatment/rehabilitation following sport-related concussion: a systematic review. Br J Sports Med 2017; 51(12):930–4.
34. De kruijk JR, Leffers P, Meerhoff S, et al. Effectiveness of bed rest after mild traumatic brain injury: a randomised trial of no versus six days of bed rest. J Neurol Neurosurg Psychiatry 2002;73(2):167–72.
35. Thomas DG, Apps JN, Hoffmann RG, et al. Benefits of strict rest after acute concussion: a randomized controlled trial. Pediatrics 2015;135(2):213–23.
36. Varner CE, Mcleod S, Nahiddi N, et al. Cognitive rest and graduated return to usual activities versus usual care for mild traumatic brain injury: a randomized controlled trial of emergency department discharge instructions. Acad Emerg Med 2017;24(1):75–82.
37. Mcleod TC, Lewis JH, Whelihan K, et al. Rest and return to activity after sport-related concussion: a systematic review of the literature. J Athl Train 2017; 52(3):262–87.
38. Marshall S, Bayley M, Mccullagh S, et al. Updated clinical practice guidelines for concussion/mild traumatic brain injury and persistent symptoms. Brain Inj 2015; 29(6):688–700.

39. Davis GA, Anderson V, Babl FE, et al. What is the difference in concussion management in children as compared with adults? A systematic review. Br J Sports Med 2017;51(12):949–57.
40. Alves W, Macciocchi SN, Barth JT. Postconcussive symptoms after uncomplicated mild head injury. J Head Trauma Rehabil 1993;8(3):48–59.
41. Bell KR, Hoffman JM, Temkin NR, et al. The effect of telephone counselling on reducing post-traumatic symptoms after mild traumatic brain injury: a randomised trial. J Neurol Neurosurg Psychiatry 2008;79(11):1275–81.
42. Ponsford J, Willmott C, Rothwell A, et al. Impact of early intervention on outcome after mild traumatic brain injury in children. Pediatrics 2001;108(6):1297–303.
43. Ponsford J, Willmott C, Rothwell A, et al. Impact of early intervention on outcome following mild head injury in adults. J Neurol Neurosurg Psychiatry 2002;73(3):330–2.
44. Eliyahu L, Kirkland S, Campbell S, et al. The effectiveness of early educational interventions in the emergency department to reduce incidence or severity of postconcussion syndrome following a concussion: a systematic review. Acad Emerg Med 2016;23(5):531–42.
45. Whittaker R, Kemp S, House A. Illness perceptions and outcome in mild head injury: a longitudinal study. J Neurol Neurosurg Psychiatry 2007;78(6):644–6.
46. Mccrory P, Davis G, Makdissi M. Second impact syndrome or cerebral swelling after sporting head injury. Curr Sports Med Rep 2012;11(1):21–3.
47. Covassin T, Stearne D, Elbin R. Concussion history and postconcussion neurocognitive performance and symptoms in collegiate athletes. J Athl Train 2008;43(2):119–24.
48. Guskiewicz KM, Mccrea M, Marshall SW, et al. Cumulative effects associated with recurrent concussion in collegiate football players: the NCAA Concussion Study. JAMA 2003;290(19):2549–55.
49. King D, Brughelli M, Hume P, et al. Assessment, management and knowledge of sport-related concussion: systematic review. Sports Med 2014;44(4):449–71.
50. Majerske CW, Mihalik JP, Ren D, et al. Concussion in sports: postconcussive activity levels, symptoms, and neurocognitive performance. J Athl Train 2008;43(3):265–74.
51. Leddy JJ, Haider MN, Ellis M, et al. Exercise is medicine for concussion. Curr Sports Med Rep 2018;17(8):262–70.
52. Makdissi M, Schneider KJ, Feddermann-demont N, et al. Approach to investigation and treatment of persistent symptoms following sport-related concussion: a systematic review. Br J Sports Med 2017;51(12):958–68.
53. Iverson GL, Gardner AJ, Terry DP, et al. Predictors of clinical recovery from concussion: a systematic review. Br J Sports Med 2017;51(12):941–8.
54. Zuckerman SL, Yengo-kahn AM, Buckley TA, et al. Predictors of postconcussion syndrome in collegiate student-athletes. Neurosurg Focus 2016;40(4):E13.
55. Ban VS, Madden CJ, Bailes JE, et al. The science and questions surrounding chronic traumatic encephalopathy. Neurosurg Focus 2016;40(4):E15.
56. Gardner A, Iverson GL, Mccrory P. Chronic traumatic encephalopathy in sport: a systematic review. Br J Sports Med 2014;48(2):84–90.
57. Manley G, Gardner AJ, Schneider KJ, et al. A systematic review of potential long-term effects of sport-related concussion. Br J Sports Med 2017;51(12):969–77.
58. Guskiewicz KM, Marshall SW, Bailes J, et al. Association between recurrent concussion and late-life cognitive impairment in retired professional football players. Neurosurgery 2005;57(4):719–26.

59. Fralick M, Thiruchelvam D, Tien HC, et al. Risk of suicide after a concussion. CMAJ 2016;188(7):497–504.
60. Gardner RC, Byers AL, Barnes DE, et al. Mild TBI and risk of Parkinson disease: a chronic effects of neurotrauma consortium study. Neurology 2018;90(20): e1771–9.
61. Kerr ZY, Marshall SW, Harding HP, et al. Nine-year risk of depression diagnosis increases with increasing self-reported concussions in retired professional football players. Am J Sports Med 2012;40(10):2206–12.
62. Kerr ZY, Evenson KR, Rosamond WD, et al. Association between concussion and mental health in former collegiate athletes. Inj Epidemiol 2014;1(1):28.
63. Lehman EJ, Hein MJ, Baron SL, et al. Neurodegenerative causes of death among retired National Football League players. Neurology 2012;79(19):1970–4.
64. Lumba-brown A, Yeates KO, Sarmiento K, et al. Centers for Disease Control and Prevention guideline on the diagnosis and management of mild traumatic brain injury among children. JAMA Pediatr 2018;172:e182853.
65. Dunning J, Daly JP, Lomas JP, et al. Derivation of the children's head injury algorithm for the prediction of important clinical events decision rule for head injury in children. Arch Dis Child 2006;91(11):885–91.
66. Kuppermann N, Holmes JF, Dayan PS, et al. Identification of children at very low risk of clinically-important brain injuries after head trauma: a prospective cohort study. Lancet 2009;374(9696):1160–70.
67. Osmond MH, Klassen TP, Wells GA, et al. CATCH: a clinical decision rule for the use of computed tomography in children with minor head injury. CMAJ 2010; 182(4):341–8.
68. Babl FE, Oakley E, Dalziel SR, et al. Accuracy of clinician practice compared with three head injury decision rules in children: a prospective cohort study. Ann Emerg Med 2018;71(6):703–10.
69. Easter JS, Bakes K, Dhaliwal J, et al. Comparison of PECARN, CATCH, and CHALICE rules for children with minor head injury: a prospective cohort study. Ann Emerg Med 2014;64(2):145–52, 152.e1-5.
70. Halstead ME, Eagan brown B, Mcavoy K. Cognitive rest following concussions: rethinking 'cognitive rest'. Br J Sports Med 2017;51(3):147.
71. Irvine A, Babul S, Goldman RD. Return to learn after concussion in children. Can Fam Physician 2017;63(11):859–62.
72. Zemek R, Barrowman N, Freedman SB, et al. Clinical risk score for persistent postconcussion symptoms among children with acute concussion in the ED. JAMA 2016;315(10):1014–25.
73. Dick RW. Is there a gender difference in concussion incidence and outcomes? Br J Sports Med 2009;43:I46–50.
74. Schneider K, Zernicke RF. Computer simulation of head impact: estimation of head-injury risk during soccer heading. Int J Sport Biomech 1988;4(4):358–71.
75. Tierney RT, Higgins M, Caswell SV, et al. Sex differences in head acceleration during heading while wearing soccer headgear. J Athl Train 2008;43(6):578–84.
76. Collins CL, Fletcher EN, Fields SK, et al. Neck strength: a protective factor reducing risk for concussion in high school sports. J Prim Prev 2014;35(5): 309–19.
77. Broshek DK, Kaushik T, Freeman JR, et al. Sex differences in outcome following sports-related concussion. J Neurosurg 2005;102(5):856–63.
78. Granite V, Carroll J. Psychological response to athletic injury: sex differences. J Sport Behav 2002;25(3):243–59.

79. Berry C, Ley E, Tillou A, et al. The effect of gender on patients with moderate to severe head injuries. J Trauma 2009;67(5):950–3.

80. Brotfain E, Gruenbaum SE, Boyko M, et al. Neuroprotection by estrogen and progesterone in traumatic brain injury and spinal cord injury. Curr Neuropharmacol 2016;14(6):641–53.

81. Broglio SP, Williams RM, O'connor KL, et al. Football players' head-impact exposure after limiting of full-contact practices. J Athl Train 2016;51(7):511–8.

82. Cobb BR, Urban JE, Davenport EM, et al. Head impact exposure in youth football: elementary school ages 9-12 years and the effect of practice structure. Ann Biomed Eng 2013;41(12):2463–73.

83. Emery CA, Kang J, Shrier I, et al. Risk of injury associated with body checking among youth ice hockey players. J Am Med Assoc 2010b;303(22):2265–72.

84. Emery CA, Black AM, Kolstad A, et al. What strategies can be used to effectively reduce the risk of concussion in sport? A systematic review. Br J Sports Med 2017;51(12):978–84.

85. Covassin T, Elbin RJ, Sarmiento K. Educating coaches about concussion in sports: evaluation of the CDC's "Heads Up: concussion in youth sports" initiative. J Sch Health 2012;82(5):233–8.

86. Chrisman SP, Schiff MA, Rivara FP. Physician concussion knowledge and the effect of mailing the CDC's "Heads Up" toolkit. Clin Pediatr (Phila) 2011;50(11): 1031–9.

87. Sawyer RJ, Hamdallah M, White D, et al. High school coaches' assessments, intentions to use, and use of a concussion prevention toolkit: Centers for Disease Control and Prevention's heads up: concussion in high school sports. Health Promot Pract 2010;11(1):34–43.

88. Viano DC, Halstead D. Change in size and impact performance of football helmets from the 1970s to 2010. Ann Biomed Eng 2012;40(1):175–84.

89. Hedlund J. Risky business: safety regulations, risk compensation, and individual behavior. Inj Prev 2000;6(2):82–90.

90. Viano DC, Withnall C, Wonnacott M. Effect of mouthguards on head responses and mandible forces in football helmet impacts. Ann Biomed Eng 2012;40(1): 47–69.

91. CPSC. Public playground safety handbook 2010. Available at: http://www.cpsc. gov/PageFiles/107329/325.pdf. Accessed March 25, 2013.

92. Fuller CW, Dick RW, Corlette J, et al. Comparison of the incidence, nature and cause of injuries sustained on grass and new generation artificial turf by male and female football players. Part 1: match injuries. Br J Sports Med 2007; 41(Suppl I):i20–6.

93. Meyers MC. Incidence, mechanisms, and severity of game-related college football injuries on FieldTurf versus natural grass: a 3-year prospective study. Am J Sports Med 2010;38(4):687–97.

Pain Management for Orthopedic Injuries

Nupur Nischal, DO[a], Evangeline Arulraja, MD[a], Stephen P. Shaheen, MD, CAQSM[b],*

KEYWORDS

- Pain • Pain management • Orthopedic injuries • Analgesia • NSAID

KEY POINTS

- Orthopedic injuries encompass a large breadth of disorders, which requires an individual clinical approach based on mechanism, subjective and objective patient evaluation, and expected course of healing.
- Nonsteroidal antiinflammatory drugs and acetaminophen work synergistically and represent a good foundation for most minor to moderate musculoskeletal injuries.
- Local infiltration of anesthetics, as well as regional and hematoma blocks, should be considered in appropriate situations. They are safe to administer, often provide complete relief, and decrease the amount of systemic medication required for analgesia.
- Opioids are effective and should be used judiciously with a focus on route of administration and length of treatment. They have significant side effects in addition to their abuse potential.
- Pain control continues after the discharge and can be augmented with proper expectations, adjuncts, and follow-up appointments.

INTRODUCTION

Pain is the most common chief complaint in the emergency department (ED), making its appropriate evaluation and management an important skill for providers to master.[1] However, the achievement of adequate pain control remains a challenge because of changing practice patterns and systemic protocols, and the education surrounding societal complications of commonly prescribed medications.[2]

Pain can be described as a sensation and an emotion. When acute, it is most often associated with a stress response manifested by vital sign (ie, hypertension, tachycardia) and physiologic changes (eg, local muscle contraction, pupillary dilatation).[3]

Disclosure: The authors have no financial or academic conflicts of interests to report.
[a] Division of Emergency Medicine, Duke University Medical Center, Durham, NC, USA;
[b] Emergency Medicine and Orthopedic Surgery, Division of Emergency Medicine, Department of Orthopedic Surgery, Duke University Medical Center, DUMC Box 3096, Durham, NC 27710, USA
* Corresponding author.
E-mail address: Stephen.shaheen@duke.edu

Emerg Med Clin N Am 38 (2020) 223–241
https://doi.org/10.1016/j.emc.2019.09.013

Management is predicated on appropriate assessment, which includes a clinical review of verbal subjective descriptions and a physical examination. When possible, pain control should be designed to treat the source, as opposed to an attempt to simply mask symptoms.

Pain Assessment Tools

Pain still remains difficult to quantify and a failure to properly assess it is the largest barrier to providing adequate control.[2] Formal methods of evaluation, however limited in scope, improve management and reduce return ED visits.[4] For this reason, numerous tools have been created to assist clinicians in developing a quantitative assessment and a means to appraise intervention responsiveness.[5]

Examples of pain assessment tools:

- Visual analog scale: patients rate pain on a 100-mm marked scale. Extremes of the scale are labeled as the least and worst possible pain. It is rated during 1-minute intervals.
- Numerical rating scale: patients are verbally asked to choose a number on a numerical scale (usually 1–10) that reflects the intensity of their symptoms.
- Verbal descriptor scale: patients select a phrase, usually of a few given choices, that best describes their pain.
- Faces rating scale: patients pick a picture of a face that best relates to their level of pain (see the Wong Baker Pain Scale at https://wongbakerfaces.org/)

However, no assessment tool has been proved to be more efficacious than another. All methods of quantifying pain, especially when used with pretreatment and posttreatment comparisons on the same scale, provide assistance in the elimination of provider bias and improvement of treatment satisfaction.

Pathophysiology of Pain, in Brief

Pain can be divided into 3 major categories: somatic, visceral, and neuropathic. Consideration of the type may help drive the appropriate choice of therapy. Somatic pain tends to be localized and sharp (eg, lacerations). Visceral pain is complex, often accompanied by autonomic symptoms such as nausea and vomiting; it is described as generalized, achy, pressurelike, or sharp. Neuropathic pain is elicited when there is injury or dysfunction in the central or peripheral nervous system (eg, limb amputation).

Pain receptors signal the central nervous system of noxious stimuli, which include temperature extremes, mechanical disruption (eg, blunt or penetrating trauma), and chemical irritants. Inflammatory mediators such as bradykinin, nerve-growth factor, prostaglandins, and leukotrienes contribute to peripheral and central sensitization by lowering the threshold for activating pain receptors and increasing the frequency of firing for all stimulus intensities. Prostaglandins, especially, function in pain production; to a lesser extent they inhibit platelet aggregation and gastric acid secretion, which contribute to its pharmacologic side effect profiles. Because of the aforementioned, inflammation is a key mediator of acute pain.

In addition, the subjective perception of the same mechanism can vary dramatically among individuals; the brain's pain modulation circuits play an implicit role in creating this variance, and this is another factor to consider when determining modalities to achieve adequate pain control.[3]

Early treatment of pain is paramount because it can amplify with duration. The initial response to a stimulus is generally short-lived and causes a sharp, localized sensation. It is followed by a longer phase that is interpreted as a dull, diffuse pain. Prolonged tissue injury can cause sensitization of nerves, which leads to persistent symptoms that last long after initial conditions have resolved. If the noxious neural cascade is halted, there are studies that suggest the development of chronic pain may be prevented.[6]

PHARMACOLOGIC INTERVENTIONS FOR ACUTE ORTHOPEDIC PAIN

As with any medication, the lowest effective dose should be used to limit side effects. The route of administration is determined based on symptom severity, access, and the rapidity with which analgesia needs to be realized. In general, mild to moderate pain can be treated with oral medication. In patients with moderate to severe pain, the intravenous (IV) route can be considered for ease of titration. It is preferable to limit the total number of different medications administered so as to limit confusion about the most efficacious form of treatment, and more importantly, limit side effects from polypharmacy.[7]

Acetaminophen

Acetaminophen (APAP) is a centrally acting analgesic; it does not have significant antiinflammatory properties. APAP is thought to weakly inhibit cyclooxygenase (COX)-1 and COX-2 (COX-2 to a greater extent) enzymes to inhibit central prostaglandin synthesis and increase the pain threshold. Different from nonsteroidal antiinflammatory drugs (NSAIDs), it has limited gastrointestinal (GI) effects and poor antiplatelet activity; the most severe side effect is dose-dependent hepatotoxicity, found with inappropriate administration (>4 g in a 24-hour period).[8]

Nonsteroidal Antiinflammatory Drugs

NSAIDs are used to reduce inflammation from acute injury, thus providing analgesia. They impede the synthesis of prostaglandins through the inhibition of enzymes COX-1 (platelets, stomach, kidney) and COX-2 (synovial fluid). Because of this, some of the more common side effects of prolonged NSAID use include increased bleeding times, gastric ulcers, and decreased kidney function. COX-2 selective inhibitors, although sparing gastrointestinal complications, are associated with an increased risk of myocardial infarction and thrombotic events. These risks are mediated via COX-2 inhibition, which reduces prostacyclin factors involved in vasodilation.[9]

Topical NSAIDs have been shown to provide similar pain relief to oral agents in acute sprains, strains, and overuse injuries; gel formulations of diclofenac, ibuprofen, and ketoprofen, along with diclofenac patches, provide the best effects[10] (Table 1).

For acute pain, a combination of acetaminophen and ibuprofen has been shown to provide greater analgesic effect than solitary treatment with either alone.[11] In addition, some patient-blinded studies have indicated a decrease in reported pain when using a combination therapy of acetaminophen and ibuprofen in comparison with opioids alone in the acute pain setting. Nonopioid medications should be used as first-line therapy given the extensive side effects of narcotics, which are reviewed later.

Special mention: nonsteroidal antiinflammatory drugs for fractures
Note that there is controversy surrounding the use of NSAIDs for fractures because there is a hypothetical risk that they hinder union.[12] It is thought that COX-2, which is inhibited by NSAIDs, mediates a primary role in fracture repair.[13] There are limitations in the current understanding of their effects on bone healing. However, retrospective studies on humans have failed to definitively link nonunion to NSAIDs.[14,15] Although it is beneficial to be aware of this potential risk, it is not wrong to prescribe them; withholding use does not have an evidence-based benefit and may even cause harm by increasing narcotic requirements. The authors recommend a discussion and

Table 1
Commonly administered nonsteroidal antiinflammatory drugs

Medication	Adult Dosage	Comments and Side Effects
Acetaminophen (paracetamol)	PO, 650–1000 mg every 4–6 h; maximum daily dose 4g, PR, 650–1000 mg every 4–6 h; maximum daily dose, 3900 mg daily IV: <50 kg, 12.5 mg/kg every 4 h or 15 mg/kg every 6 h; maximum single dose, 15 mg/kg/dose ($\leq$750 mg/dose); maximum daily dose, 75 mg/kg/d ($\leq$3.75 g/d) $\geq$50 kg, 650 mg every 4 h or 1000 mg every 6 h; maximum single dose, 1000 mg/dose; maximum daily dose, 4 g/d	Liver dysfunction and necrosis
Aspirin	PO, 325–650 mg as needed every 4 h or 975 mg as needed every 6 h or 500–1000 mg as needed every 4–6 h for no more than 10 d or as directed by health care provider; maximum daily dose, 4 g/d	GI irritation and mucosal bleeding Platelet dysfunction Tinnitus, CNS toxicity, metabolic acidosis
Ibuprofen	PO, 200–800 mg 3–4 times daily; usual dose, 400 mg; usual daily dose: 1200–2400 mg/ d maximum, 3200 mg/d	GI upset, platelet dysfunction, renal dysfunction
Naproxen	PO, initially 500 mg, followed by 500 mg every 12 h or 250 mg every 6–8 h; maximum daily dose, day 1, 1250 mg; subsequent daily doses should not exceed 1000 mg	GI upset, platelet dysfunction, renal dysfunction
Indomethacin	PO, 25–50 mg every 8 h Maximum dose is 200 mg per day	GI upset, platelet dysfunction, renal dysfunction
Ketorolac	PO: >50 kg 20 mg, followed by 10 mg every 4–6 h as needed; maximum, 40 mg/d; oral dosing is intended to be a continuation of IM or IV therapy only <50 kg 10 mg, followed by 10 mg every 4–6 h as needed; maximum, 40 mg/d; oral dosing is intended to be a continuation of IM or IV therapy only	GI upset, platelet dysfunction, renal dysfunction, bronchospasm Greater risk of GI bleeding than ibuprofen

(continued on next page)

Table 1 (continued)		
Medication	Adult Dosage	Comments and Side Effects

	IM:
	  >50 kg
	  30 mg as a single dose or 15 mg
	    every 6 h (maximum, 60 mg/d)
	  <50 kg
	  30 mg as a single dose or
	    15 mg every 6 h (maximum,
	    60 mg/d); alternatively, an
	    initial dose of 10 mg (as a
	    single dose) and then every
	    4–6 h as needed has been
	    recommended
	  Maximum, 60 mg/d
	IV:
	  >50 kg
	  15 mg as a single dose or 15 mg
	    every 6 h (maximum, 60 mg/d)
	  <50 kg
	  15 mg as a single dose or 15 mg
	    every 6 h (maximum, 60 mg/d)	

Abbreviations: CNS, central nervous system; IM, intramuscular; PO, by mouth; PR, per rectum.
  Data from Lexicomp Online, LexiDrugs, Wolters Kluwer Health, Inc. Riverwoods, IL; 2013; April 15, 2013.

consensus with the team that follows the patient after discharge from the ED as to any preferences on NSAID use in fractures.

Opioids Opioids (including partial opioid agonists) are a class of medications that carry analgesic and sedative properties. They modulate nociception at both the central and peripheral nervous system, and gastrointestinal tract, by acting as agonists at the 3 primary opioid receptors: mu, kappa, and delta. Potency is generally noted to be: mu>kappa>delta. Mu receptor effects include respiratory depression, cough suppression, and euphoria. When kappa receptors are acted on, downstream actions include dysphoria and hallucinations. In addition, delta receptors decrease respiration and GI motility. Opioids vary in their potency per their individualized specificity and affinity for each class of receptor.[16]

When choosing an opioid, emergency providers should consider the following:

- Desired onset of action
- Available routes of administration
- How frequently the drug needs to be, and can be, delivered
- Use of nonopioid medications as adjuncts
- Incidence and risks associated with side effects, especially those potentiated by other medications the patient is currently taking
- Ability to continue the opioid of choice on discharge
- Prior prescriptions for a similar class of medication (**Table 2**)

Recently, opioid medications have been at the center of much national and media attention. The number of deaths related to opioid misuse has led to a nationwide epidemic and has resulted in guidelines and laws regarding prescription and use. However, it is important to remember that many patients seeking care in the ED are

Table 2
Commonly administered opioids

Medication	Adult Dosage	Onset	Peak Effect	Duration of Action	Comments and Side Effects
Fentanyl	IV, 1.0 µg/kg every 30–60 min as needed	IV, 1 min	IV, 2–5 min	IV, 30–60 min	Short acting No histamine release High doses may cause chest wall stiffness Available in transdermal patch and oral form
Morphine	PO, 10–30 mg every 4 h as needed IM, 5–10 mg every 4 h as needed; usual dosage range, 5–15 mg every 4 h as needed IV: 2.5–5 mg (OR 0.1 mg/kg) every 1–4 h	PO, ~30 min IM, 10–15 min IV, 1–2 min	PO, 60 min IM, 15–30 min IV, 3–5 min	PO, 3–5 h IM, 3–4 h IV, 1–2 h	May cause transient nausea/emesis, hypotension caused by histamine release May cause myoclonus in patients with renal failure
Hydromorphone	PO, 2–4 mg every 4–6 h as needed IV, 0.2–1 mg every 2–3 h as needed; higher doses may be used for opioid tolerance or significant pain	PO, 15–30 min IV, 5 min	PO, 30–60 min IV, 10–20 min	PO, 3–4 h IV, 3–4 h	Potent Good choice for patients with renal failure
Oxycodone	PO, 5–15 mg every 4–6 h as needed	PO, 10–15 min	PO, 30–60 min	PO, 3–6 h	—
Tramadol	PO, 25–50 mg every 4–6 h as needed	PO, 1 h	PO, 2–3 h	PO, 6–8 h	CNS side effects Partial opioid

Data from Lexicomp Online, LexiDrugs, Wolters Kluwer Health, Inc. Riverwoods, IL; 2013; April 15, 2013.

presenting with true, severe pain (acute or chronic). Emergency providers should continue to deliver excellent care and alleviate pain in the most efficacious, safe, and direct method. It is for this reason that opioid medications remain crucial for treatment of severe pain in the ED.

Ketamine

Ketamine is a unique phencyclidine derivative that has dose-dependent analgesic and dissociative activity. It can be used in the treatment of acute and chronic pain.[17] Ketamine is a known N-methyl-D-aspartate (NMDA) receptor blocker; however, the drug's precise mechanism of action remains elusive. Its side effects include sedation and increased sympathetic activity, rarely causing respiratory depression or vocal cord dysfunction; it is more hemodynamically stable than other similar agents.[18] Especially in the pediatric population, there is a low, but notable, chance of an emergence reaction. Emergence reactions are a state of agitation or delirium on exit from the dissociative state. There is some evidence that this may be directly tied to the predosing environment; because of this, some clinicians coadminister small doses of benzodiazepines to decrease sensory stimulation. Benzodiazepines are also the treatment of choice for ketamine-induced vocal cord dysfunction or laryngospasm. There has been concern that ketamine can cause increased intracranial pressures via its activation of endogenous catecholamines but studies are inconclusive, with many trials debunking this theory.[19]

Although a fairly new addition to the emergency medicine pain armamentarium, there are good recent data supporting the use of ketamine for acute pain, as standalone treatment or an adjunct to opioids.[20]

Ketamine does not have a typical dose-response continuum with progressive titration. At doses lower than threshold (which vary by patient), analgesia and sedation occur; once the critical threshold is exceeded (usually around 1–1.5 mg/kg IV), the dissociative state is elicited. It may be administered intramuscularly and intranasally, which can be beneficial in pediatric patients (**Table 3**).

Neuropathic medications

Because pain sensation is processed by the central nervous system, endogenous opioids (ie, enkephalin and dynorphin), serotonin, and norepinephrine are released. Antidepressants work by preventing the reuptake of serotonin and norepinephrine and therefore seem to have a potential role in therapy. Anticonvulsants or membrane stabilizers (eg, carbamazepine, gabapentin) exert their function at the peripheral nerve by blocking transmission through increased production of gamma-aminobutyric acid (GABA), an inhibitory neurotransmitter. Specifically, subjective complaints of burning pain may be alleviated by antidepressants, whereas shooting pain can respond to anticonvulsants.[6]

Table 3 Ketamine administration		
Medication	**Adult Dosage**	**Comments and Side Effects**
Ketamine	Intranasal (IN), 0.5–1 mg/kg; may repeat in 10–15 min with 0.25– 0.5 mg/kg if necessary IM, 2–4 mg/kg IV, 0.2–0.8 mg/kg bolus.	No renal or hepatic adjustment Consider the concomitant use of a benzodiazepine (eg, lorazepam) to prevent or reduce psychotomimetic effects

Data from Lexicomp Online, LexiDrugs, Wolters Kluwer Health, Inc. Riverwoods, IL; 2013; April 15, 2013.

Skeletal muscle relaxants

Relaxants are often used to treat muscle spasms but major symptom relief may come from their centrally mediated sedative properties; studies have shown that they can be effective in the acute setting (<1 week) but prolonged treatment benefit is still in question.[21–23] They are valuable in conjunction with NSAIDs as adjunctive therapy but there is no evidence that there is greater efficacy than NSAIDs when prescribed alone.[21,23]

PHARMACOLOGY OF PROCEDURAL SEDATION

Procedural sedation is commonly used during painful orthopedic manipulations to provide a depressed level of consciousness while maintaining cardiorespiratory function. Sedation is often coadministered with analgesia.[24] Ideal pharmacologic agents are those that are short acting and have limited, or no, respiratory and hemodynamic depression.

Commonly administered medications are discussed next.

Ketamine

Ketamine offers the most stable safety profile overall but it can increase sympathetic surge. It is the only sedative that maintains a patient's intrinsic ventilatory effort with limited hemodynamic impact.[25] It may be administered intramuscularly and intranasally, which can be beneficial in pediatric patients without intravenous access.

Propofol

Level A recommendation for use in both pediatric and adult populations.[25]

Propofol is easy to titrate and is associated with fewer complications compared with other sedatives.[26] It is often a preferred medication in the ED because of its short duration of action, allowing decreased recovery times and overall length of stay.[27–29] Notably, it does cause respiratory depression so emergency medicine physicians need to be prepared to assist ventilation and even intubate if needed.[30] Hypotension may develop, secondary to its action as negative inotrope and vasodilator.

Propofol/Ketamine (Ketofol)

Level B recommendation for use in both pediatric and adult populations.[25]

When ketamine and propofol are combined to achieve analgesia and sedation, the most commonly used ratio dosing is 1:1 (0.5–0.75 mg/kg of each). They can be prepared in a single syringe or separately.

This decreased individual dosing provides the advantage of reducing the adverse effects of both agents. It is theorized that the side effect profiles mirror each other (ie, ketamine-induced increases in circulatory norepinephrine mitigate propofol-associated hypotension and respiratory depression; ketamine-associated nausea is limited by the antiemetic properties of propofol).[27,31–36]

Midazolam and Fentanyl

Midazolam is a short-acting benzodiazepine that is used for sedation, often coadministered with fentanyl for pain control. With midazolam, up to 15% of patients can have a paradoxic agitation reaction. One downside to using these medications together is that they potentiate the risk of significant respiratory depression. When this happens, flumazenil is available as a reversal agent (avoided in chronic benzodiazepine users). Midazolam can be an interesting choice because it offers an additional route of administration, intranasal, that most other sedatives do not.[37]

Although this is a common combination of benzodiazepine and opioid, there are multiple others used with similar effect. Any benzodiazepine can be combined with a narcotic, although the preference is to keep with shorter half-life medications to limit the time the patient needs one-on-one monitoring by a nurse and physician.

Dexmedetomidine

Dexmedetomidine, initially approved for use as a sedative, is under investigation as a pain medication because of its unique properties.[38] It is a selective and specific alpha-2 adrenergic receptor agonist, similar to clonidine, and has analgesic and anxiolytic characteristics that have been shown to be beneficial in orthopedic pain management, potentially as a single agent.[39,40]

Etomidate

Etomidate is a sedative-hypnotic with rapid onset (within 30 seconds) and a short half-life (~5 min). Compared with other sedatives, it causes similar respiratory depression but has improved hemodynamic stability. Etomidate is used in the ED for procedural sedation because of its low rate of reported complications (10%–15% overall) and rapid recovery to patient baseline.[41–45] Of note, although this figure may seem high, it includes all complications, even those that are minor, including prolonged sedation, snoring, and mild changes in oxygenation (90%–95%) requiring supplemental oxygen. It is often administered with fentanyl for pain management (**Table 4**).

PHARMACOLOGY OF LOCAL ANESTHESIA

Local anesthesia is a method of providing targeted pain control to a specific location. It can often decrease the amount of overall systemic medication needed and, in some cases, preclude the need for sedation altogether, resulting in simplified procedures.

Profound complications secondary to the delivery of local anesthetics are rare. The most insidious complication of local anesthetic use is systemic toxicity; this can range from minor neurologic symptoms to seizures, and includes cardiac arrhythmias and arrest.[46] The odds of occurrence are minimized further through familiarity with maximum dosages, proper administration, and review of patient allergy profiles.[47] Toxicity is related to progression of sodium channel blockade in tissues beyond those of intention.[48,49]

Local anesthetics can be administered topically, intradermally, or subdermally, or infiltrated near peripheral nerves. When considering each approach, many factors should be taken into account. In the setting of wound management, these factors include the patient (ie, age, anticipated pain tolerance, comorbidities), wound characteristics (ie, location, depth, contamination status, concomitant neurovascular injury), and technical components (ie, anticipated time requirement, clinician experience).

Dosing of these medications varies significantly, depending on many of the factors listed earlier. As a general guide, lidocaine has the shortest onset and duration of action; ropivacaine is at the opposite end of the spectrum, with effects often lasting beyond 5 hours. Bupivacaine is in the middle.

Providers may also choose to have additives combined with analgesics to fortify their effect.

- Epinephrine causes vasoconstriction, decreasing the diffusion of anesthetic. This action allows an increased maximum dose, a faster onset of action, and an wider safety window.
- Sodium bicarbonate has several potential effects through its changes to solution pH. First, it may decrease the time to complete sensory block. Evidence also

Table 4
Commonly administered medications for sedation

Medication	Adult Dosage	Peak Action	Duration of Action	Comments and Side Effects
Ketamine	IV, 1–2 mg/kg bolus; 0.5–1 mg/kg PRN after bolus dose	IV, 1–3 min	IV, 15–30 min	Nausea, laryngospasm
	IM, 4–5 mg/kg followed by 2–4 mg/kg IM if first dose is unsuccessful	IM, 5–20 min	IM, 30–60 min	
Propofol	IV, 0.5–1 mg/kg bolus, followed by 0.5 mg/kg every 3 min, if needed	30–60 s	5–6 min	Hypotension, respiratory depression
Ketofol	IV, 1:1 ratio 0.5 mg/kg for each agent mixed in a syringe or given separately Starting dose, 0.5 mg/kg followed by another 0.5 mg/kg, as needed, after 30–60 s Maintenance, 0.25 mg/kg as needed	30–60 s	15 min	Similar side effects to propofol and ketamine but much reduced
Fentanyl/ midazolam	IV, dose fentanyl first, 1–2 µg/kg; follow with 0.1 mg/kg midazolam	2–3 min	1 h	—
Fentanyl/ etomidate	IV, dose fentanyl first, 0.5–1 µg/kg; then etomidate 0.15 mg/kg (8–10 mg average)	—	6 min	Myoclonus and adrenal suppression
Dexmedetomidine	1 µg/kg loading dose followed by 0.2–1 µg/kg/h maintenance dose	—	—	Bradycardia and hypotension Avoid in patients with heart blocks
Etomidate	0.1 mg/kg 1-time dosing	—	—	Minimal respiratory depression, hypotension, bradycardia

Abbreviation: PRN, as needed.
   Data from Lexicomp Online, LexiDrugs, Wolters Kluwer Health, Inc. Riverwoods, IL; 2013; April 15, 2013.

supports that injections are perceived as less painful to patients.[50,51] Adding 1 mL of sodium bicarbonate 8.4% (1 mEq/mL) to 9 mL of 1% lidocaine (literature cites ratios from 1:5 to 1:15) effectively buffers the preparation.[52] However, the inclusion of bicarbonate precipitates the anesthetic agent (especially bupivacaine) and accelerates the degradation of epinephrine; as a result, it should not be added unless it is to be immediately used.

- Clonidine shows promise as a time-augmenting agent; a dose of 0.5 µg/kg (maximal dose, 150 µg) can be mixed to prolong the duration of anesthesia by greater than 50%.[53] However, it may also cause hypotension, limiting its usefulness.[54]
- The addition of dexmedetomidine has a similar effect to that of clonidine (alpha-2 adrenoceptor agonist), but it is more selective and shorter acting. It is still controversial and subject to ongoing research.[38,39]

Hematoma Block

Anesthetic injected into a hematoma around the site of a fractured bone drives medication into the sensitive periosteum and blankets surrounding sensory nerves. It is easily performed and proper location is confirmed by aspiration of blood into the syringe before injection. Studies have shown faster time to reduction, no significant difference in pain control, and similar rates of reduction displacement at 1 week compared with propofol-assisted procedural sedation.[55]

Regional Anesthesia

For increased area of effect, medication can be placed more proximally, surrounding a peripheral nerve (or plexus); this produces downstream anesthesia in a specific sensory locale. Nerve blocks, especially when used in conjunction with parenteral opioids, have been proved to decrease pain intensity and the need for repeated dosing, in addition to having limited adverse events.[56–60] They are an acceptable alternative in patient populations in which procedural sedation is contraindicated.

A recent Cochrane Review revealed that the use of ultrasonography decreases complications associated with nerve blocks and improves performance duration and quality.[61,62]

Studies have suggested that peripheral nerve blocks are underused in the emergency setting; they are in the scope of practice for trained providers and should be considered more frequently as a means of analgesia in the ED.[58,59,63]

Methods of nerve blocks include peripheral (eg, femoral nerve block), nerve plexus (eg, cervical plexus blocks), and neuraxial blocks (eg, epidural). Although there are multiple sites and injection methods for most nerves, a complete list is outside the purview of this article. Providers should consult their state medical boards, and hospital protocols, for guidance before their use.

Examples of common nerve blocks:

- Femoral nerve block
  - Femoral nerve blocks can be performed for injury (eg, femur fractures) in the distribution of its namesake (anterior and lateral lower extremity).[64] In the United Kingdom and Australia, select emergency services administer them in the field.[65] They are well tolerated and easy to administer.
- Digital block
  - This block provides pain relief to a single digit, distal to injection of the anesthetic. There are several methods, the most common being the ring and

transthecal (ie, flexor tendon sheath). In the latter, anesthetic is injected above the digital flexor tendon sheath, typically at the palmar crease, near the base of the finger. Medication disperses longitudinally along its course, numbing the entirety of the targeted digit. Although traditional teaching was to avoid epinephrine in fingers, it is unsupported by data and is now known to be safe.[66–69]

Intra-articular Injections

For successful intra-articular relief, analgesic (usually bupivacaine or lidocaine), sometimes combined with steroid, is injected directly into the synovial space. The best approach provides maximal access to the synovial cavity with minimal obstruction; this can vary and is best chosen according to each patient's bony anatomy. Although less commonly used, injection of morphine is another method of providing analgesia; typical dosing guidelines recommend 1 to 5 mg, diluted in sterile normal saline. Between these two variations, morphine seems to be more effective in providing extended pain relief, only eclipsed by combination with a local anesthetic.[70–72]

Bier Block

Although this method is effective, it requires specialized training and equipment and is most often performed by anesthesiologists in the operating room. The affected extremity is first exsanguinated through the use of a double pneumatic cuff, applied proximally. A small IV catheter is placed at the distal portion of the extremity. Local anesthetic (eg, 1.5–3 mg/kg of 0.5% lidocaine) is administered. Pain control is most potent in the extremity for 30 minutes following injection, after which the cuff should be deflated; the remaining medication (minimal) is cleared systemically.

Topical Anesthetics

Lidocaine patches were approved by the US Food and Drug Administration for postherpetic neuralgia but have since been used in patients with a variety of other pain, including musculoskeletal. Some research provides evidence that they may even be beneficial in the treatment of osteoarthritis when used as monotherapy.[6] Small, nonrandomized studies have shown improvement in pain scores with lidocaine patch use.[73] They are well tolerated, with few systemic side effects, and can provide adjunctive analgesia to patients who are receiving multimodal treatment (or are on multiple medications) without increasing risks for adverse drug interactions.[6]

Topical NSAIDs, such as diclofenac and ketoprofen, have recently seen increased use because there seems to be efficacy for the relief of acute muscular and chronic osteoarthritic pain. In reviews, oral versus topical NSAIDs have had similar reported pain reduction benefit. One advantage of topical NSAIDs is the decreased GI side effect profile.[74]

NONPHARMACOLOGIC INTERVENTIONS

In addition to known pharmaceuticals, there are other commonly used and proven methods of relief, such as physical therapy and range-of-motion exercises. Rest, ice, compression, and elevation (RICE) is a widely accepted starting point for pain control in most orthopedic injuries.

Other alternate treatment modalities are sometimes dismissed in the ED secondary to the time and effort they take to properly explain. However, these interventions should be considered as adjuncts for pain management on an individual basis. These treatments include, but are not limited to, cognitive behavior therapy, transcutaneous electrical nerve stimulation, music, acupuncture, meditation, biofeedback, hypnosis, and distraction.[75] Specialized training may be necessary before they can be appropriately administered or prescribed. Literature support, as expected, varies significantly as to the degree of effectiveness for each.

PAIN CONTROL STRATEGIES FOR SELECT ORTHOPEDIC INJURIES
Fractures

Fractures can be caused by direct trauma, overuse, or osteoporosis. Ice, compression, and elevation of the injury above the level of the heart, prevents excessive local edema, a potential cause of worsening pain.

Primary management should focus on definitive treatment, which is often simply stabilizing the fracture site through casting or splinting.

Analgesic medication recommendations

For minor fractures, acetaminophen and NSAIDs offer appropriate analgesia. With major or comminuted fractures, the addition of opioid medications may be necessary.[76] Short-acting opioids in combination with acetaminophen/NSAIDs cause fewer side effects and allow smaller doses to provide equivalent relief.[77]

Acute pain can vary depending on the fracture class and type but typically lasts from a few days to several weeks; any opioid prescriptions for breakthrough relief should reflect this. It is unusual to have severe, or worsening, fracture pain greater than 7 days after the primary insult; this may represent a complication and warrants further investigation.

Dislocations

Joint dislocations are most commonly caused by trauma and result in significant damage to surrounding tendons, ligaments, muscles, and nerves.[78] Definitive management of associated pain is with reduction, but this must be approached cautiously.

The longer the delay from time of injury, the more difficult and painful it is to achieve a closed reduction. Reduction provides pain relief by relieving tension on nerves and vessels stretched during the dislocation, subsequently bringing cessation to the risk of injury exacerbation (eg, conversion of a closed fracture with skin tenting to an open fracture or restoring circulation in an emergent pulseless extremity).[79] Delays may also increase the risk of adverse events because of prolonged compression of neurovascular structures, muscle spasm, and contracture, making it imperative to minimize time to reduction whenever possible.[80] Of note, some reductions can be done rapidly or painlessly without sedation (eg, radial head subluxation) or by using secondary techniques (eg, Cunningham method for anterior shoulder dislocations).

An alternative to sedation for reduction is local anesthesia via hematoma blocks, regional nerve blocks, or intra-articular injections. When intra-articular injection was compared with IV sedation of a dislocation-reduction, it provided similar pain relief with fewer complications and shorter duration of hospitalization.[81] Specifics on bracing, splinting, and casting for stabilizing discharge pain control are discussed in previous articles.

Muscular Sprains/Strains/Spasms

Sprains, strains, and contusions are common soft tissue injuries seen in the ED. By definition, acute insult to muscle fibers is a strain, and ligaments, a sprain; however, in practice, they often coexist. These mechanisms result in pain primarily through the inflammatory pathway and cascade. Hence, to treat the source in the acute setting

(<7 days), antiinflammatories such as NSAIDs are the most effective therapy; opioids have not been shown to have greater clinical efficacy.[82]

In contrast, muscle spasms are often treated with muscle relaxants. The evidence suggests using them in combination with NSAIDs for pain relief in the acute setting.[21–23] As for individual selection of therapy, there has been no difference in performance among the various medications.

Infections

Infectious causes of discomfort with relation to orthopedics include septic joints, cellulitis, necrotizing infections, and osteomyelitis. This subset of pain is primarily mediated through the inflammatory pathway, making treatment of the infection (ie, antibiotics) and source control (ie, drainage or washout) the optimal management in these scenarios. NSAIDs are not commonly used when operative management is an option because they are physiologically associated with increased bleeding times via inhibition of platelet aggregation. Direct data are insufficient regarding overall risk and morbidity of significant bleeding associated with NSAIDs in the perioperative setting.[83] Provided the patient has stable hemodynamics, opioids are a reasonable choice for therapy.

SUMMARY

Orthopedic pain management needs be tailored to the needs of the individual patient with respect to the underlying condition, expected healing timeline, comorbidities, and current medications. This article exposes providers to new and alternative forms of therapy; they should prescribe pharmaceutical agents that are within their scope of practice and comfort zone.

In general, the pain of minor orthopedic injuries is often controlled with NSAIDs and acetaminophen. If this is not enough, oral, then IV, opioids can be used. The authors recommend always using the lowest appropriate dosage first, with a plan for escalation of therapy as needed. Opioids have a role, but care must be taken because of their side effect profile and abuse potential.

REFERENCES

1. Todd KH, Ducharme J, Choiniere M, et al. Pain in the emergency department: results of the pain and emergency medicine initiative (PEMI) multicenter study. J Pain 2007;8(6):460–6.
2. Vuille M, Foerster M, Foucault E, et al. Pain assessment by emergency nurses at triage in the emergency department: a qualitative study. J Clin Nurs 2018; 27(3–4):669–76.
3. Rathmell JP, Fields HL. Pain: pathophysiology and management. In: Jameson JL, Fauci AS, Kasper DL, et al, editors. Harrison's principles of internal medicine, 20e. New York: McGraw-Hill Education; 2018. Available at: http://accessmedicine. mhmedical.com/content.aspx?aid=1160046913. Accessed January 20, 2019.
4. Lee JS. Pain measurement: understanding existing tools and their application in the emergency department. Emerg Med (Fremantle) 2001;13(3):279–87.
5. Hawker GA, Mian S, Kendzerska T, et al. Measures of adult pain: visual analog scale for pain (VAS pain), numeric rating scale for pain (NRS pain), McGill pain questionnaire (MPQ), short-form McGill pain questionnaire (SF-MPQ), chronic pain grade scale (CPGS), short form-36 bodily pain scale (SF-36 BPS), and measure of intermittent and constant osteoarthritis pain (ICOAP). Arthritis Care Res (Hoboken) 2011;63(Suppl 11):S240–52.

6. Miner JR, Todd KH. Pain management in the emergency department. In: Benzon HT, Raj PP, editors. Raj's practical management of pain. Philadelphia: Mosby-Elsevier; 2008. p. 1143–50. https://doi.org/10.1016/B978-032304184-3.50066-2.

7. Pescatore R, Nyce A. Managing shoulder injuries in the emergency department: fracture, dislocation, and overuse. Emerg Med Pract 2018;20(6):1–28.

8. Negm AA, Furst DE. Nonsteroidal anti-inflammatory drugs, disease-modifying antirheumatic drugs, nonopioid analgesics, & drugs used in gout. In: Katzung BG, editor. Basic & clinical pharmacology, 14e. New York: McGraw-Hill Education; 2017. Available at: http://accessmedicine.mhmedical.com/content.aspx?aid=1148438488. Accessed January 26, 2019.

9. Conaghan PG. A turbulent decade for NSAIDs: update on current concepts of classification, epidemiology, comparative efficacy, and toxicity. Rheumatol Int 2012;32(6):1491–502.

10. Derry S, Moore RA, Gaskell H, et al. Topical NSAIDs for acute musculoskeletal pain in adults. Cochrane Database Syst Rev 2015;(6):CD007402.

11. Moore RA, Wiffen PJ, Derry S, et al. Non-prescription (OTC) oral analgesics for acute pain - an overview of Cochrane reviews. Cochrane Database Syst Rev 2015;(11):CD010794.

12. Beck A, Krischak G, Sorg T, et al. Influence of diclofenac (group of nonsteroidal anti-inflammatory drugs) on fracture healing. Arch Orthop Trauma Surg 2003;123(7):327–32.

13. Vane JR, Botting RM. Mechanism of action of nonsteroidal anti-inflammatory drugs. Am J Med 1998;104(3A):2S–8S [discussion: 21S].

14. Richards CJ, Graf KW, Mashru RP. The effect of opioids, alcohol, and nonsteroidal anti-inflammatory drugs on fracture union. Orthop Clin North Am 2017;48(4):433–43.

15. Marquez-Lara A, Hutchinson ID, Nuñez F, et al. Nonsteroidal anti-inflammatory drugs and bone-healing: a systematic review of research quality. JBJS Rev 2016;4(3). https://doi.org/10.2106/JBJS.RVW.O.00055.

16. Burillo-Putze G, Miro O. Opioids. In: Tintinalli JE, Stapczynski JS, Ma OJ, et al, editors. Tintinalli's emergency medicine: a comprehensive study guide, 8e. New York: McGraw-Hill Education; 2016. Available at: http://accessmedicine.mhmedical.com/content.aspx?aid=1121499663. Accessed January 26, 2019.

17. Duman RS, Li N, Liu R-J, et al. Signaling pathways underlying the rapid antidepressant actions of ketamine. Neuropharmacology 2012;62(1):35–41.

18. Sleigh J, Harvey M, Voss L, et al. Ketamine – More mechanisms of action than just NMDA blockade. Trends in Anaesthesia and Critical Care 2014;4(2–3):76–81.

19. Roberts DJ, Hall RI, Kramer AH, et al. Sedation for critically ill adults with severe traumatic brain injury: a systematic review of randomized controlled trials. Crit Care Med 2011;39(12):2743–51.

20. Schwenk ES, Viscusi ER, Buvanendran A, et al. Consensus guidelines on the use of intravenous ketamine infusions for acute pain management from the american society of regional anesthesia and pain medicine, the american academy of pain medicine, and the american society of anesthesiologists. Reg Anesth Pain Med 2018;43(5):456–66.

21. van Tulder MW, Touray T, Furlan AD, et al. Muscle relaxants for non-specific low back pain. Cochrane Database Syst Rev 2003;(2):CD004252.

22. Abdel Shaheed C, Maher CG, Williams KA, et al. Efficacy and tolerability of muscle relaxants for low back pain: systematic review and meta-analysis. Eur J Pain 2017;21(2):228–37.

23. Chou R, Deyo R, Friedly J, et al. Systemic pharmacologic therapies for low back pain: a systematic review for an american college of physicians clinical practice guideline. Ann Intern Med 2017;166(7):480–92.

24. Godwin SA, Caro DA, Wolf SJ, et al. Clinical policy: procedural sedation and analgesia in the emergency department. Ann Emerg Med 2005;45(2):177–96.

25. Godwin SA, Burton JH, Gerardo CJ, et al. Clinical policy: procedural sedation and analgesia in the emergency department. Ann Emerg Med 2014;63(2): 247–58.e18.

26. Miner JR, Biros M, Krieg S, et al. Randomized clinical trial of propofol versus methohexital for procedural sedation during fracture and dislocation reduction in the emergency department. Acad Emerg Med 2003;10(9):931–7.

27. Uri O, Behrbalk E, Haim A, et al. Procedural sedation with propofol for painful orthopaedic manipulation in the emergency department expedites patient management compared with a midazolam/ketamine regimen: a randomized prospective study. J Bone Joint Surg Am 2011;93(24):2255–62.

28. Rahman NHNA, Hashim A. Is it safe to use propofol in the emergency department? A randomized controlled trial to compare propofol and midazolam. Int J Emerg Med 2010;3(2):105–13.

29. Lee Y-K, Chen C-C, Lin H-Y, et al. Propofol for sedation can shorten the duration of ED stay in joint reductions. Am J Emerg Med 2012;30(8):1352–6.

30. Burton JH, Miner JR, Shipley ER, et al. Propofol for emergency department procedural sedation and analgesia: a tale of three centers. Acad Emerg Med 2006; 13(1):24–30.

31. Willman EV, Andolfatto G. A prospective evaluation of "ketofol" (ketamine/propofol combination) for procedural sedation and analgesia in the emergency department. Ann Emerg Med 2007;49(1):23–30.

32. Andolfatto G, Willman E. A prospective case series of pediatric procedural sedation and analgesia in the emergency department using single-syringe ketamine-propofol combination (ketofol). Acad Emerg Med 2010;17(2):194–201.

33. Shah A, Mosdossy G, McLeod S, et al. A blinded, randomized controlled trial to evaluate ketamine/propofol versus ketamine alone for procedural sedation in children. Ann Emerg Med 2011;57(5):425–33.e2.

34. Phillips W, Anderson A, Rosengreen M, et al. Propofol versus propofol/ketamine for brief painful procedures in the emergency department: clinical and bispectral index scale comparison. J Pain Palliat Care Pharmacother 2010;24(4):349–55.

35. Sharieff GQ, Trocinski DR, Kanegaye JT, et al. Ketamine-propofol combination sedation for fracture reduction in the pediatric emergency department. Pediatr Emerg Care 2007;23(12):881–4.

36. Nejati A, Moharari RS, Ashraf H, et al. Ketamine/propofol versus midazolam/fentanyl for procedural sedation and analgesia in the emergency department: a randomized, prospective, double-blind trial. Acad Emerg Med 2011;18(8):800–6.

37. Tintinalli's Emergency Medicine. A Comprehensive Study Guide, 8e | AccessMedicine | McGraw-Hill Medical. Available at: https://accessmedicine-mhmedical-com.proxy.lib.duke.edu/book.aspx?bookid=1658. Accessed January 30, 2019.

38. Zhang X, Bai X. New therapeutic uses for an alpha2 adrenergic receptor agonist–dexmedetomidine in pain management. Neurosci Lett 2014;561:7–12.

39. Rahimzadeh P, Faiz SHR, Imani F, et al. Comparative addition of dexmedetomicine and fentanyl to intrathecal bupivacaine in orthopedic procedure in lower limbs. BMC Anesthesiol 2018;18(1):62.

40. Swami SS, Keniya VM, Ladi SD, et al. Comparison of dexmedetomidine and clonidine ($\alpha 2$ agonist drugs) as an adjuvant to local anaesthesia in

supraclavicular brachial plexus block: a randomised double-blind prospective study. Indian J Anaesth 2012;56(3):243–9.

41. Bordo D, Chan SB, Shin P. Patient satisfaction and return to daily activities using etomidate procedural sedation for orthopedic injuries. West J Emerg Med 2008; 9(2):86–90.

42. Denny MA, Manson R, Della-Giustina D. Propofol and etomidate are safe for deep sedation in the emergency department. West J Emerg Med 2011;12(4):399–403.

43. Zed PJ, Mabasa VH, Slavik RS, et al. Etomidate for rapid sequence intubation in the emergency department: is adrenal suppression a concern? CJEM 2006;8(5): 347–50.

44. Miner JR, Danahy M, Moch A, et al. Randomized clinical trial of etomidate versus propofol for procedural sedation in the emergency department. Ann Emerg Med 2007;49(1):15–22.

45. Cicero M, Graneto J. Etomidate for procedural sedation in the elderly: a retrospective comparison between age groups. Am J Emerg Med 2011;29(9):1111–6.

46. Di Gregorio G, Neal JM, Rosenquist RW, et al. Clinical presentation of local anesthetic systemic toxicity. Reg Anesth Pain Med 2010;35(2):181–7.

47. Auroy Y, Benhamou D, Bargues L, et al. Major complications of regional anesthesia in France: The SOS Regional Anesthesia Hotline Service. Anesthesiology 2002;97(5):1274–80.

48. Butterworth JF. Models and mechanisms of local anesthetic cardiac toxicity. Reg Anesth Pain Med 2010;35(2):167–76.

49. French J, Sharp LM. Local anaesthetics. Ann R Coll Surg Engl 2012;94(2):76–80.

50. Hanna MN, Elhassan A, Veloso PM, et al. Efficacy of bicarbonate in decreasing pain on intradermal injection of local anesthetics: a meta-analysis. Reg Anesth Pain Med 2009;34(2):122–5.

51. Brummett CM, Williams BA. Additives to local anesthetics for peripheral nerve blockade. Int Anesthesiol Clin 2011;49(4):104–16.

52. Cepeda MS, Tzortzopoulou A, Thackrey M, et al. Adjusting the pH of lidocaine for reducing pain on injection. Cochrane Database Syst Rev 2010;(12):CD006581.

53. McCartney CJL, Duggan E, Apatu E. Should we add clonidine to local anesthetic for peripheral nerve blockade? A qualitative systematic review of the literature. Reg Anesth Pain Med 2007;32(4):330–8.

54. Pöpping DM, Elia N, Marret E, et al. Clonidine as an adjuvant to local anesthetics for peripheral nerve and plexus blocks: a meta-analysis of randomized trials. Anesthesiology 2009;111(2):406–15.

55. Myderrizi N, Mema B. The hematoma block an effective alternative for fracture reduction in distal radius fractures. Med Arh 2011;65(4):239.

56. Beaudoin FL, Haran JP, Liebmann O. A comparison of ultrasound-guided three-in-one femoral nerve block versus parenteral opioids alone for analgesia in emergency department patients with hip fractures: a randomized controlled trial. Acad Emerg Med 2013;20(6):584–91.

57. Wathen JE, Gao D, Merritt G, et al. A randomized controlled trial comparing a fascia iliaca compartment nerve block to a traditional systemic analgesic for femur fractures in a pediatric emergency department. Ann Emerg Med 2007;50(2): 162–71, 171.e1.

58. Pennington N, Gadd RJ, Green N, et al. A national survey of acute hospitals in England on their current practice in the use of femoral nerve blocks when splinting femoral fractures. Injury 2012;43(6):843–5.

59. Ritcey B, Pageau P, Woo MY, et al. Regional nerve blocks for hip and femoral neck fractures in the emergency department: a systematic review. CJEM 2016; 18(1):37–47.
60. Riddell M, Ospina M, Holroyd-Leduc JM. Use of femoral nerve blocks to manage hip fracture pain among older adults in the emergency department: a systematic review. CJEM 2016;18(4):245–52.
61. Walker KJ, McGrattan K, Aas-Eng K, et al. Ultrasound guidance for peripheral nerve blockade. Cochrane Database Syst Rev 2009;(4):CD006459.
62. Ganesh A, Gurnaney HG. Ultrasound guidance for pediatric peripheral nerve blockade. Anesthesiol Clin 2009;27(2):197–212.
63. Zewdie A, Debebe F, Azazh A, et al. A survey of emergency medicine and orthopaedic physicians' knowledge, attitude, and practice towards the use of peripheral nerve blocks. Afr J Emerg Med 2017;7(2):79–83.
64. Mutty CE, Jensen EJ, Manka MA, et al. Femoral nerve block for diaphyseal and distal femoral fractures in the emergency department. J Bone Joint Surg Am 2007;89(12):2599–603.
65. Hards M, Brewer A, Bessant G, et al. efficacy of prehospital analgesia with fascia iliaca compartment block for femoral bone fractures: a systematic review. Prehosp Disaster Med 2018;33(3):299–307.
66. Welch JL, Cooper DD. Should I use lidocaine with epinephrine in digital nerve blocks? Ann Emerg Med 2016;68(6):756–7.
67. Chowdhry S, Seidenstricker L, Cooney DS, et al. Do not use epinephrine in digital blocks: myth or truth? Part II. A retrospective review of 1111 cases. Plast Reconstr Surg 2010;126(6):2031–4.
68. Lalonde DH, Lalonde JF. Discussion. Do not use epinephrine in digital blocks: myth or truth? Part II. A retrospective review of 1111 cases. Plast Reconstr Surg 2010;126(6):2035–6.
69. Waterbrook AL, Germann CA, Southall JC. Is epinephrine harmful when used with anesthetics for digital nerve blocks? Ann Emerg Med 2007;50(4):472–5.
70. VanNess SA, Gittins ME. Comparison of intra-articular morphine and bupivacaine following knee arthroscopy. Orthop Rev 1994;23(9):743–7.
71. Xie D-X, Zeng C, Wang Y-L, et al. A single-dose intra-articular morphine plus bupivacaine versus morphine alone following knee arthroscopy: a systematic review and meta-analysis. PLoS One 2015;10(10):e0140512.
72. Ho ST, Wang TJ, Tang JS, et al. Pain relief after arthroscopic knee surgery: intravenous morphine, epidural morphine, and intra-articular morphine. Clin J Pain 2000;16(2):105–9.
73. Galer BS, Gammaitoni AR, Oleka N, et al. Use of the lidocaine patch 5% in reducing intensity of various pain qualities reported by patients with low-back pain. Curr Med Res Opin 2004;20(Suppl 2):S5–12.
74. Adili A, Bhandari M. Cochrane in CORR®: topical nsaids for chronic musculoskeletal pain in adults. Clin Orthop Relat Res 2018;476(11):2128–34.
75. Oncel M, Sencan S, Yildiz H, et al. Transcutaneous electrical nerve stimulation for pain management in patients with uncomplicated minor rib fractures. Eur J Cardiothorac Surg 2002;22(1):13–7.
76. Bear DM, Friel NA, Lupo CL, et al. Hematoma block versus sedation for the reduction of distal radius fractures in children. J Hand Surg Am 2015;40(1):57–61.
77. Hartling L, Ali S, Dryden DM, et al. How safe are common analgesics for the treatment of acute pain for children? A systematic review. Pain Res Manag 2016;2016:5346819.

78. Smith RL, Brunolli J. Shoulder kinesthesia after anterior glenohumeral joint dislocation. J Orthop Sports Phys Ther 1990;11(11):507–13.
79. Menkes JS. Initial evaluation and management of orthopedic injuries. In: Tintinalli JE, Stapczynski JS, Ma OJ, et al, editors. Tintinalli's emergency medicine: a comprehensive study guide, 8e. New York: McGraw-Hill Education; 2016. Available at: http://accessmedicine.mhmedical.com/content.aspx?aid=1121517100. Accessed February 7, 2019.
80. Kanji A, Atkinson P, Fraser J, et al. Delays to initial reduction attempt are associated with higher failure rates in anterior shoulder dislocation: a retrospective analysis of factors affecting reduction failure. Emerg Med J 2016;33(2):130–3.
81. Cheok CY, Mohamad JA, Ahmad TS. Pain relief for reduction of acute anterior shoulder dislocations: a prospective randomized study comparing intravenous sedation with intra-articular lidocaine. J Orthop Trauma 2011;25(1):5–10.
82. Jones P, Dalziel SR, Lamdin R, et al. Oral non-steroidal anti-inflammatory drugs versus other oral analgesic agents for acute soft tissue injury. Cochrane Database Syst Rev 2015;(7):CD007789.
83. Kelley BP, Bennett KG, Chung KC, et al. Ibuprofen may not increase bleeding risk in plastic surgery: a systematic review and meta-analysis. Plast Reconstr Surg 2016;137(4):1309–16.

Ultrasound Imaging of Orthopedic Injuries

Robert Simard, MD, FRCPC[a,b,*]

KEYWORDS

- Musculoskeletal ultrasound • Point-of-care ultrasound • Fracture • Dislocation
- Tendon injury • Ligament injury

KEY POINTS

- Musculoskeletal (MSK) point-of-care ultrasound (POCUS) is readily available in many acute care settings and has shown to be useful in diagnosing many common orthopedic injuries.
- POCUS can aid or guide management of orthopedic injuries, such as confirming reduction, preventing repeated sedations, and safely guiding regional analgesia.
- POCUS training is variable; thus, studies show a wide range of sensitivities and specificities in diagnosing orthopedic injuries.
- MSK ultrasound studies are limited to case reports and studies with small sample sizes. Few large studies or randomize control trials exist.

 Video content accompanies this article at http://www.emed.theclinics.com.

INTRODUCTION

Ultrasound (US) has become increasingly mobile and portable, leading to its use by specialties other than radiologists. Point-of-care US (POCUS) is now a popularized term, given the increasing use of physicians performing a US at the patient bedside. Emergency medicine (EM) POCUS is a core competency in both the Royal College of Physicians and Surgeons of Canada and Accreditation Council for Graduate Medical Education emergency medicine residencies along with the Canadian College of Family Physicians training programs.[1] Its use by emergency physicians, orthopedic and plastic surgeons, rheumatologists, and sports medicine specialists can be helpful in diagnosing a variety of musculoskeletal (MSK) conditions.

Disclosure Statement: No disclosures.
[a] Emergency Department, Sunnybrook Health Sciences Centre, 2075 Bayview Avenue C7-53, Toronto, Ontario M4N 3M5, Canada; [b] Emergency Department, North York General Hospital, Toronto, Ontario, Canada
* Emergency Department, Sunnybrook Health Sciences Centre, 2075 Bayview Avenue C7-53, Toronto, Ontario M4N 3M5, Canada.
E-mail address: Robert.simard@sunnybrook.ca

Emerg Med Clin N Am 38 (2020) 243–265
https://doi.org/10.1016/j.emc.2019.09.009
0733-8627/20/© 2019 Elsevier Inc. All rights reserved.

Many modalities exist to determine orthopedic injuries, including plain radiographs, computed tomography (CT) scans, and magnetic resonance imaging (MRI). US has many advantages over other imaging modalities, including being a point-of-care tool capable of real-time image acquisition, having a low cost of procurement that makes it available in many centers, and being void of any harmful radiation. It can be used to avoid radiation in pediatric and obstetric patients and eliminates the need for numerous radiographs of an entire limb in patient populations that are unable to localize the pain to solely the area of injury.[2] It not only diagnoses MSK injuries but also can be used to assist in interventional procedures, such as fracture reductions, hematoma blocks, and arthrocentesis. US has been proved to improve patient safety, especially compared with performing blind procedures.[3]

The equipment required to perform the majority of MSK US includes a US machine equipped with linear and curvilinear probes. The linear probe (**Fig. 1**) has a flat footprint for its contacting surface. The advantage of this high-frequency probe

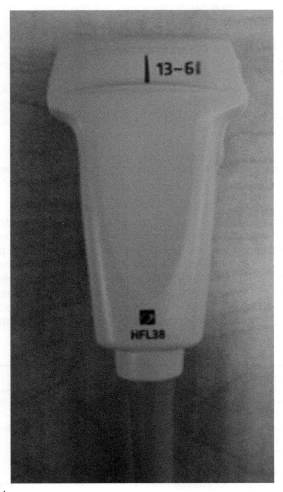

Fig. 1. Linear probe.

is the ability to see superficial structures with high resolution. Bones, joints, ligaments, and tendons that are near the skin's surface are best evaluated with this probe. Deeper structures, such as the femur and hip joint, are best seen with the curvilinear probe (**Fig. 2**). The curvilinear probe has a curved footprint for its contacting surface and has a lower frequency, thus allowing it to generate images of deeper structures. The majority of MSK US can be performed with the linear probe.

Most commonly, orthopedic injuries are evaluated using US in both the long-axis view and short-axis view. The long-axis view (**Fig. 3**) is generated by placing the probe parallel to the central axis of the orthopedic injury. The short-axis view (**Fig. 4**) is generated by placing the probe perpendicular to the central axis of the orthopedic injury, which is usually 90° from the long-axis view. The majority of MSK US for orthopedic injuries is performed in the long-axis view.

Many orthopedic injuries can be identified with US, including fractures, dislocations, tendon injuries, and ligamentous injuries. In addition, US is beneficial in guiding MSK interventions, including fracture and dislocation reduction, hematoma blocks, nerve blocks, and arthrocentesis. US can be utilized to evaluate essentially any bone, joint, ligament, and tendon in the body. Although US does have good sensitivity and specificity for some orthopedic injuries, other imaging modalities are still used for orthopedic injuries where US is impractical, requires significant additional training, or is inferior. US does not replace plain radiographs in the diagnosis of orthopedic injuries,

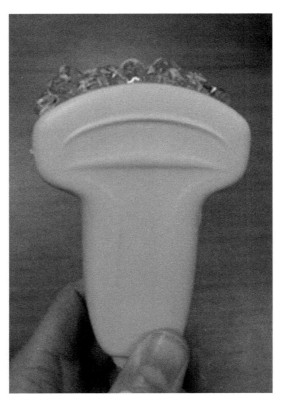

Fig. 2. Curvilinear probe.

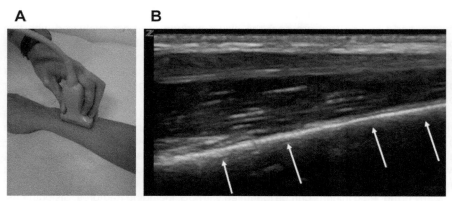

Fig. 3. (*A*) Long-axis view on skin of probe parallel to radius; (*B*) POCUS image of radius (*arrows*) in long-axis view.

where it has traditionally been used, but it can aid in the diagnosis of orthopedic injuries and other concomitant injuries.[4]

The remainder of this article describes the common US usages in orthopedic injuries. Most of the literature on POCUS in MSK injuries has small sample sizes or is case reports. Few systematic reviews and even fewer randomized control trials exist. Many studies in the use of US for orthopedic injury conclude that more extensive research is needed. There is also a varying degree of training by the sonographers in the literature, with some training only occurring in online tutorials, single bedside teaching sessions, or a generalized POCUS course. It is possible that more detailed training may improve the accuracy of POCUS in the evaluation of MSK injuries.

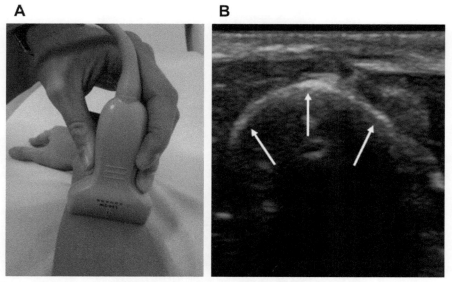

Fig. 4. (*A*) Short-axis view on skin of probe perpindicular to radius; (*B*) POCUS image of radius (*arrows*) in short-axis view.

FRACTURES

Although fractures are traditionally diagnosed with plain radiographs, fracture identification is one of the common uses of MSK US. Plain radiographs are not universal to all areas of the world and are even unavailable in some large centers after hours.[5] The linear probe is used most commonly; however, the curvilinear probe likely is needed for evaluating deeper bones (eg, femur). The technique is similar for all fractures and consists of placing the probe in long-axis view over the injured bone and sliding the probe from side to side to generate the best view of the boney cortex (Video 1). To minimize the patient's discomfort, the probe should be placed gently on a generous layer of US gel. On the US screen, the boney cortex appears echogenic (eg, white). Because US waves do not pass through bone, a shadow artifact that is anechoic (eg, black) is generated on the screen far field to the echogenic boney cortex. Rotating the probe into the short-axis view is sometimes helpful to identify bone from other echogenic structures on the screen (Video 2). Each suspected fracture site should be evaluated in both the long-axis view and short-axis view. A second orthogonal plane is needed to evaluate all fractures with US, similar to obtaining multiple views of bones with plain radiographs.[6]

When evaluating a bone for fracture on US, look for a discontinuity in the cortex. A normal bone has a smooth, continuous contour. A fracture has an obvious interruption in the contour of the bone (**Fig. 5**). In addition, a hematoma at the site of the discontinuity in the cortex of the bone can assist in identifying fractures. The hematoma appears as an echolucent area on the screen (**Fig. 6**). Whenever in doubt, imaging the contralateral side may be helpful in distinguishing normal anatomy versus a fracture.

Angulation and displacement of the bones can be assessed on US. Angulation is best seen in the long-axis view, where the angle of the proximal and distal bone created by the fracture site can be measured (**Fig. 7**). Displacement is also best seen in the long-axis view, where the step-off deformity from the proximal to distal portion of the bones can be measured (**Fig. 8**).

Another advantage of evaluating fractures with US is in the plain radiograph occult fracture. Scaphoid,[7] sternum,[8] and rib[9] fractures are difficult to see in the acute setting on plain films but can be detected on US. It also has utility in detecting occult fractures in children, where cartilaginous pediatric bone makes identifying fractures on plain radiographs difficult.[10]

Some of the more superficial bones, such as the bones of the hands and feet, may be difficult to see secondary to the dead space in the near field of the US probe. The dead space is the first few millimeters at the near field of the screen that is

A   **B**

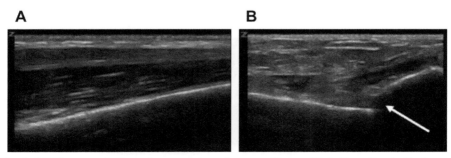

Fig. 5. (*A*) The smooth, linear boney cortex of a normal bone; (*B*) A disruption in the boney cortex indicative of a fracture (*arrow*).

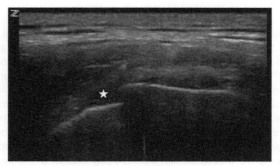

Fig. 6. Hematoma (*star*) at the site of the fracture.

uninterpretable. Using plenty of gel to eliminate the dead space is one technique (**Fig. 9**); however, the use of a water bath is a better technique.[11] This technique involves filling a container with fluid and submerging the affected body part in water (**Fig. 10**). By placing the footprint of the probe in the water a short distance from the affected body part, the water creates an acoustic window that brings pathologic findings out of the dead space to an area farther field on the US screen that can be visualized.

Reductions also can be imaged in real time using POCUS. Although point-of-care fluoroscopy is advocated to assist in fracture reduction, its cost, size, radiation, and need for health care providers to wear lead protectors make it less practical. POCUS is a safer alternative compared with bedside fluoroscopy for fracture reduction and is considered an acceptable alternative.[12] Due to the swelling at the site of fractures, clinical examination of the fracture site during reduction may not be reliable and may lead to repeated sedation attempts once postreduction radiographs are obtained to assess the reduction.[13] POCUS use during a reduction can aid in identifying the adequacy of the reduction before splinting to optimize reduction success on postreduction plain radiographs (**Figs. 11** and **12**) Once the POCUS images show a satisfactory reduction, the patient can be immobilized in a splint and plain radiographs obtained to confirm continuity of the reduction.

Hematoma blocks can also be performed under US guidance. Visualizing the needle in the long-axis view going directly into the fracture segment is helpful in patients when the fracture site is not easily determined by the palpation method.[14] Body habitus, soft tissue swelling, and pain on palpation of the fracture site can make the palpation method challenging. In addition, US-guided hematoma blocks may be used in patients where it is unsafe to provide sedation or opioids.[15] Although procedural

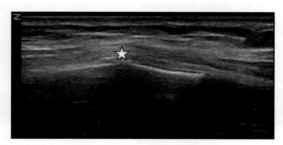

Fig. 7. Fracture (*star*) with angulation of the distal fragment.

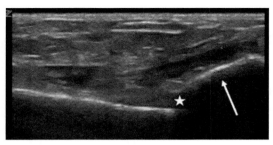

Fig. 8. Fracture (*star*) with displacement of the distal fragment (*arrow*).

sedation has the benefit of providing muscle relaxation and analgesia during fracture reduction, adverse events, such as hypotension and apnea, may occur.[16] During procedural sedation, very close monitoring of the respiratory rate, heart rate, heart rhythm, and blood pressure is necessary.[17] The presence of 2 physicians, a dedicated nurse, and a respiratory therapist may be required at some hospitals for emergency department (ED) procedure sedations, consuming many personnel resources. These additional requirements are not needed with hematoma blocks.

To perform a hematoma block, use the linear probe and identify the fracture site. Ensure the probe is positioned in the long-axis view of the bone. Clean the skin with a cleaning solution (eg, chlorhexidine). Insert a 20-gauge needle in-plane with the probe and visualize the needle on the US screen. The needle can be followed in real time as it enters the fracture site. Aspirate a small amount of hematoma, as in the blind technique, to ensure that the needle tip is in the correct place. Then the anesthetic can be injected to provide the hematoma block.

Finally, US-guided nerve blocks can be used to provide analgesia in patients with fractures. Traditionally, nerve blocks have been performed blind or by using a nerve stimulator, which is not commonly found in the ED.[18] Furthermore, although a nerve stimulator was considered the gold standard for peripheral nerve blocks, a systematic review suggested that US was more successful, faster, provided longer blocks, and reduced the risk of vascular puncture compared with nerve stimulators.[19] Also, US-guided nerve blocks have been performed successfully after traditional non–US-guided regional anesthesia attempts have failed in superobese patients.[20]

US-guided nerve blocks can provide pain relief by real-time visualization of local anesthetic being deposited around the nerve. The technique includes using the linear

A   **B**

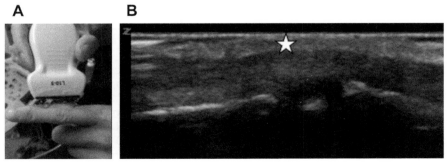

Fig. 9. (*A*) Using copious amounts of gel on the finger; (*B*) image of the phalynx is far field to the dead space (*star*) secondary to the copious amounts of gel.

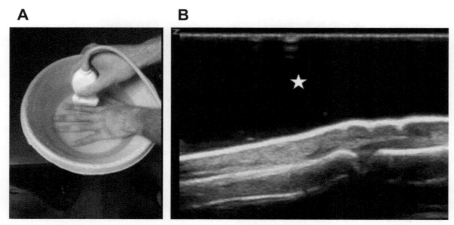

Fig. 10. (*A*) Placing the hand in a water bath and floating the probe on top of the water. (*B*) POCUS image of the finger with the anechoic water (*star*) visible in the near field.

probe to identify the nerve that innervates the bone that is fractured (eg, femoral nerve in a patient with a hip fracture). Once the nerve is identified, if feasible, insert the 20-gauge needle in-plane with the linear probe (**Fig. 13**). In areas where performing in-plane technique would cause harm or is not feasible (eg, Achilles tendon and tibia preventing the in-plane approach for the posterior tibial nerve), an out-of-plane approach is needed (**Fig. 14**). Following the needle tip toward the nerve in real time with US helps prevent rogue locations of the needle, essentially preventing vascular puncture and nerve puncture. Once the needle tip is adjacent to the appropriate nerve, aspiration of the syringe should be performed to ensure the needle is not in a vessel, followed by injection of the local anesthetic around the nerve. Although many peripheral nerves that can be identified on US can be anesthetized, the risks and practicality of performing a nerve block need to be addressed.

Tips

- Ensure plenty of gel is applied over fracture sites for patient comfort.
- Gently place the probe on gel over injuries to minimize patient discomfort.
- Always evaluate fractures in 2 orthogonal planes.
- Compare the image of the site of injury to the patient's contralateral side.
- POCUS can guide reduction attempts, hematoma blocks, and nerve blocks.

Long Bone Fractures

Long bone fractures (LBFs), including the humerus, radius, ulna, femur, tibia, and fibula, are common in the ED. One systematic review on LBFs of 2982 pooled patients with 1200 LBFs revealed that US had sensitivity of greater than 90% (range 64.7%–100%), specificity of greater than 90% (range 79.2%–100%), Likelihood ratio (LR)+ above 10 (range 3.11 to infinity), and LR− below 0.1 (range 0 to 0.45) in detecting the fracture in the majority of the included studies.[13] The same investigators performed a meta-analysis showing sensitivity of 93.1%, specificity of 92.9%, LR+ 14.1, and LR− 0.08 for detection of pediatric forearm fractures and sensitivity of

A   B

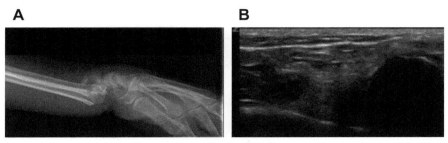

Fig. 11. (A) Prereduction radiograph of a distal radius fracture; (B) prereduction POCUS image of the same distal radius fracture.

89.5%, specificity of 94.2%, LR+ 16.4, and LR− 0.12 for ankle fractures in adults. These values reveal that POCUS can be a useful tool for detecting LBFs.

POCUS also was helpful in determining angulation, step-off deformity, and the type of fracture (eg, linear, comminuted, or fissure fracture) in tibia and fibula fractures.[21] POCUS also was found to be accurately performed with minimal training to rule out LBFs.[22,23] Because neurovascular compromise leads to morbidity and mortality in orthopedic injuries, POCUS rapidly and reliably diagnoses LBFs, leading to early treatment and disposition.[24] In pediatric patient populations, POCUS had a significantly lower pain score compared with plain radiographs for distal radius fractures and was able to diagnose buckle fractures.[25] It was also successful in diagnosing greenstick fractures[26] and Salter-Harris I fractures.[27] Finally, after POCUS diagnoses the LBF, it can be used to help guide nerve blocks for pain relief[28] and aid in confirming the reduction.[29] A study by Socransky and colleagues[30] showed that after initial clinical satisfaction of distal radius fracture reduction, POCUS led to greater physician certainty in the initial reduction attempt, and 40% of cases required repeated reduction attempts. Multiple articles also support the role of POCUS in guiding pediatric LBF reduction.[29,31,32]

Scaphoid Fractures

With the scaphoid susceptible to nonunion and avascular necrosis, it is essential to identify scaphoid fractures. With occult scaphoid fractures being common, it is helpful to have an easily accessible diagnostic image to rule out scaphoid fractures and prevent unnecessary immobilization.

US can be used in multiple planes to assess the scaphoid. On the dorsal surface of the wrist, the scaphoid appears like a pyramid (**Fig. 15**). On the volar surface of the

A   B

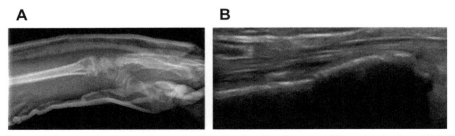

Fig. 12. (A) Postreduction radiograph of a distal radius fracture; (B) postreduction POCUS image of the same distal radius fracture prior to splinting.

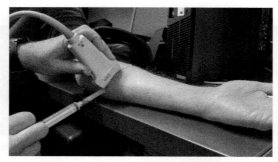

Fig. 13. The needle is being inserted in-plane to the probe.

wrist, the scaphoid appears like a peanut (**Fig. 16**). A disruption in the cortex of the bone is consistent with a fracture (**Fig. 17**).

US outperforms plain films in the early diagnosis of scaphoid fractures.[33] MSK radiologists have been able to reliably assess occult fractures with US,[7,34] but high-spatial-resolution sonography is not readily available in all centers. In a recent systematic review, US was found to have a moderate accuracy of diagnosing occult scaphoid fractures, with pooled sensitivity of 85.6% and specificity of 83.3%, but most of the studies were performed by MSK radiologists.[35] MRI is considered the superior test compared with CT, bone scan, US, plain radiographs, and physical examination,[36] but it has limited availability. Although it is possible for POCUS to detect scaphoid fractures, POCUS is not consistently sensitive or specific enough to rule out scaphoid fractures.

Metacarpal and Phalange Fractures

The use of a water bath is helpful when examining the metacarpal and phalanges for fractures. Multiple studies showed that POCUS for metacarpal fractures has good sensitivity (92.5%–97.4%), specificity (92.9%–98.3), positive predictive value (PPV) (92.6%–97.4%), and negative predictive value (NPV) (95%–98%).[37–39] Similar values were obtained when using POCUS for phalange fractures.[40] POCUS also has the advantage of aiding in US-guided ulnar nerve blocks in fifth metacarpal fractures[41] and can confirm reductions of metacarpal and phalange fractures.[42]

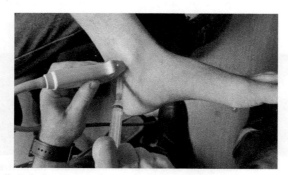

Fig. 14. The needle is being inserted out-of-plane to the probe.

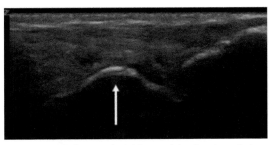

Fig. 15. Pyramid appearance of the scaphoid (*arrow*) in the dorsal view.

Hip Fractures

Not all hip fractures are visualized on plain radiographs. Delaying operative management of hip fractures by missing a diagnosis of hip fracture by more than 2 days doubles the 1-year mortality.[43] POCUS was shown to have value in quickly and correctly diagnosing an occult hip fracture in an elderly patient.[44] This may be valuable in settings where CT or MRI is unavailable.

Knee Fractures

A lipohemarthrosis results from an intra-articular fracture. Although US may not identify the fracture in the setting of acute knee trauma, it has sensitivity of 97%, specificity of 100%, PPV of 100%, and NPV of 94% for detecting lipohemarthrosis.[45] Two case reports demonstrate that POCUS detected a lipohemarthrosis, which led to a diagnosis of intra-articular tibial plateau fracture.[46,47] To assess the knee joint for lipohemarthrosis, the probe is placed in the long-axis view proximal to the patella. The quadriceps tendon and femur are identified by sliding the probe side to side. Once identified, the probe is moved distally until a portion of the patella is visible on the screen (Video 3) An anechoic area near field to the femur and far field of the quadriceps tendon represents a joint effusion (**Fig. 18**). A layer of effusion and fat is a lipohemarthrosis (**Fig. 19**) and represents an intra-articular fracture until proved otherwise.

Foot Fractures

As with US for bone fractures of the hand and fingers, foot fractures may also be technically difficult to visualize. Using a water bath may help. A study using MRI as the gold standard showed that when plain radiographs were normal, US detection of metatarsal fractures had sensitivity of 83%, specificity of 76%, and negative predictive value of 92%.[48]

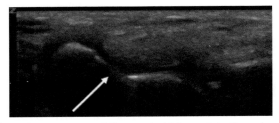

Fig. 16. Peanut-shaped appearance of the scaphoid (*arrow*) in the volar view.

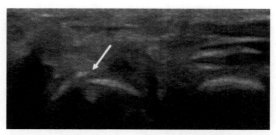

Fig. 17. Disruption in the cortex of the scaphoid (*arrow*) consistent with a scaphoid fracture.

Clavicle Fractures

US to assess for clavicle fractures can be used in the pediatric patient population to avoid radiation. One study showed US had sensitivity of 95%, specificity of 96%, LR+ 27, LR− 0.05, PPV of 95%, and NPV of 96% compared with plain radiographs.[49] Another study demonstrated that with minimal training to diagnose clavicle fractures, US did not worsen patient pain and potentially reduced the length of stay with sensitivity of 89.7%, specificity of 89.5%, LR+ 8.33, LR− 0.11, PPV of 94.6%, and NPV of 81.0%.[50]

Rib and Sternal Fractures

Rib and sternal fractures are notoriously difficult to see on plain films in the acute setting. POCUS can be used over a patient's area of maximal pain to identify rib fractures (**Fig. 20**, Video 4). A systematic review revealed that US for diagnosing rib fractures was superior to plain films.[51] In another study, US for sternal fractures also was considered superior to plain films.[52] Both rib and sternal fractures seem to have a high specificity (98% and 97%, respectively) and only moderate sensitivity (67% and 83%, respectively).[53]

DISLOCATIONS

Traditionally, plain radiographs are obtained to diagnose dislocations. Due to the discomfort of radiographs, time, and radiation risk, US can be used as an adjunct

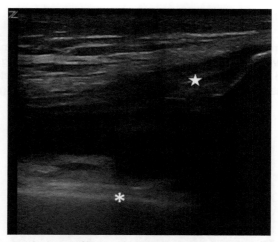

Fig. 18. POCUS image of a knee effusion (*black*) located between the near-field quadriceps tendon (*star*) and the far-field femur (*asterisk*).

A   B

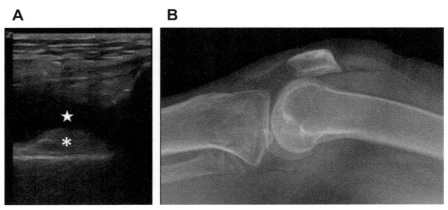

Fig. 19. (*A*) Knee POCUS showing a layer of fat (*asterisk*) and effusion (*star*) consistent with a lipohemarthrosis. (*B*) Corresponding knee radiograph showing the lipohemarthrosis.

for diagnosis. Commonly, the linear probe or curvilinear probe is used depending on the depth of the joint. Dislocations appear as loss of continuity of adjacent bony joint structures on US.[40] Comparing the bony joint structures on one side of the body to its contralateral joint helps determine if a dislocation is present.

Once reduction has been attempted, POCUS can be used to confirm the reduction. In addition to diagnosing and confirming reductions in dislocations, US-guided regional anesthesia can be performed to provide analgesia to facilitate reduction. POCUS can improve success with intra-articular injections for shoulder reduction.[54] There are case reports of POCUS use with femoral nerve blocks for hip dislocation[55] and a patellar dislocation[56] and an infraclavicular brachial plexus block for an elbow dislocation.[57] Several studies comparing US-guided interscalene nerve blocks versus procedural sedation in shoulder reductions showed that ED length of stay was shorter in the nerve block group and fewer personal resources were used; however, the difference in pain scores varied in the 2 studies.[58,59]

Glenohumeral Joint

The glenohumeral joint is the most common dislocation seen in the acute care setting. There are multiple US approaches to diagnose shoulder dislocations, including anterior, lateral, and posterior approach.

For the anterior approach (**Fig. 21**), the patient is seated or laying down, and the probe is placed over the coracoid process in the transverse orientation generating a view of the coracoid and humeral head.[60] In the same article, the investigators

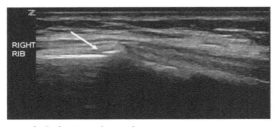

Fig. 20. POCUS image of rib fracture (*arrow*).

describe a lateral approach, where the probe is placed laterally on the patient in the longitudinal position just below the acromion, generating a view of the acromion and humeral head. A posterior approach is also described, where the patient is seated upright and the US probe is placed in transverse orientation with glenoid rim and humeral head visualized on the screen to measure the glenohumeral separation distance.[61] Once reduced, the US probe can be placed back on the patient to confirm the reduction (**Fig. 22**).

POCUS can be used as a tool in diagnosing posterior shoulder dislocations.[62,63] A 2017 systematic review found that all studies were 100% specific; however, there was a varying degrees of sensitivity.[64] Although these studies show that POCUS can be used for the detection of shoulder dislocations and confirmation of their reductions further validation of these findings is needed.

Elbow Joint

Subluxation of the radial head (pulled elbow or nursemaid's elbow) is a frequent presentation to the ED in young children. Children poorly localize their pain, and frequently a history is provided by a caregiver that the patient is not moving the entire arm. A case series showed how POCUS can be used to diagnose a subluxed radial head by finding the hook sign, and POCUS also can be used to confirm reduction.[65]

TENDON INJURIES AND LIGAMENT INJURIES

Although best found on MRI, the high cost and low availability for the high incidence of ligament and tendon injuries make this modality impractical. US can be utilized to diagnose tendinopathy as well as partial and complete tendon and ligament ruptures.[66] To identify the tendon, the linear probe is placed over the tendon in either the long-axis

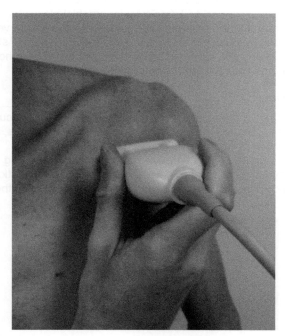

Fig. 21. The probe placement for the anterior approach of a dislocated shoulder.

A   B

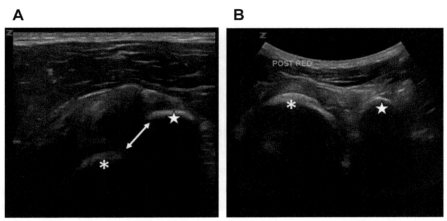

Fig. 22. (A) POCUS image showing the separation (*arrow*) of the humeral head (asterisk) from the glenoid (*star*) consistent with anterior shoulder dislocation. (B) POCUS image showing reduction of this distance consistent with a successful shoulder reduction.

view or short-axis view. By sliding the probe along the entire length of the tendon, it can be evaluated for areas of injury. In the long-axis view, the tendon appears rectangular as many parallel fibers emanating from a muscle and terminating on a bone (**Fig. 23**). In the short-axis view, the tendon appears circular or oval as many dots and lines (**Fig. 24**). Tendons are best seen when the US probe is completely perpendicular; otherwise, it may appear more echolucent in areas. This loss of echogenic appearance is known as anisotropy (Video 5).

In acute tendinopathy, the tendon appears thickened with hypoechoic areas around the tendon and anechoic fluid, but the tendon remains completely intact. In partial tears of the tendon, part of the tendon remains intact, but the area that is torn appears as a hypoechoic space with disruption of some of the tendon's fibers. In a complete tear of the tendon, there is a discontinuation of the tendon with anechoic fluid separating the two (2) ends (**Fig. 25**). Wu and colleagues[67] demonstrated that POCUS is more sensitive and specific for diagnosing tendon injuries and was more efficient than traditional diagnostic techniques.

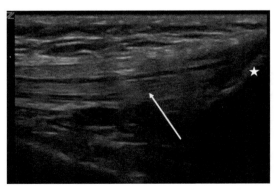

Fig. 23. Parallel fibers representing the long-axis view of the quadriceps tendon (*arrow*) attaching to the patella (*star*)

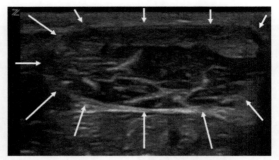

Fig. 24. Oval appearance of the Achilles tendon (*arrows*) in short-axis view.

Ligaments are structurally very similar on US but appear less echogenic compared with tendons. They also are susceptible to anisotropy; thus, the probe should always be completely perpendicular to the ligament to obtain the best view. Ligamentous tears also appear as an abrupt discontinuation with hypoechoic fluid separating the ends. One major advantage of US over other imaging modalities is the ability to perform a dynamic assessment, such as ranging a ligament or tendon with POCUS, to determine the extent of a tear.[68]

Acromioclavicular Joint

By placing the linear probe such that the footprint of the probe is partially on the acromion and partially on the clavicle, the acromioclavicular (AC) joint can be assessed (**Fig. 26**). US can be accurate and reliable at evaluating the AC joint by assessing the distance from the acromion and clavicle, periarticular ligaments, and effusion.[69]

Ulnar Collateral Ligament

Traditionally, diagnosis of an ulnar collateral ligament (UCL) injury of the thumb is clinical and consists of valgus strain causing pain.[70] One study performed by a radiologist showed an overall accuracy of 80% in detecting traumatic UCL injuries[71]; however, another study showed that emergency physicians correctly identified the rupture of the UCL in only 45% of cases.[72]

Rotator Cuff

A systematic review showed that rotator cuff US is most accurate for complete tears and less accurate for partial tears.[73] The rotator cuff is considered an advanced US scan that requires significant training to determine the injury.[74] It does not seem

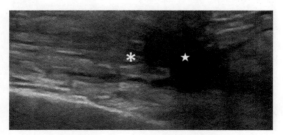

Fig. 25. POCUS image showing discontinuity of the quadriceps tendon (*asterisk*) with an anechoic area (*star*) consistent with tendon rupture.

practical for average POCUS users in the acute care setting unless they have considerable training.

Cruciate Ligament

Traditionally, patients presenting in acute pain with cruciate ligament injuries are diagnosed by physical examination and follow-up with diagnostic imaging, such as MRI. The diagnostic accuracy of the physical examination rarely rules in or rules out knee pathology.[75] A systematic review found that for anterior cruciate ligament injuries, US had sensitivity of 90%, specificity of 97%, LR+ 31.08, and LR− 0.11.[76] Case reports have shown that POCUS can help diagnose both anterior and posterior cruciate ligament injuries.[77,78]

Quadriceps and Achilles Tendon

Complete tears of the quadriceps and Achilles tendons are detectable with POCUS. Multiple case reports identify quadriceps tendon ruptures[79–81] and Achilles tendon ruptures[82–84] on POCUS. Visualizing the abrupt disruption of the tendon and the hypoechoic fluid surrounding the 2 ends allows for the diagnosis (see **Fig. 25**).

COMMON ERRORS

There are a few common errors when performing MSK US. The first is the failure to compare the affected side to the contralateral side. Normal angulation of boney contours and cartilage in joints have been mistaken for pathology. It is essential to

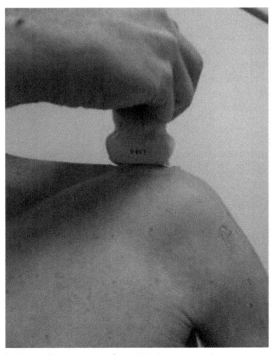

Fig. 26. Location of the probe to assess for AC joint separation.

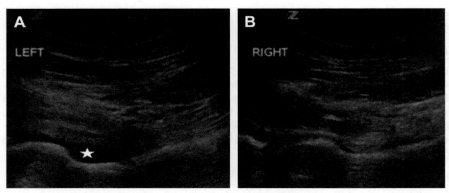

Fig. 27. Side-by-side comparison of a hip joint showing (*A*) a joint effusion (*star*) on the left and (*B*) a normal hip on the right.

compare the anatomy on the contralateral side to prevent an incorrect diagnosis. It is helpful to use the dual-screen or split-screen function on the US machine, where an image of each side can be stored on 1 screen for side-by-side comparison (**Fig. 27**).

Also, knowledge of normal anatomy is essential when performing US. Commonly, new learners identify joint spaces as fracture sites (**Fig. 28**). Because the near-field portion of the screen is the dead space, representing where the probe contacts the skin, cautious interpretations of any structures should occur in this area. It is best to either use a stand-off pad or water bath to eliminate structures in the dead space and optimize image generation and interpretation. A stand-off pad (eg, a fluid-filled saline bag with its air removed) can be placed over the orthopedic injury and the US probe placed on top.

Finally, anisotropy is a US artifact that is seen when interrogating ligaments and tendons. When sound waves reflect off a ligament or tendon, they can be reflected away from the probe. This leads to the appearance of a hypoechoic area on the screen. If the probe is placed perpendicular to the tendon, it appears more echogenic and more accurately assessed for injury (see Video 5). Lack of knowledge of anisotropy can lead to an image of a ligament or tendon appearing like it is ruptured or injured. Altering

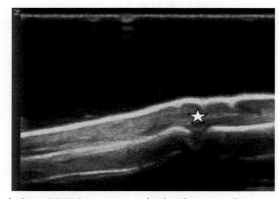

Fig. 28. Normal phalanx POCUS in a water bath. The normal joint space (*star*) can be mistaken for a fracture.

the angle of the probe due to anisotropy may be necessary to generate an adequate image for interpretation.

SUMMARY

With the high cost and limited availability of gold standard imaging modalities, US has emerged as a readily available point-of-care test in many acute care settings. It can detect many orthopedic injuries, including fractures, dislocation, and tendon and ligament injuries. It also can aid in confirming reductions of fractures and dislocations and guide regional anesthesia. Its accuracy is dependent on the training and experience of the operator.

SUPPLEMENTARY DATA

Supplementary data related to this article can be found online at https://doi.org/10.1016/j.emc.2019.09.009.

REFERENCES

1. Fischer LM, Woo MY, Lee AC, et al. Emergency medicine point-of-care ultrasonography: a national needs assessment of competencies for general and expert practice. CJEM 2015;17(1):74–88.
2. Watson NA, Ferrier GM. Diagnosis of femoral shaft fracture in pregnancy by ultrasound. J Accid Emerg Med 1999;16(5):380.
3. Arienti V, Camaggi V. Clinical applications of bedside ultrasonography in internal and emergency medicine. Intern Emerg Med 2011;6(3):195–201.
4. Lyon M, Blaivas M. Evaluation of extremity trauma with sonography. J Ultrasound Med 2003;22(6):625–30.
5. Sippel S, Muruganandan K, Levine A, et al. Use of ultrasound in the developing world. Int J Emerg Med 2011;4(1):72.
6. Saul T, Ng L, Lewiss RE. Point-of-care ultrasound in the diagnosis of upper extremity fracture-dislocation. A pictorial essay. Med Ultrason 2013;15(3):230–6.
7. Hauger O, Bonnefoy O, Moinard M, et al. Occult fractures of the waist of the scaphoid: early diagnosis by high-spatial-resolution sonography. AJR Am J Roentgenol 2002;178(5):1239–45.
8. Fenkl R, Knaepler H. Emergency diagnosis of sternum fracture with ultrasound. Unfallchirurg 1992;95(8):375–9.
9. Griffith JF, Rainer TH, Ching AS, et al. Sonography compared with radiography in revealing acute rib fracture. AJR Am J Roentgenol 1999;173(6):1603–9.
10. Warkentine FH, Horowitz R, Pierce MC. The use of ultrasound to detect occult or unsuspected fractures in child abuse. Pediatr Emerg Care 2014;30(1):43–6.
11. Javadzadeh HR, Davoudi A, Davoudi F, et al. Diagnostic value of "bedside ultrasonography" and the "water bath technique" in distal forearm, wrist, and hand bone fractures. Emerg Radiol 2014;21(1):1–4.
12. Auten JD, Naheedy JH, Hurst ND, et al. Comparison of pediatric post-reduction fluoroscopic-and ultrasound forearm fracture images. Am J Emerg Med 2019;37(5):832–8.
13. Chartier LB, Bosco L, Lapointe-Shaw L, et al. Use of point-of-care ultrasound in long bone fractures: a systematic review and meta-analysis. CJEM 2017;19(2):131–42.
14. Gottlieb M, Cosby K. Ultrasound-guided hematoma block for distal radial and ulnar fractures. J Emerg Med 2015;48(3):310–2.

15. Lovallo E, Mantuani D, Nagdev A. Novel use of ultrasound in the ED: ultrasound-guided hematoma block of a proximal humeral fracture. Am J Emerg Med 2015; 33(1):130.e1-2.

16. Roback MG, Wathen JE, Bajaj L, et al. Adverse events associated with procedural sedation and analgesia in a pediatric emergency department: a comparison of common parenteral drugs. Acad Emerg Med 2005;12(6):508–13.

17. Godwin SA, Burton JH, Gerardo CJ, et al. Clinical policy: procedural sedation and analgesia in the emergency department. Ann Emerg Med 2014;63(2): 247–58.

18. Urmey WF. Using the nerve stimulator for peripheral or plexus nerve blocks. Minerva Anestesiol 2006;72(6):467–71.

19. Abrahams MS, Aziz MF, Fu RF, et al. Ultrasound guidance compared with electrical neurostimulation for peripheral nerve block: a systematic review and meta-analysis of randomized controlled trials. Br J Anaesth 2009;102(3):408–17.

20. Kilicaslan A, Topal A, Erol A, et al. Ultrasound-guided multiple peripheral nerve blocks in a superobese patient. Case Rep Anesthesiol 2014;2014:1–4.

21. Kozaci N, Ay MO, Avci M, et al. The comparison of point-of-care ultrasonography and radiography in the diagnosis of tibia and fibula fractures. Injury 2017;48(7): 1628–35.

22. Marshburn TH, Legome E, Sargsyan A, et al. Goal-directed ultrasound in the detection of long-bone fractures. J Trauma 2004;57(2):329–32.

23. Hedelin H, Tingström C, Hebelka H, et al. Minimal training sufficient to diagnose pediatric wrist fractures with ultrasound. Crit Ultrasound J 2017;9(1):11.

24. Patel RM, Tollefson BJ. Bedside ultrasound detection of long bone fractures. J Miss State Med Assoc 2013;54(6):159–62.

25. Poonai N, Myslik F, Joubert G, et al. Point-of-care ultrasound for nonangulated distal forearm fractures in children: test performance characteristics and patient-centered outcomes. Acad Emerg Med 2017;24(5):607–16.

26. Herren C, Sobottke R, Ringe MJ, et al. Ultrasound-guided diagnosis of fractures of the distal forearm in children. Orthop Traumatol Surg Res 2015;101(4):501–5.

27. Taggart I, Voskoboynik N, Shah S, et al. ED point-of-care ultrasound in the diagnosis of ankle fractures in children. Am J Emerg Med 2012;30(7):1328.e1-3.

28. Atkinson P, Lennon R. Use of emergency department ultrasound in the diagnosis and early management of femoral fractures. Emerg Med J 2003;20(4):395.

29. Chen L, Kim Y, Moore CL. Diagnosis and guided reduction of forearm fractures in children using bedside ultrasound. Pediatr Emerg Care 2007;23(8):528–31.

30. Socransky S, Skinner A, Bromley M, et al. Ultrasound-assisted distal radius fracture reduction. Cureus 2016;8(7):e674.

31. Scheier E, Balla U. Ultrasound-assisted reduction of displaced and shortened fractures by pediatric emergency physicians. Pediatr Emerg Care 2017;33(9): 654–6.

32. Patel DD, Blumberg SM, Crain EF. The utility of bedside ultrasonography in identifying fractures and guiding fracture reduction in children. Pediatr Emerg Care 2009;25(4):221–5.

33. Jain R, Jain N, Sheikh T, et al. Early scaphoid fractures are better diagnosed with ultrasonography than X-rays: a prospective study over 114 patients. Chin J Traumatol 2018;21(4):206–10.

34. Fusetti C, Poletti PA, Pradel PH, et al. Diagnosis of occult scaphoid fracture with high-spatial-resolution sonography: a prospective blind study. J Trauma 2005; 59(3):677–81.

35. Kwee RM, Kwee TC. Ultrasound for diagnosing radiographically occult scaphoid fracture. Skeletal Radiol 2018;4:1–8.

36. Carpenter CR, Pines JM, Schuur JD, et al. Adult scaphoid fracture. Acad Emerg Med 2014;21(2):101–21.

37. Kocaoğlu S, Özhasenekler A, İçme F, et al. The role of ultrasonography in the diagnosis of metacarpal fractures. Am J Emerg Med 2016;34(9):1868–71.

38. Kozaci N, Ay MO, Akcimen M, et al. The effectiveness of bedside point-of-care ultrasonography in the diagnosis and management of metacarpal fractures. Am J Emerg Med 2015;33(10):1468–72.

39. Aksay E, Yesilaras M, Kılıc TY, et al. Sensitivity and specificity of bedside ultrasonography in the diagnosis of fractures of the fifth metacarpal. Emerg Med J 2015; 32(3):221–5.

40. Tayal VS, Antoniazzi J, Pariyadath M, et al. Prospective use of ultrasound imaging to detect bony hand injuries in adults. J Ultrasound Med 2007;26(9):1143–8.

41. Ünlüer EE, Karagöz A, Ünlüer S, et al. Ultrasound-guided ulnar nerve block for boxer fractures. Am J Emerg Med 2016;34(8):1726–7.

42. McManus JG, Morton MJ, Crystal CS, et al. Use of ultrasound to assess acute fracture reduction in emergency care settings. Am J Disaster Med 2008;3(4): 241–7.

43. Zuckerman JD, Skovron ML, Koval KJ, et al. Postoperative complications and mortality associated with operative delay in older patients who have a fracture of the hip. J Bone Joint Surg Am 1995;77(10):1551–6.

44. Colon RM, Chilstrom ML. Diagnosis of an occult hip fracture by point-of-care ultrasound. J Emerg Med 2015;49(6):916–9.

45. Bonnefoy O, Diris B, Moinard M, et al. Acute knee trauma: role of ultrasound. Eur Radiol 2006;16(11):2542–8.

46. Aponte EM, Novik JI. Identification of lipohemarthrosis with point-of-care emergency ultrasonography: case report and brief literature review. J Emerg Med 2013;44(2):453–6.

47. Rippey J. Ultrasound for knee effusion: lipohaemarthrosis and tibial plateau fracture. Australas J Ultrasound Med 2014;17(4):159–66.

48. Banal F, Gandjbakhch F, Foltz V, et al. Sensitivity and specificity of ultrasonography in early diagnosis of metatarsal bone stress fractures: a pilot study of 37 patients. J Rheumatol 2009;36(8):1715–9.

49. Cross KP, Warkentine FH, Kim IK, et al. Bedside ultrasound diagnosis of clavicle fractures in the pediatric emergency department. Acad Emerg Med 2010;17(7): 687–93.

50. Chien M, Bulloch B, Garcia-Filion P, et al. Bedside ultrasound in the diagnosis of pediatric clavicle fractures. Pediatr Emerg Care 2011;27(11):1038–41.

51. Battle C, Hayward S, Eggert S, et al. Comparison of the use of lung ultrasound and chest radiography in the diagnosis of rib fractures: a systematic review. Emerg Med J 2019;36(3):185–90.

52. Racine S, Drake D. BET 3: bedside ultrasound for the diagnosis of sternal fracture. Emerg Med J 2015;32(12):971–2.

53. Kozaci N, Avci M, Ararat E, et al. Comparison of ultrasonography and computed tomography in the determination of traumatic thoracic injuries. Am J Emerg Med 2019;37(5):864–8.

54. Stone MB, Sutijono D. Intraarticular injection and closed glenohumeral reduction with emergency ultrasound. Acad Emerg Med 2009;16(12):1384–5.

55. Carlin E, Stankard B, Voroba A, et al. Ultrasound-guided femoral nerve block to facilitate the closed reduction of a dislocated hip prosthesis. Clin Pract Cases Emerg Med 2017;1(4):333.

56. Eksert S, Akay S, Kaya M, et al. Ultrasound-guided femoral nerve blockage in a patellar dislocation: an effective technique for emergency physicians. J Emerg Med 2017;52(5):699–701.

57. Akay S, Eksert S, Kaya M, et al. Case report: ultrasound-guided infraclavicular brachial plexus block for a case with posterior elbow dislocation. J Emerg Med 2017;53(2):232–5.

58. Doost ER, Heiran MM, Movahedi M, et al. Ultrasound-guided interscalene nerve block vs procedural sedation by propofol and fentanyl for anterior shoulder dislocations. Am J Emerg Med 2017;35(10):1435–9.

59. Blaivas M, Adhikari S, Lander L. A prospective comparison of procedural sedation and ultrasound-guided interscalene nerve block for shouder reduction in the emergency department. Acad Emerg Med 2011;18(9):922–7.

60. Abbasi S, Molaie H, Hafezimoghadam P, et al. Diagnostic accuracy of ultrasonographic examination in the management of shoulder dislocation in the emergency department. Ann Emerg Med 2013;62(2):170–5.

61. Lahham S, Becker B, Chiem A, et al. Pilot study to determine accuracy of posterior approach ultrasound for shoulder dislocation by novice sonographers. West J Emerg Med 2016;17(3):377.

62. Mackenzie DC, Liebmann O. Point-of-care ultrasound facilitates diagnosing a posterior shoulder dislocation. J Emerg Med 2013;44(5):976–8.

63. Beck S, Chilstrom M. Point-of-care ultrasound diagnosis and treatment of posterior shoulder dislocation. Am J Emerg Med 2013;31(2):449.e3-5.

64. Gottlieb M, Russell F. Diagnostic accuracy of ultrasound for identifying shoulder dislocations and reductions: a systematic review of the literature. West J Emerg Med 2017;18(5):937.

65. Güngör F, Kılıç T. Point-of-care ultrasonography to assist in the diagnosis and management of subluxation of the radial head in pediatric patients: a case series. J Emerg Med 2017;52(5):702–6.

66. Hodgson RJ, O'connor PJ, Grainger AJ. Tendon and ligament imaging. Br J Radiol 2012;85(1016):1157–72.

67. Wu TS, Roque PJ, Green J, et al. Bedside ultrasound evaluation of tendon injuries. Am J Emerg Med 2012;30(8):1617–21.

68. Situ-LaCasse E, Grieger RW, Crabbe S, et al. Utility of point-of-care musculoskeletal ultrasound in the evaluation of emergency department musculoskeletal pathology. World J Emerg Med 2018;9(4):262.

69. Iovane A, Midiri M, Galia M, et al. Acute traumatic acromioclavicular joint lesions: role of ultrasound versus conventional radiography. Radiol Med 2004;107(4):367–75.

70. Avery DM, Caggiano NM, Matullo KS. Ulnar collateral ligament injuries of the thumb: a comprehensive review. Orthop Clin North Am 2015;46(2):281–92.

71. Shekarchi B, Dashti MM, Shahrezaei M, et al. The accuracy of ultrasonography in detection of ulnar collateral ligament of thumb injuries; a cross-sectional study. Emerg (Tehran) 2018;6(1):e15.

72. Jones MH, England SJ, Muwanga CL, et al. The use of ultrasound in the diagnosis of injuries of the ulnar collateral ligament of the thumb. J Hand Surg Br 2000;25(1):29–32.

73. Smith TO, Back T, Toms AP, et al. Diagnostic accuracy of ultrasound for rotator cuff tears in adults: a systematic review and meta-analysis. Clin Radiol 2011; 66(11):1036–48.
74. McCormack RA, Nayyar S, Jazrawi L. Physician training: ultrasound and accuracy of diagnosis in rotator cuff tears. Bull Hosp Jt Dis 2016;74(3):207.
75. Décary S, Ouellet P, Vendittoli PA, et al. Diagnostic validity of physical examination tests for common knee disorders: an overview of systematic reviews and meta-analysis. Phys Ther Sport 2017;23:143–55.
76. Wang J, Wu H, Dong F, et al. The role of ultrasonography in the diagnosis of anterior cruciate ligament injury: a systematic review and meta-analysis. Eur J Sport Sci 2018;18(4):579–86.
77. Lee SH, Yun SJ. Diagnosis of simultaneous acute ruptures of the anterior cruciate ligament and posterior cruciate ligament using point-of-care ultrasound in the emergency department. J Emerg Med 2018;54(3):335–8.
78. Karabay N, Sugun TS, Toros T. Ultrasonographic diagnosis of the posterior cruciate ligament injury in a 4-year-old child: a case report. Emerg Radiol 2009;16(5): 415–7.
79. LaRocco BG, Zlupko G, Sierzenski P. Ultrasound diagnosis of quadriceps tendon rupture. J Emerg Med 2008;35(3):293–5.
80. Nesselroade RD, Nickels LC. Ultrasound diagnosis of bilateral quadriceps tendon rupture after statin use. West J Emerg Med 2010;11(4):306.
81. Carter K, Nesper A, Gharahbaghian L, et al. Ultrasound detection of patellar fracture and evaluation of the knee extensor mechanism in the emergency department. West J Emerg Med 2016;17(6):814.
82. Adhikari S, Marx J, Crum T. Point-of-care ultrasound diagnosis of acute Achilles tendon rupture in the ED. Am J Emerg Med 2012;30(4):634.e3-4.
83. Lee WJ, Tsai WS, Wu RH. Focused ultrasound for traumatic ankle pain in the emergency department. J Emerg Med 2013;44(2):476–7.
84. Odom M, Haas N, Phillips K. Bedside ultrasound diagnosis of complete achilles tendon tear in a 25-year-old man with calf injury. J Emerg Med 2018; 54(5):694–6.

Moving?

Make sure your subscription moves with you!

To notify us of your new address, find your **Clinics Account Number** (located on your mailing label above your name), and contact customer service at:

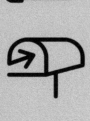

Email: journalscustomerservice-usa@elsevier.com

800-654-2452 (subscribers in the U.S. & Canada)
314-447-8871 (subscribers outside of the U.S. & Canada)

Fax number: 314-447-8029

Elsevier Health Sciences Division
Subscription Customer Service
3251 Riverport Lane
Maryland Heights, MO 63043

*To ensure uninterrupted delivery of your subscription, please notify us at least 4 weeks in advance of move.

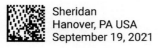